Hypersomnolence

Editor

AHMED S. BAHAMMAM

SLEEP MEDICINE CLINICS

www.sleep.theclinics.com

Consulting Editor
TEOFILO LEE-CHIONG Jr

September 2017 • Volume 12 • Number 3

ELSEVIER

1600 John F. Kennedy Boulevard • Suite 1800 • Philadelphia, Pennsylvania, 19103-2899

http://www.theclinics.com

SLEEP MEDICINE CLINICS Volume 12, Number 3
September 2017, ISSN 1556-407X, ISBN-13: 978-0-323-54572-3

Editor: Katie Pfaff
Developmental Editor: Donald Mumford

Sleep Medicine Clinics (ISSN 1556-407X) is published quarterly by Elsevier Inc., 360 Park Avenue South, New York, NY 10010-1710. Months of issue are March, June, September and December. Business and Editorial Offices: 1600 John F. Kennedy Blvd., Ste. 1800, Philadelphia, PA 19103-2899. Customer Service Office: 3251 Riverport Lane, Maryland Heights, MO 63043. Periodicals postage paid at New York, NY and additional mailing offices. Subscription prices are $203.00 per year (US individuals), $100.00 (US students), $476.00 (US institutions), $244.00 (Canadian and international individuals), $135.00 (Canadian and international students), $540.00 (Canadian institutions) and $529.00 (International institutions). Foreign air speed delivery is included in all *Clinics* subscription prices. All prices are subject to change without notice. **POSTMASTER:** Send change of address to *Sleep Medicine Clinics*, Elsevier Health Sciences Division, Subscription Customer Service, 3251 Riverport Lane, Maryland Heights, MO 63043. Customer Service: **Tel: 1-800-654-2452 (U.S. and Canada); 314-447-8871 (outside U.S. and Canada). Fax: 314-447-8029. E-mail: journalscustomerservice-usa@elsevier.com (for print support); journalsonline support-usa@elsevier.com (for online support).**

Reprints. For copies of 100 or more of articles in this publication, please contact the Commercial Reprints Department, Elsevier Inc., 360 Park Avenue South, New York, NY 10010-1710. Tel.: 212-633-3874; Fax: 212-633-3820; E-mail: reprints@elsevier.com.

Sleep Medicine Clinics is covered in *MEDLINE/PubMed (Index Medicus)*.

PROGRAM OBJECTIVE

The goal of *Sleep Clinics of North America* is to keep practicing physicians up to date with current clinical practice by providing timely articles reviewing the state of the art in patient care.

TARGET AUDIENCE

All practicing physicians and other healthcare professionals.

LEARNING OBJECTIVES

Upon completion of this activity, participants will be able to:

1. Review various causes and comorbidities of hypersomnia.
2. Discuss pharmacological and non-pharmacological management of hypersomnia.
3. Recognize the presentation and assessment of hypersomnia in children, adults, and the elderly.

ACCREDITATION

The Elsevier Office of Continuing Medical Education (EOCME) is accredited by the Accreditation Council for Continuing Medical Education (ACCME) to provide continuing medical education for physicians.

The EOCME designates this enduring material for a maximum of 15 *AMA PRA Category 1 Credit*(s)™. Physicians should claim only the credit commensurate with the extent of their participation in the activity.

All other healthcare professionals requesting continuing education credit for this enduring material will be issued a certificate of participation.

DISCLOSURE OF CONFLICTS OF INTEREST

The EOCME assesses conflict of interest with its instructors, faculty, planners, and other individuals who are in a position to control the content of CME activities. All relevant conflicts of interest that are identified are thoroughly vetted by EOCME for fair balance, scientific objectivity, and patient care recommendations. EOCME is committed to providing its learners with CME activities that promote improvements or quality in healthcare and not a specific proprietary business or a commercial interest.

The planning committee, staff, authors and editors listed below have identified no financial relationships or relationships to products or devices they or their spouse/life partner have with commercial interest related to the content of this CME activity:

Imran M. Ahmed, MD; Hammam Akil, MD; Saad M. Al Suwayri, MD, MHPE, SBIM; Aljohara S. Almeneessier, MD, ABFM; Ahmed S. BaHammam, MD, FRCP, FACP; Lucie Barateau, MD; Sushanth Bhat, MD; Arina Bingeliene, MD; Sudhansu Chokroverty, MD, FRCP, FACP; Matthew R. Ebben, PhD; Elisa Evangelista, MD; Anjali Fortna; Namni Goel, PhD; Ravi Gupta, MD, PhD; Fang Han, MD; Ken He, MD; Seung Bong Hong, MD, PhD; Vishesh K. Kapur, MD, MPH; Régis Lopez, MD, PhD; Roah A. Merdad, MD, MSc; Renee Monderer, MD; Gustavo Antonio Moreira, MD, PhD; Brian James Murray, MD, FRCPC, D,ABSM; Seiji Nishino, MD, PhD; J.F. Pagel, MS, MD; Katie Pfaff; Marcia Pradella-Hallinan, MD, PhD; Colin Shapiro, MBBCh, MRC Psych, FRCP (C), PhD; Shahrad Taheri, MSc, MB BS (hons), PhD, FRCP; Shinichi Takenoshita, MD, MPH; Michael Thorpy, MD; Lynn Marie Trotti, MD, MSc; Rajakumar Venkatesan; Siraj Omar Wali, MBBS, FACP, FCCP, FRCPC; Katie Widmeier; Dora Zalai, MD; Jun Zhang, MD.

The planning committee, staff, authors and editors listed below have identified financial relationships or relationships to products or devices they or their spouse/life partner have with commercial interest related to the content of this CME activity:

Yves Dauvilliers, MD, PhD is on the speakers' bureau for UCB, Inc; Bioprojet; Jazz Pharmaceuticals; and Theranexus, is a consultant/advisor for Flamel, and has research support from UCB, Inc and Jazz Pharmaceuticals.

Teofilo Lee-Chiong Jr, MD is a consultant/advisor for Elsevier and CareCore International, has stock ownsership in and an employment affiliation with Elsevier, and receieves royalties/patents from Lippincott; Oxford University Press; CreateSpace, a DBA of On-Demand Publishing, LLC; and John Wiley & Sons, Inc.

Seithikurippu R. Pandi-Perumal, MSc has stock ownership in Somnogen Canada Inc, and receives royalties/patents from Springer-Verlag GmbH.

Yoshihiro Urade, PhD is on the speakers' bureau for, has research support from, and receives royalties/patents from Lion Co. Ltd, is on the speakers' bureau for, is a consultant/advisor for, and receives research support from Watanabe Oyster Laboratory Co. Ltd, and receives research support from Nisshin Seifun Group Inc.

UNAPPROVED/OFF-LABEL USE DISCLOSURE

The EOCME requires CME faculty to disclose to the participants:

1. When products or procedures being discussed are off-label, unlabelled, experimental, and/or investigational (not US Food and Drug Administration [FDA] approved); and
2. Any limitations on the information presented, such as data that are preliminary or that represent ongoing research, interim analyses, and/or unsupported opinions. Faculty may discuss information about pharmaceutical agents that is outside of FDA-approved labelling. This information is intended solely for CME and is not intended to promote off-label use of these

medications. If you have any questions, contact the medical affairs department of the manufacturer for the most recent pre-scribing information.

TO ENROLL
To enroll in the Sleep Medicines Clinic Continuing Medical Education program, call customer service at 1-800-654-2452 or sign up online at http://www.theclinics.com/home/cme. The CME program is available to subscribers for an additional annual fee of USD $140.

METHOD OF PARTICIPATION
In order to claim credit, participants must complete the following:
1. Complete enrolment as indicated above.
2. Read the activity.
3. Complete the CME Test and Evaluation. Participants must achieve a score of 70% on the test. All CME Tests and Evaluations must be completed online.

CME INQUIRIES/SPECIAL NEEDS
For all CME inquiries or special needs, please contact elsevierCME@elsevier.com.

SLEEP MEDICINE CLINICS

THE CLINICS ARE AVAILABLE ONLINE!
Access your subscription at:
www.theclinics.com

Contributors

CONSULTING EDITOR

TEOFILO LEE-CHIONG Jr, MD
Professor of Medicine, National Jewish Health,
School of Medicine, University of Colorado
Denver, Denver, Colorado, USA; Chief Medical
Liaison, Philips Respironics, Monroeville,
Pennsylvania, USA

EDITOR

AHMED S. BaHAMMAM, MD, FRCP, FACP
Professor of Medicine and Director,
University Sleep Disorders Center, Department
of Medicine, College of Medicine, King
Saud University, Strategic Technologies
Program, National Plan for Sciences and
Technology and Innovation, Riyadh,
Saudi Arabia

AUTHORS

IMRAN M. AHMED, MD
Sleep-Wake Disorders Center, Department
of Neurology, Montefiore Medical Center,
Albert Einstein College of Medicine, Bronx,
New York, USA

HAMMAM AKIL, MD
Department of Pediatrics, Jeddah
Maternity and Children's Hospital, Jeddah,
Saudi Arabia

SAAD M. AL SUWAYRI, MD, MHPE, SBIM
Assistant Professor, Department of Internal
Medicine, College of Medicine, Al Imam
Mohammad Ibn Saud Islamic University
(IMSIU), Riyadh, Saudi Arabia

ALJOHARA S. ALMENEESSIER, MD, ABFM
Department of Family and Community
Medicine, College of Medicine, King Saud
University, Riyadh, Saudi Arabia

AHMED S. BaHAMMAM, MD, FRCP, FACP
Professor of Medicine and Director,
University Sleep Disorders Center, Department
of Medicine, College of Medicine, King
Saud University, Strategic Technologies
Program, National Plan for Sciences and
Technology and Innovation, Riyadh,
Saudi Arabia

LUCIE BARATEAU, MD
National Reference Center for Orphan
Disease, Narcolepsy and Hypersomnia,
Sleep Disorder Unit, Gui de Chauliac
Hospital, University of Montpellier, Montpellier,
France

SUSHANTH BHAT, MD
Division of Sleep Medicine, Department
of Neuroscience, JFK Neuroscience
Institute, Seton Hall University, Edison,
New Jersey, USA

ARINA BINGELIENE, MD
Department of Neurology, University Health
Network, Toronto, Ontario, Canada

SUDHANSU CHOKROVERTY, MD, FRCP, FACP
Professor and Director of Research for
Sleep Medicine, Co-Chair Emeritus of
Neurology, Division of Sleep Medicine,
Department of Neuroscience, JFK
Neuroscience Institute, Seton Hall
University, Edison, New Jersey, USA

YVES DAUVILLIERS, MD, PhD
National Reference Center for Orphan
Disease, Narcolepsy and Hypersomnia,
Sleep Disorder Unit, Gui de Chauliac
Hospital, University of Montpellier,
Montpellier, France

MATTHEW R. EBBEN, PhD
Associate Professor, Department of
Neurology, Center for Sleep Medicine, Weill
Cornell Medical College of Cornell University,
New York, New York, USA

ELISA EVANGELISTA, MD
National Reference Center for Orphan
Disease, Narcolepsy and Hypersomnia,
Sleep Disorder Unit, Gui de Chauliac
Hospital, University of Montpellier,
Montpellier, France

NAMNI GOEL, PhD
Associate Professor, Division of Sleep and
Chronobiology, Department of Psychiatry,
Perelman School of Medicine, University of
Pennsylvania, Philadelphia, Pennsylvania, USA

RAVI GUPTA, MD, PhD
Department of Psychiatry and Sleep Clinic,
Himalayan Institute of Medical Sciences,
Doiwala, Dehradun, India

FANG HAN, MD
Department of Respiratory Medicine, Peking
University People's Hospital, Beijing, China

KEN HE, MD
Clinical Instructor, Division of General Internal
Medicine, University of Washington, Clinical
Instructor, Hospital and Sleep Medicine
Sections, VA Puget Sound Health Care
System, Seattle, Washington, USA

SEUNG BONG HONG, MD, PhD
Professor, Department of Neurology,
Samsung Medical Center, Samsung
Advanced Institute for Health Sciences and
Technology, Sungkyunkwan University School
of Medicine, Samsung Biomedical Research
Institute, Seoul, Republic of Korea

VISHESH K. KAPUR, MD, MPH
Professor, Division of Pulmonary, Critical Care
and Sleep Medicine, University of Washington,
Seattle, Washington, USA

RÉGIS LOPEZ, MD, PhD
National Reference Center for Orphan
Disease, Narcolepsy and Hypersomnia,
Sleep Disorder Unit, Gui de Chauliac
Hospital, University of Montpellier,
Montpellier, France

ROAH A. MERDAD, MD, MSc
Department of Family and Community
Medicine, Faculty of Medicine, King
Abdulaziz University, Jeddah, Saudi Arabia;
Department of Community Health and
Epidemiology, Faculty of Medicine,
Dalhousie University, Halifax, Nova Scotia,
Canada

RENEE MONDERER, MD
Sleep-Wake Disorders Center, Department
of Neurology, Montefiore Medical Center,
Albert Einstein College of Medicine, Bronx,
New York, USA

GUSTAVO ANTONIO MOREIRA, MD, PhD
Departments of Psychobiology and Pediatrics,
Universidade Federal de São Paulo, São Paulo,
São Paulo, Brazil

BRIAN JAMES MURRAY, MD, FRCPC, D,ABSM
Associate Professor, Neurology and Sleep
Medicine, Sunnybrook Health Sciences
Centre, University of Toronto, Toronto,
Ontario, Canada

SEIJI NISHINO, MD, PhD
Director, Sleep and Circadian Neurobiology
Laboratory, Professor, Department of
Psychiatry and Behavioral Sciences, Stanford
University School of Medicine, Stanford
University, Palo Alto, California, USA

J.F. PAGEL, MS, MD
Director, Rocky Mountain Sleep Disorders
Center, Associate Clinical Professor, Southern
Colorado Family Medicine Residency
Program, Department of Family Medicine,
University of Colorado School of Medicine,
Pueblo, Colorado, USA

SEITHIKURIPPU R. PANDI-PERUMAL, MSc
Somnogen Canada Inc, Toronto, Ontario,
Canada

MARCIA PRADELLA-HALLINAN, MD, PhD
Department of Psychobiology, Universidade
Federal de São Paulo, São Paulo, São Paulo,
Brazil

**COLIN SHAPIRO, MBBCh, MRC Psych,
FRCP (C), PhD**
Professor in Psychiatry and Ophthalmology,
Department of Neurology, University Health
Network, Toronto, Ontario, Canada

**SHAHRAD TAHERI, MSc, MB BS (hons),
PhD, FRCP**
Professor, Department of Medicine, Weill
Cornell Medicine, New York, New York, USA;
Professor, Department of Medicine,
Weill Cornell Medicine Qatar, Qatar
Foundation–Education City, Doha, Qatar

SHINICHI TAKENOSHITA, MD, MPH
Visiting Assistant Professor, Sleep and
Circadian Neurobiology Laboratory,
Department of Psychiatry and Behavioral
Sciences, Stanford University School of
Medicine, Stanford University, Palo Alto,
California, USA

MICHAEL THORPY, MD
Sleep-Wake Disorders Center, Department
of Neurology, Montefiore Medical Center,
Albert Einstein College of Medicine, Bronx,
New York, USA

LYNN MARIE TROTTI, MD, MSc
Associate Professor, Department of Neurology
and Sleep Center, Emory University School of
Medicine, Atlanta, Georgia, USA

YOSHIHIRO URADE, PhD
Professor, International Institute of Integrative
Sleep Medicine, Tsukuba University, Tsukuba,
Ibaraki, Japan

**SIRAJ OMAR WALI, MBBS, FACP, FCCP,
FRCPC**
Professor of Medicine, College of Medicine,
Consultant in Pulmonary and Sleep Medicine,
Director, Sleep Medicine and Research
Center, King Abdulaziz University Hospital,
King Abdulaziz University, Jeddah,
Saudi Arabia

DORA ZALAI, MD
PhD Candidate, Department of Psychology,
Ryerson University, Toronto, Ontario,
Canada

JUN ZHANG, MD
Department of Neurology, Peking University
People's Hospital, Beijing, China

Contents

Neurobiological Basis of Hypersomnia   265

Yoshihiro Urade

Narcolepsy is the most well-characterized hypersomnia in both clinical and basic research fields. Narcolepsy is caused by degeneration of hypocretin-producing neurons in the hypothalamus. Although hypocretin receptor antagonists have been developed as sleep-inducing drugs, a high dose of suvorexant, a hypocretin receptor antagonist, inhibits gene expression of prepro-hypocretin to induce narcoleptic attack in wild-type mice. Prostaglandin D_2 is the most potent endogenous sleep-promoting substance. Overproduction of prostaglandin D_2 is involved in hypersomnia in patients with mastocytosis and African sleeping sickness or in mice after a pentylenetetrazole-induced seizure. Commercialized sleep-promoting supplements also may induce hypersomnia in humans.

The Immune Basis of Narcolepsy: What Is the Evidence?   279

Shahrad Taheri

Narcolepsy is a chronic neurologic sleep disorder. Type 1 narcolepsy (narcolepsy-cataplexy) is associated with the destruction of lateral hypothalamic hypocretin neurons. It is thought that the loss of hypocretin neurons is autoimmune mediated. This is because of the close relationship between type 1 narcolepsy and HLA DQB1*0602 and the onset of narcolepsy at a young age. Evidence suggests that streptococcal and H1N1 influenza infections (and H1N1 vaccination) may be involved in the pathogenesis of narcolepsy. There are suggestions from genetic and immune studies that the immune system plays a key role in narcolepsy.

Genetic Markers of Sleep and Sleepiness   289

Namni Goel

The circadian clock interacts with the sleep homeostatic drive in humans. Chronotype and sleep parameters show substantial heritability, underscoring a genetic component to these measures. This article reviews the genetic underpinnings of chronotype and of sleep, including sleepiness, sleep quality and latency, and sleep timing and duration in healthy adult sleepers, drawing on candidate gene and genome-wide association studies. Notably, both circadian and noncircadian genes associate with individual differences in chronotype and in sleep parameters. The article concludes with a brief discussion of future research directions.

Evaluation of the Sleepy Patient: Differential Diagnosis   301

Renee Monderer, Imran M. Ahmed, and Michael Thorpy

Excessive daytime sleepiness is defined as the inability to maintain wakefulness during waking hours, resulting in unintended lapses into sleep. It is important to distinguish sleepiness from fatigue. The evaluation of a sleep patient begins with a careful clinical assessment that includes a detailed sleep history, medical and psychiatric history, a review of medications, as well as a social and family history. Physical examination should include a general medical examination with careful attention to the upper airway and the neurologic examination. Appropriate objective testing with a polysomnogram and a multiple sleep latency test if needed will help confirm the diagnosis and direct the appropriate treatment plan.

studies, next-generation genetics, multimodal functional imaging, biomarker discovery, and clinical drug trials. A centralized registry of afflicted individuals must be established. Disease uniformity should make the identification of associated genetic or imaging biomarkers easier, but clinical efforts require laboratory-based research to model the disease and generate preclinical data for clinical translation.

various mood disorders, such as major depressive disorder, bipolar disorder, or seasonal affective disorder. Assessment of hypersomnolence is challenging in depressed patients, with objective tests often in the normal range despite a high level of sleepiness complaint. On the other hand, many patients with central hypersomnias reported depressive symptoms. The self-assessment of mood symptoms in patients with central hypersomnias may overdiagnose depression with an overlap between both conditions.

tauopathies, synucleinopathies, and other conditions. Common nocturnal sleep problems that may result in daytime hypersomnia are delineated. A clinical approach to hypersomnia in patients with neurodegenerative diseases, recommended diagnostic testing, and available treatment options are also discussed.

Preface
Hypersomnolence

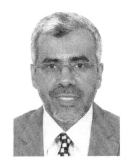

Ahmed S. BaHammam, MD, FRCP, FACP
Editor

The feeling of sleepiness when you are not in bed, and can't get there, is the meanest feeling in the world.
—*Edgar Watson Howe (1853–1937)*

Sleep and its functions have intrigued scholars and scientists from different cultures throughout written history. Although everyone agrees that sleep is important, hypersomnolence (excessive sleepiness) has been associated with significant costs and complications. Excessive daytime sleepiness refers to the inability to stay awake and alert during the day, even after having attained adequate or prolonged sleep. While the term "hypersomnolence" refers to the symptom of excessive sleepiness, hypersomnia indicates specific disorders, such as idiopathic hypersomnia. Primary causes of hypersomnolence, such as narcolepsy and idiopathic hypersomnia, are less common than secondary causes, such as insufficient sleep syndrome and sleep-disordered breathing. Although hypersomnolence in itself presents a great challenge to practicing physicians, another major challenge is differentiation between sleepiness and fatigue, as both are very common in the general population.

This issue of *Sleep Medicine Clinics* covers both hypersomnolence and hypersomnia. From basic concepts to new developments in the field, this issue explores hypersomnolence in depth, while also addressing its various causes. The choice of topics included in this issue was based on the importance of the covered disorders and the availability of new data, although most authors point out the need for further research. As the studies in this issue reveal, there is undoubtedly much work to be done in the field of hypersomnolence and hypersomnia.

The topics chosen are diverse and represent most causes of hypersomnolence. Topics include the basic concepts behind sleepiness, new genetic data, clinical approaches to the diagnosis and treatment of excessive sleepiness, primary and secondary causes of hypersomnolence, hypersomnolence in different age groups, hypersomnolence in neurodegenerative and psychiatric disorders, driving while sleepy, treatment options, and recent imaging findings in central hypersomnia disorders. Likewise, authors featured in this issue are from various locations around the world, each representing a particular area of expertise in sleep and sleepiness research.

This *Sleep Medicine Clinics* issue is an excellent reference for sleep medicine practitioners and physicians in training as well as primary care and general physicians. I am grateful to the authors who devoted their time and expertise to contributing to this issue amidst densely packed schedules.

I dedicate this issue to my wife, whose love and encouragement has inspired me throughout my career.

Ahmed S. BaHammam, MD, FRCP, FACP
University Sleep Disorders Center
Department of Medicine
College of Medicine
King Saud University
Box 225503
Riyadh 11324, Saudi Arabia

E-mail addresses:
ashammam2@gmail.com
ashammam@ksu.edu.sa

Sleep Med Clin 12 (2017) xvii
http://dx.doi.org/10.1016/j.jsmc.2017.06.002
1556-407X/17/© 2017 Published by Elsevier Inc.

Neurobiological Basis of Hypersomnia

Yoshihiro Urade, PhD

KEYWORDS

- Hypocretin • Narcolepsy • Suvorexant • Prostaglandin D2 • Adenosine • Cytokines
- Sleep-promoting supplement • Gene-knockout mice

KEY POINTS

- Narcolepsy is the most well-characterized hypersomnia and is caused by the degeneration of hypocretin-producing neurons in the hypothalamus, which are important for maintenance of wakefulness.
- Hypocretin receptor antagonist Suvorexant is a recently developed sleep-inducing drug but induces narcoleptic attack in wild-type mice by suppressing the gene expression of prepro-hypocretin.
- Prostaglandin D_2 is the most potent endogenous sleep-promoting substance, and the action mechanism of sleep induction is best characterized at neurologic and molecular levels.
- Overproduction of prostaglandin D_2 is associated with hypersomnia in patients with mastocytosis and African sleeping sickness or in mice after a pentylenetetrazole-induced seizure.
- Hypersomnia is also caused by cytokines produced during bacterial or viral infection and in various neurodegenerative diseases, and by intake of some sleep-promoting supplements.

CLINICAL DEFINITION OF HYPERSOMNIA

According to the International Classification of Sleep Disorders-3, central hypersomnia is classified into the following 6 categories: (1) Narcolepsy type 1 (previously narcolepsy with cataplexy); (2) Narcolepsy type 2 (previously narcolepsy without cataplexy); (3) Idiopathic hypersomnia; (4) Klein-Levin syndrome; (5) Hypersomnia due to medical disorder, medication, or substance abuse; and (6) Insufficient sleep syndrome (**Box 1**). This classification is based on the clinical diagnosis based on polysomnography, multiple sleep latency tests, sleep diary, and so forth. The cause, diagnosis, and treatment of each of these sleep disorders are described in other sections of this issue. In this article, the author summarizes the neurobiology of hypersomnia from the molecular and biochemical points of view, mainly based on his research studies of hypocretin (Hcrt), prostaglandin (PG) D_2, and adenosine.

NARCOLEPSY AND THE HYPOCRETIN/OREXIN SYSTEM

Among the hypersomnias, narcolepsy has been the most well characterized in both clinical and basic research fields. Narcolepsy is diagnosed

This study was supported in part by Japan Society for the Promotion of Science grant JP16H01881; by a grant from the Research Project on Development of Agricultural Products and Foods with Health-promoting benefits (NARO), Japan; and by funding from Korean Food Research Institute; Mizkan Holding Co, Ltd; Ezaki Glico Co, Ltd; Ajinomoto Co, Ltd; Lion Co Ltd; Fujifilm Co, Ltd; ONO Pharmaceutical Co, Ltd; and Takeda Science Foundation.
International Institute of Integrative Sleep Medicine, Tsukuba University, 1-1-1 Tennodai, Tsukuba, Ibaraki 305-8575, Japan
E-mail address: urade.yoshihiro.ft@u.tsukuba.ac.jp

Sleep Med Clin 12 (2017) 265–277
http://dx.doi.org/10.1016/j.jsmc.2017.03.003
1556-407X/17/© 2017 Elsevier Inc. All rights reserved.

by excessive daytime sleepiness, cataplexy, sleep-onset rapid eye movement sleep (SOREM), and sleep paralysis or hallucination,[1,2] and it is now known to be a disease caused by the degeneration of Hcrt-producing neurons.[3]

Discovered in 1998 by the research team of T. Kilduff at Stanford University, Hcrt was found to be a functionally unknown neuropeptide selectively expressed in the hypothalamus.[4] This group subsequently identified the gene encoding the prepropeptide of Hcrt, the biosynthetic pathway of isopeptide-1 and -2, and 2 subtypes of receptors for Hcrt, 1 and 2 (**Fig. 1**). These isopeptides were also independently isolated in 1998 as an orphan ligand for GPCR, HFGAN72, by T. Sakurai and M. Yanagisawa, University of Texas Southwestern, and termed orexins, because these

researchers assumed that these peptides were involved in orexinergic regulation of feeding behavior.[5] Hcrt and orexin are the same peptide.

In 1999, the year following of the discovery of Hcrt and the identification of Hcrt receptors, the research team of E. Migno, Stanford University, showed that the Hcrt receptor gene is mutated in dogs with inherited canine narcolepsy,[6] the colony of which was established and maintained by Kilduff and Migno's mentor, Professor William C. Dement. The narcoleptic attack, involving SOREM and cataplexy-like behavior, was then reported to occur in the Hcrt/orexin gene knockout (KO) mice.[7] These 2 animal studies strongly suggested that abnormality of the Hcrt system causes human narcolepsy. In 2000, the research team of J.M. Siegel at University of California, Los Angeles, and of S. Nishino and E. Migno at Stanford University finally demonstrated that the Hcrt-producing neurons had disappeared in the hypothalamus of autopsied brain tissue from narcolepsy patients.[3,8,9] They measured the Hcrt content in the cerebrospinal fluid (CSF) of healthy volunteers and hypersomnia patients diagnosed as having narcolepsy or other neurodegenerative diseases and found that the Hcrt content was selectively and markedly decreased in those patients with narcolepsy, especially in most of the patients classified as having the cataplexy-associated type 1 narcolepsy.[10] Today, a decreased CSF level of Hcrt is used as an important marker for the diagnosis of narcolepsy. Epidemiologic studies

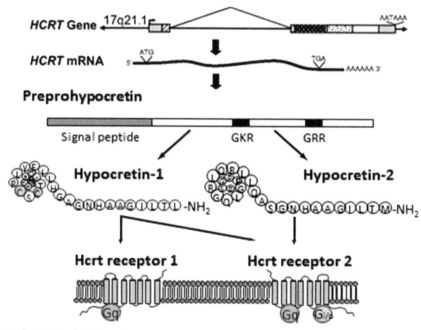

Fig. 1. Hcrt production and receptors.

strongly suggest that Hcrt-producing neurons are probably decreased in number in patients with narcolepsy, the loss being due to an autoimmune disease against some unidentified self-antigen. Although the neural networks of Hcrt-producing neurons and the distribution of Hcrt receptors have been extensively studied, the molecular mechanism responsible for the accumulation of excessive sleepiness caused by this loss of function remains to be elucidated.

HYPOCRETIN ANTAGONIST-INDUCED NARCOLEPSY

The intracerebroventricular (ICV) infusion of Hcrt into wild-type (WT) mice increases arousal to almost the level of complete insomnia, indicating that the Hcrt system is involved in the maintenance of wakefulness. The intensive awake-induction activity caused by the Hcrt infusion is completely abolished in histamine H1 receptor KO mice.[11] Therefore, Hcrt receptor antagonists are predicted to be useful to act as a sleep-inducing drug, similar to the histamine H1 receptor blocker present in over-the-counter sleep-aid pills. Based on this assumption, several Hcrt receptor antagonists

have been developed as sleep-inducing drugs. Among them, Suvorexant (**Fig. 2**A) has already been commercialized in the United States and Japan.[12–14]

The loss of Hcrt-producing neurons or Hcrt receptors induces narcolepsy in humans, dogs, and mice, as described above. To assess the ability of Hcrt receptor antagonists to induce narcoleptic symptoms, the author's team orally administered a high dose (100 mg/kg) of Suvorexant 3 times at 6-hour intervals to (WT) mice and then measured the messenger RNA (mRNA) for prepro-Hcrt and the Hcrt content in the brain and found that the high-dose administration of Suvorexant inhibited strongly the production of Hcrt (M. Kaushik, Y. Urade, unpublished results, 2017). The prepro-Hcrt mRNA level was decreased in the brain to less than 20% at 4 hours after the last administration of Suvorexant. The Hcrt content measured by use of a radioimmunoassay kit was decreased to almost undetectable levels at 1 day after the last Suvorexant administration. These results suggest that Hcrt production is controlled by autoreceptors, which are blocked by Suvorexant to stop the transcription of prepro-Hcrt and that the turnover of Hcrt stored within

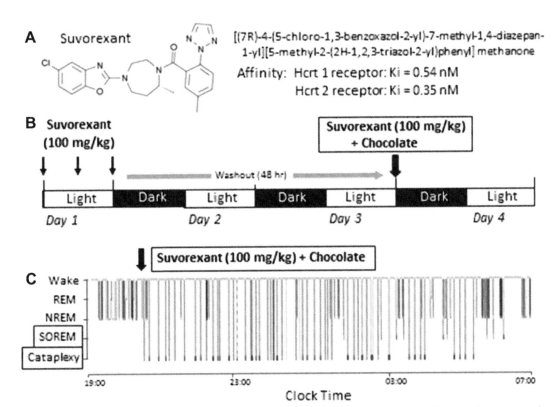

Fig. 2. Suvorexant-induced narcolepsy in WT mice. (*A*) Chemical structure and binding affinities of Suvorexant for Hcrt receptor-1 and -2. (*B*) Experimental protocol. (*C*) Hypnogram of narcoleptic attack induced by rechallenge with Suvorexant together with chocolate to a WT mouse.

Hcrt-producing neurons is relatively rapid, for the stored Hcrt is used up within 1 day in the presence of a high dose of Suvorexant.

In the absence or the presence of a very low level of an endogenous ligand, an exogenous antagonist should show intensive antagonistic action. To examine this possibility, the author's team performed electroencephalogram (EEG), electromyogram (EMG), and behavioral observation by video recording of (WT) mice after a rechallenge with Suvolexant following 2 days of antagonist washout. In narcolepsy patients and in the canine model, cataplexy is caused by a positive emotion such as laughing in patients and by delicious dog food in the canine model. In the mouse model of narcolepsy, chocolate is effective to induce cataplexy.[15] So the author gave chocolate to Suvorexant-pretreated mice at the rechallenge period (**Fig. 2**B). As expected, a Suvorexant rechallenge induced severe SOREM and cataplexy in all of the WT mice used in this experiment (**Fig. 2**C).

It is still unclear how much loss of Hcrt neurons must occur to induce narcolepsy. Even if the Hcrt content in the CSF decreases to 20% to 30%, some people remain healthy and do not develop narcolepsy.[16,17] Those people may be more sensitive to the Hcrt antagonist–induced narcolepsy. To avoid the risk of Hcrt antagonist–induced narcolepsy, it is important to monitor the endogenous Hcrt production by the drug user.

SLEEP SUBSTANCES INVOLVED IN HYPERSOMNIA

Involvement of Prostaglandin D₂ in Hypersomnia

In terms of the molecular basis of sleepiness, many endogenous sleep substances have been proposed. Among them, PGD_2 is the most potent of sleep-promoting substance, and the action mechanism of sleep induction by it is the best characterized. Several review articles on this prostanoid have already been reported.[18–21]

In 1982, the research team of the author's mentor, the late Professor O. Hayaishi, discovered that PGD_2 is the major prostanoid produced in the brain of rats[22] and humans[23] and that it induces dose-dependent non–rapid eye movement (NREM) sleep in freely moving rats after ICV administration of it.[24] In 1988, the NREM sleep induction by PGD_2 was confirmed in monkeys, in which the PGD_2-induced sleep was shown to be indistinguishable from physiologic sleep and clearly different from benzodiazepine-induced sleep as judged by the behavioral observation and EEG spectral analyses.[25] In both rats and monkeys, PGD_2-induced sleep is easily interrupted by sound stimulation, such as hand clapping, and the power spectrum of EEG is almost the same as that of physiologic sleep.

The involvement of PGD_2 in hypersomnia has been reported in 2 types of diseases, mastocytosis[26] and African sleeping sickness.[27] In the former case, the plasma concentration of a PGD_2 metabolite was reported to increase during sleep attacks in patients with mastocytosis. Mast cells release several inflammatory mediators, such as histamine, PGD_2, and leukotrienes. The sleep attack is not prevented by antihistaminergic drugs, but it is effectively suppressed by administration of aspirin, which inhibits the production of all prostanoids including PGD_2 in mammals. African sleeping sickness is caused by infection with pathogenic protozoan parasites, that is, *Trypanosoma brucei gambienze* or *rhodesiense*. These single-cell protozoa are transmitted to humans by a blood-sucking fly, the tsetse fly. In the early stage of transfection, the trypanosoma infection is limited to the peripheral circulation, such that the symptom is not severe; however, in the advanced stage, trypanosomes enter the central nervous system, making the individual enter into a deep sleep as seen in a coma. During this advanced stage, the PGD_2 concentration in the CSF of patients increases 500-fold or more. The author's team then found that *Trypanosoma brucei* produces prostanoids de novo from arachidonic acid by unique enzymes that are not inhibited by aspirin or indomethacin.[28,29]

Molecular Mechanism of Prostaglandin D₂-Induced Sleep

Two distinct types of PGD synthase (PGDS) exist in the brain[30,31]: one is lipocalin-type PGDS (L-PGDS),[32] mainly localized in the arachnoid membrane, choroid plexus, and oligodendrocytes[33–35] and secreted into CSF as beta-trace, a major human CSF protein,[36] and the other, hematopoietic PGDS (H-PGDS[37]), found in microglial cells.[38] There are 2 distinct types of receptors for PGD_2: one is the DP1 (DP) receptor coupled to a Gs protein and belonging to the gene family of prostanoid receptors,[39] and the other, DP2 (CRTH2, GPR44), is coupled to Gi/Gq protein and a member of chemoattractant receptor family.[40,41] The author's team generated KO mice for L-PGDS, H-PGDS, DP1, and DP2 and used them for genetic dissection of PGD_2-induced NREM sleep.

For this study, the author's team developed a sleep bioassay system for measuring EEG, EMG, and locomotor activity during the continuous slow infusion (1 µL/h) of drug into the brain of freely moving mice (**Fig. 3**).[42] The vigilance state is

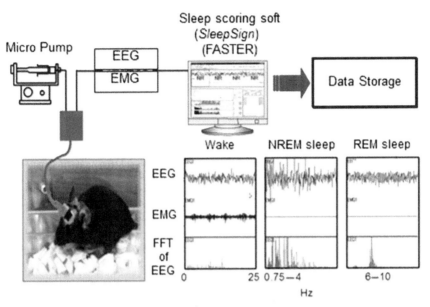

Fig. 3. Sleep bioassay system. FFT, fast Fourier transform.

classified as wakefulness, NREM sleep, or rapid eye movement (REM) sleep by using software called Sleepsign[43] or FASTER,[44] both of which are based on the EEG and EMG. By the combination of this sleep bioassay system with several types of gene-manipulated animals and various pharmacologic tools, such as enzyme inhibitors and receptor agonists/antagonists, the author's team clarified the molecular mechanism of sleep induction by PGD_2 (**Fig. 4**).[19]

PGD_2, acting as an endogenous somnogen, is produced by L-PGDS localized in the arachnoid membrane surrounding the brain, secreted into the CSF, and circulates within the brain as a kind

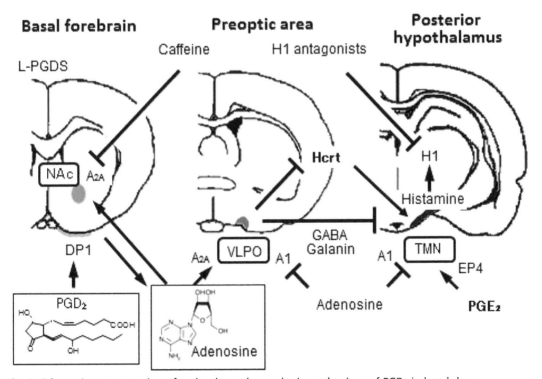

Fig. 4. Schematic representation of molecular and neurologic mechanisms of PGD_2-induced sleep.

of sleep-maintaining hormone. The PGD_2 concentration in the CSF is monitored by DP1 receptors localized in the arachnoid membrane of the ventral surface of the basal forebrain.[45,46] When PGD_2 is infused into the brain of DP1 receptor KO mice, their sleep is not increased at all, indicating that the sleep induction completely depends on DP1 receptors (**Fig. 5**). When DP1 receptors are activated, the concentration of extracellular adenosine is increased in the subarachnoid space in the basal forebrain. However, this increase was not observed when PGD_2 was infused into the basal forebrain of DP1 receptor-KO mice, indicating that the increase in extracellular adenosine occurs in a DP1 receptor-dependent manner.[46]

Adenosine has long been proposed as an endogenous somnogen.[47–50] PGD_2-induced sleep is inhibited by antagonists against adenosine A_{2A} receptors, such as KF-17837.[51] Furthermore, PGD_2-induced NREM sleep is significantly attenuated in adenosine A_{2A} receptor KO mice.[52] These results, taken together, suggest that the somnogenic information is transferred from PGD_2 to adenosine, which then diffuses into the brain parenchyma, that is, adenosine acts as a secondary somnogenic substance.

Non–Rapid Eye Movement Sleep Centers in the Preoptic Area and the Basal Ganglia

The author's team then induced NREM sleep by the ICV infusion of PGD_2 or by an agonist for adenosine A_{2A} receptors, CGS-21680, surveyed the activated neurons during NREM sleep by c-Fos staining, and found that a cluster of neurons in the ventrolateral preoptic (VLPO) area was selectively activated during NREM sleep.[53,54] The VLPO neurons are silent when animals are awake and selectively activated during NREM sleep. The number of c-Fos-positive neurons in the VLPO is positively correlated with the amount of NREM sleep during a 2-hour period before sampling the brain for c-Fos. The VLPO neurons suppress the downstream histaminergic arousal center in the tuberomammillary nucleus (TMN) through GABA'gic or galaninergic inhibitory projection.[55–57] The number of c-Fos–positive neurons in the TMN is positively correlated with the amount of wakefulness. Based on these findings, the sleep-wake cycle is proposed to be regulated by a flip-flop mechanism between the VLPO and TMN.[58] The inhibition of TMN neurons induced by infusion of PGD_2 or an adenosine A_{2A} receptor agonist, such as CGS-21680, suppresses the various downstream arousal centers to induce finally NREM sleep in the whole brain.

In the brain parenchyma, adenosine deaminase, an enzyme that catabolizes adenosine to inosine, is dominantly localized in the TMN, indicating that the histaminergic neurons are actively regulated by adenosine. Histaminergic neurons project from the TMN to most of the central nervous system and promote wakefulness through histamine H_1 receptors. The extracellular histamine level in the frontal cortex was 3.8 times higher during wake episodes than during sleep episodes, being positively correlated ($r = 0.845$) with the time spent in wakefulness, as examined by an in vivo microdialysis study using freely moving rats.[59] The

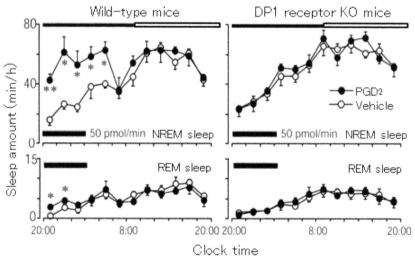

Fig. 5. PGD_2-induced sleep in WT and DP1 receptor KO mice. *$P<.05$; **$P<.01$ versus vehicle (artificial CSF)-injected group. (*Data from* Mizoguchi A, Eguchi N, Kimura K, et al. Dominant localization of prostaglandin D receptors on arachnoid trabecular cells in mouse basal forebrain and their involvement in the regulation of non-rapid eye movement sleep. Proc Natl Acad Sci U S A 2001;98:11674–9.)

histaminergic neurons in the TMN express inhibitory adenosine A_1 receptors, but not A_{2A} receptors. Bilateral injection of adenosine, coformycin (an adenosine deaminase inhibitor), or N(6)-cyclopentyladenosine (an A_1 receptor agonist) into the rat TMN decreased histamine release in the frontal cortex and increased NREM sleep (Fig. 6), both of which were completely abolished by coadministration of 1,3-dimethyl-8-cyclopenthylxanthine, a selective A_1 receptor antagonist, indicating that endogenous adenosine in the TMN suppresses the histaminergic system via A_1 receptors to promote NREM sleep.[60] The adenosine A_1 receptor-mediated inhibition of histaminergic arousal neurons may be associated with hypersomnia.

In 2011, the author's team identified another sleep center, one in the nucleus accumbens (NAc) shell of the basal ganglia, as the target site of caffeine-induced arousal.[61] When adenosine A_{2A} receptors were selectively deleted from the NAc shell of rats, the animals became completely insensitive to caffeine. These results indicate that activation of adenosine A_{2A} receptor-possessing neurons of NAc shell must be activated by endogenous adenosine to maintain sleep, because caffeine induces arousal by acting as an antagonist of adenosine A_{2A} receptors.[62] Because the NAc shell is anatomically assigned as being a center of motivation, the NAc shell is considered to be important for motivation-driven arousal.[63–65] Adenosine A_{2A} receptors and dopamine D_2 receptors are colocalized at the same synapses of the indirect pathway of the basal ganglia and counteract each other to activate and inhibit, respectively, the postsynaptic transmission. Therefore, unbalancing of the indirect pathway may be involved in hypersomnia.

Hypersomnia Caused by Increased Prostaglandin D_2 in the Brain

Inorganic tetravalent selenium compounds, such as $SeCl_4$, are relatively specific and reversible inhibitors of L-PGDS.[66] Microinfusion of $SeCl_4$ into the third ventricle of rats inhibits sleep almost completely. This effect is reversible, because when the infusion is interrupted, sleep is restored. Furthermore, the inhibition can be reversed by the simultaneous infusion of SH compounds such as dithiothreitol and glutathione, similar to the in vitro enzyme activity.[67] The intraperitoneal (IP) injection of $SeCl_4$ into WT mice decreases the PGD_2 content in the brain without affecting the amounts of other prostanoids such as PGE_2 and $PGF_{2\alpha}$. It inhibits sleep dose dependently and immediately after the administration during the light period when mice normally sleep. This $SeCl_4$-induced insomnia was observed in H-PGDS KO mice but not at all in L-PGDS KO, H-/L-PGDS double KO, or DP1 receptor KO mice.[68] Furthermore, the DP1 receptor antagonist ONO-4127Na reduces sleep of rats by 30% during infusion at 200 pmol/min into the subarachnoid space under the rostral basal forebrain in a dose-dependent manner.[68] These results clearly indicate that the L-PGDS/PGD$_2$/DP1 receptor system plays pivotal roles in the regulation of physiologic sleep.

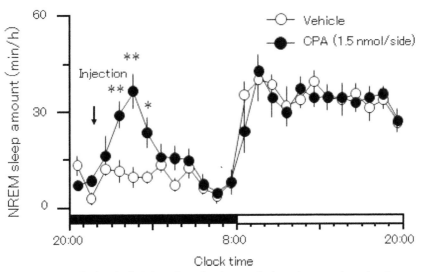

Fig. 6. NREM sleep induction by local administration of cyclopentyl adenosine, an adenosine A_1 receptor agonist, into the TMN of rats. *$P<.05$; **$P<.01$ versus vehicle (artificial CSF)-injected group. (Data from Oishi Y, Huang ZL, Fredholm BB, et al. Adenosine in the tuberomammillary nucleus inhibits the histaminergic system via A1 receptors and promotes non-rapid eye movement sleep. Proc Natl Acad Sci U S A 2008;105:19992–7.)

The sleep inhibition by the ICV infusion of ONO-4127Na was recently confirmed in WT and Hcrt-deficient narcoleptic mice,[69] in which the antagonist infusion into the basal forebrain promoted wakefulness in both types of mice and also suppressed the cataplexy in narcoleptic mice, suggesting that DP1 receptor antagonists may be a new class of drugs used for treatment of narcolepsy-cataplexy.

Hypersomnia induced by overproduction of endogenous PGD_2 was found in 2 animal models. One is human L-PGDS-overexpressing transgenic mice after tail clipping.[70] This hypersomnia was accidentally discovered by tail clipping used for DNA sampling from adult L-PGDS–transgenic mice. The tail clipping increased the PGD_2 content in the brain, probably due to the pain stimulation, and induced NREM sleep in these mice.

The other case is hypersomnia after a pentylenetetrazole-induced seizure.[71] Pentylenetetrazole administration to mice induces severe seizure. During the seizure, the PGD_2 content in the brain increases remarkably from 0.07 in the basal level to 88 ng per brain, and NREM sleep is induced and lasts for several hours after the seizure (**Fig. 7**). This increase in postepileptic NREM sleep is abolished in gene KO mice of L-PGDS or DP1 receptor, but remains unchanged in those of H-PGDS or DP2 receptor, suggesting that the L-PGDS/PGD_2/DP1 receptor system is involved in this type of hypersomnia.

In patients with narcolepsy, it is reported that the increase in the serum level of L-PGDS (beta-trace) is correlated with the symptom of excessive daytime sleepiness, suggesting that the sleepiness of narcoleptic patients may be caused by overproduction of PGD_2.[72] In severe obstructive sleep apnoea patients, morning urinary L-PGDS concentrations had significant correlations with the apnoea/hypopnoea index (R^2= 13.9%) but not with sleepiness.[73]

HYPERSOMNIA INDUCED BY CYTOKINES

Several cytokines, such as interleukin-1β (IL-1β), IL-6, and tumor necrosis factor-α, also induce NREM sleep in several animal models.[74–76] This cytokine-induced NREM sleep is proposed to be involved in hypersomnia during a bacterial or viral infection. The IL-1β–induced NREM sleep was previously reported to be mediated by PGD_2.[77] However, the author recently demonstrated that this IL-1β–induced increase in NREM sleep is not mediated by PGD_2, because this increase is also observed in DP1 receptor KO mice.[78]

Lipopolysaccharide (LPS), a bacterial endotoxin, induces sleep in various animals. LPS-induced sleep is slightly attenuated in KO mice lacking EP4 receptors, a Gs-coupled subtype of PGE_2 receptors, in their nervous system, but this sleep was not affected in KO mice lacking EP3 receptors (a Gi-coupled subtype of PGE_2 receptors) or microsomal PGE synthase or DP1 receptors, or in mice pretreated with a cyclooxygenase inhibitor.[79] These results suggest that the effect of LPS on sleep is partially dependent on PGs and is likely mediated mainly by other proinflammatory substances.

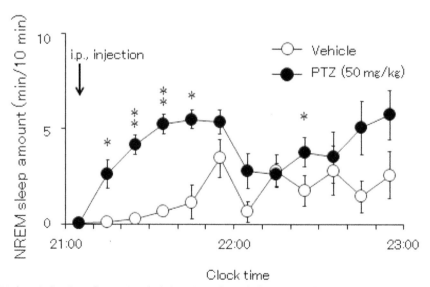

Fig. 7. NREM sleep induction after an IP administration of penthylenetetrazol to WT mice. PTZ, penthylenetetrazol. *P<.05; **P<.01 versus vehicle (saline)-injected group. (*Data from* Kaushik MK, Aritake K, Kamauchi S, et al. Prostaglandin D2 is crucial for seizure suppression and postictal sleep. Exp Neurol 2014;253:82–90.)

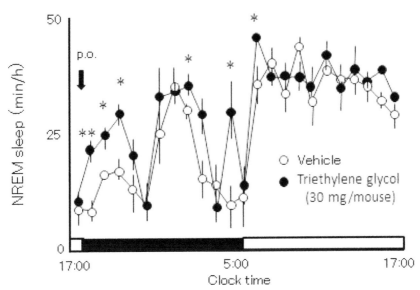

Fig. 8. NREM sleep induction by oral administration of triethylene glycol to WT mice. *$P<.05$; **$P<.01$ versus vehicle (water)-administered group. (*Data from* Kaushik MK, Kaul SC, Wadhwa R, et al. Triethylene glycol, an active component of Ashwagandha (Withania somnifera) leaves, is responsible for sleep induction. PLoS One 2017;12:e0172508.)

On the other hand, the induction of L-PGDS or H-PGDS is observed in the brain of patients with various neurodegenerative diseases and their animal models, such as subarachnoid hemorrhage,[80,81] demyelination,[82–84] lysosomal storage disease,[85] chronic multiple sclerosis,[86] hypoxic ischemic injury,[87,88] Alzheimer disease,[89] and spinal cord contusion injury,[90] the induction of which probably increases the PGD$_2$ level in the brain[91] and increases the production of various cytokines in the brain in a DP1 or DP2 receptor–dependent manner.[82]

CHEMICAL-INDUCED HYPERSOMNIA

Several natural compounds that induce NREM sleep after oral or IP administration to mice and rats have recently been identified, including hastatoside and verbenalin, which are iridoid compounds in the herbal tea Verbena[92,93]; ornithine[94]; crocin and crocetine from *Crocus sativus L* (saffron)[95]; glycine[96]; L-stepholidine,[97] honokiol,[98] and magnorol[99] from Chinese herb and medicine; polyphenols from Korean seaweed[100]; methylthioadenosine from Japanese sake yeast[101,102]; Zn-containing yeast[103,104]; and triethylene glycol from the Indian medicine Ashwagandha (**Fig. 8**).[105] Some of these compounds or materials, such as glycine, Korean seaweed polyphenol, and sake yeast, have already been commercialized as sleep-promoting supplements in Japan and Korea; they increase NREM sleep in normal, but not in sleep-deprived, animals.

Thus, it is possible that they may also induce hypersomnia in humans. Further study is necessary to examine this possibility.

ACKNOWLEDGMENTS

The author thanks Dr Mahesh Kaushik for performing the experiments on Suvorexant-induced narcolepsy and Dr Larry Frye for editing the article. Also, the author wishes to honor the memory of his dear friend and mentor, Professor Osamu Hayaishi, who passed away in December of 2015 at 95 years of age. This giant of sleep science has been and will continue to be sorely missed.

REFERENCES

1. Berro LF. Obituary: Roberto Frussa-Filho (1960-2013). Psychopharmacology (Berl) 2014;231: 1863–4.
2. Ruoff C, Rye D. The ICSD-3 and DSM-5 guidelines for diagnosing narcolepsy: clinical relevance and practicality. Curr Med Res Opin 2016;20:1–12.
3. Thannickal TC, Moore RY, Nienhuis R, et al. Reduced number of hypocretin neurons in human narcolepsy. Neuron 2000;27:469–74.
4. de Lecea L, Kilduff TS, Peyron C, et al. The hypocretins: hypothalamus-specific peptides with neuroexcitatory activity. Proc Natl Acad Sci U S A 1998;95:322–7.
5. Sakurai T, Amemiya A, Ishii M, et al. Orexins and orexin receptors: a family of hypothalamic

neuropeptides and G protein-coupled receptors that regulate feeding behavior. Cell 1998;92: 573–85.

6. Lin L, Faraco J, Li R, et al. The sleep disorder canine narcolepsy is caused by a mutation in the hypocretin (orexin) receptor 2 gene. Cell 1999;98: 365–76.

7. Chemelli RM, Willie JT, Sinton CM, et al. Narcolepsy in orexin knockout mice: molecular genetics of sleep regulation. Cell 1999;98:437–51.

8. Nishino S, Ripley B, Overeem S, et al. Hypocretin (orexin) deficiency in human narcolepsy. Lancet 2000;355:39–40.

9. Peyron C, Faraco J, Rogers W, et al. A mutation in a case of early onset narcolepsy and a generalized absence of hypocretin peptides in human narcoleptic brains. Nat Med 2000;6:991–7.

10. Dauvilliers Y, Arnulf I, Mignot E. Narcolepsy with cataplexy. Lancet 2007;369:499–511.

11. Huang ZL, Qu WM, Li WD, et al. Arousal effect of orexin A depends on activation of the histaminergic system. Proc Natl Acad Sci U S A 2001;98: 9965–70.

12. Winrow CJ, Gotter AL, Cox CD, et al. Promotion of sleep by suvorexant-a novel dual orexin receptor antagonist. J Neurogenet 2011;25:52–61.

13. Winrow CJ, Gotter AL, Cox CD, et al. Pharmacological characterization of MK-6096-a dual orexin receptor antagonist for insomnia. Neuropharmacology 2012;62:978–87.

14. Yang LP. Suvorexant: first global approval. Drugs 2014;74:1817–22.

15. Oishi Y, Williams RH, Agostinelli L, et al. Role of the medial prefrontal cortex in cataplexy. J Neurosci 2013;33:9743–51.

16. Mignot E, Lammers GJ, Ripley B, et al. The role of cerebrospinal fluid hypocretin measurement in the diagnosis of narcolepsy and other hypersomnias. Arch Neurol 2002;59:1553–62.

17. Tabuchi S, Tsunematsu T, Black SW, et al. Conditional ablation of orexin/hypocretin neurons: a new mouse model for the study of narcolepsy and orexin system function. J Neurosci 2014;34: 6495–509.

18. Hayaishi O, Urade Y. Prostaglandin D2 in sleep-wake regulation: recent progress and perspectives. Neuroscientist 2002;8:12–5.

19. Hayaishi O, Urade Y, Eguchi N, et al. Genes for prostaglandin D synthase and receptor as well as adenosine A2A receptor are involved in the homeostatic regulation of NREM sleep. Arch Ital Biol 2004; 142:533–9.

20. Huang ZL, Urade Y, Hayaishi O. Prostaglandins and adenosine in the regulation of sleep and wakefulness. Curr Opin Pharmacol 2007;7:33–8.

21. Urade Y, Hayaishi O. Prostaglandin D2 and sleep/wake regulation. Sleep Med Rev 2011;15(6):411–8.

22. Narumiya S, Ogorochi T, Nakao K, et al. Prostaglandin D2 in rat brain, spinal cord and pituitary: basal level and regional distribution. Life Sci 1982;31:2093–103.

23. Ogorochi T, Narumiya S, Mizuno N, et al. Regional distribution of prostaglandin D2, E2 and F2α and related enzymes in postmortem human brain. J Neurochem 1984;43:71–82.

24. Ueno R, Ishikawa Y, Nakayama T, et al. Prostaglandin D2 induces sleep when microinjected into the preoptic area of conscious rats. Biochem Biophys Res Commun 1982;109:576–82.

25. Onoe H, Ueno R, Fujita I, et al. Prostaglandin D2, a cerebral sleep-inducing substance in monkeys. Proc Natl Acad Sci U S A 1988;85:4082–6.

26. Roberts LJ II, Sweetman BJ, Lewis RA, et al. Increased production of prostaglandin D2 in patients with systemic mastocytosis. N Engl J Med 1980;303:1400–4.

27. Pentreath VW, Rees K, Owolabi OA, et al. The somnogenic T lymphocyte suppressor prostaglandin D2 is selectively elevated in cerebrospinal fluid of advanced sleeping sickness patients. Trans R Soc Trop Med Hyg 1990;84(6):795–9.

28. Kubata BK, Duszenko M, Kabututu Z, et al. Identification of a novel prostaglandin f(2alpha) synthase in Trypanosoma brucei. J Exp Med 2000;192: 1327–38.

29. Kubata BK, Duszenko M, Martin KS, et al. Molecular basis for prostaglandin production in hosts and parasites. Trends Parasitol 2007;23:325–31.

30. Smith WL, Urade Y, Jakobsson PJ. Enzymes of the cyclooxygenase pathways of prostanoid biosynthesis. Chem Rev 2011;111:5821–65.

31. Urade Y, Hayaishi O. Prostaglandin D synthase: structure and function. Vitam Horm 2000a;58:89–120.

32. Urade Y, Hayaishi O. Biochemical, structural, genetic, physiological, and pathophysiological features of lipocalin-type prostaglandin D synthase. Biochim Biophys Acta 2000b;1482:259–71.

33. Beuckmann CT, Lazarus M, Gerashchenko D, et al. Cellular localization of lipocalin-type prostaglandin D synthase (beta-trace) in the central nervous system of the adult rat. J Comp Neurol 2000;428:62–78.

34. Urade Y, Kitahama K, Ohishi H, et al. Dominant expression of mRNA for prostaglandin D synthase in leptomeninges, choroid plexus, and oligodendrocytes of the adult rat brain. Proc Natl Acad Sci U S A 1993;90:9070–4.

35. Yamashima T, Sakuda K, Tohma Y, et al. Prostaglandin D synthase (beta-trace) in human arachnoid and meningioma cells: roles as a cell marker or in cerebrospinal fluid absorption, tumorigenesis, and calcification process. J Neurosci 1997;17:2376–82.

36. Watanabe K, Urade Y, Mader M, et al. Identification of beta-trace as prostaglandin D synthase. Biochem Biophys Res Commun 1994;203:1110–6.

37. Kanaoka Y, Urade Y. Hematopoietic prostaglandin D synthase. Prostaglandins Leukot Essent Fatty Acids 2003;69:163–7.

38. Mohri I, Eguchi N, Suzuki K, et al. Hematopoietic prostaglandin D synthase is expressed in the developing postnatal mouse brain. Glia 2003;42: 263–74.

39. Hirata M, Kakizuka A, Aizawa M, et al. Molecular characterization of a mouse prostaglandin D receptor and functional expression of the cloned gene. Proc Natl Acad Sci U S A 1994;91(23): 11192–6.

40. Abe H, Takeshita T, Nagata K, et al. Molecular cloning, chromosome mapping and characterization of the mouse CRTH2 gene, a putative member of the leukocyte chemoattractant receptor family. Gene 1999;227(1):71–7.

41. Hirai H, Tanaka K, Yoshie O, et al. Prostaglandin D2 selectively induces chemotaxis in T helper type 2 cells, eosinophils, and basophils via seven-transmembrane receptor CRTH2. J Exp Med 2001;193(2):255–61.

42. Oishi Y, Takata Y, Taguchi Y, et al. Polygraphic recording procedure for measuring sleep in mice. J Vis Exp 2016;25(107):e53678.

43. Kohtoh S, Taguchi Y, Matsumoto N, et al. Algorithm for sleep scoring in experimental animals based on fast Fourier transform power spectrum analysis of the electroencephalogram. Sleep Biol Rhythm 2008;6:163–71.

44. Sunagawa G, Sei H, Shimba S, et al. FASTER: an unsupervised fully automated sleep staging method for mice. Genes Cells 2013;18(6):502–18.

45. Matsumura H, Nakajima T, Osaka T, et al. Prostaglandin D2-sensitive, sleep-promoting zone defined in the ventral surface of the rostral basal fore brain. Proc Natl Acad Sci U S A 1994;91: 11998–2002.

46. Mizoguchi A, Eguchi N, Kimura K, et al. Dominant localization of prostaglandin D receptors on arachnoid trabecular cells in mouse basal forebrain and their involvement in the regulation of non-rapid eye movement sleep. Proc Natl Acad Sci U S A 2001; 98:11674–9.

47. Basher R, Strecher RE, Thakkar MM, et al. Adenosine and sleep-wake regulation. Prog Neurobiol 2004;73:379–96.

48. Huang ZL, Urade Y, Hayaishi O. The role of adenosine in the regulation of sleep. Curr Top Med Chem 2011;11:1047–57.

49. Porkka-Heiskanen T, Strecker RE, Thakkar M, et al. Adenosine: a mediator of the sleep-inducing effects of prolonged wakefulness. Science 1997; 276:1265–8.

50. Porkka-Heiskanen T, Kalinchuk AV. Adenosine, energy metabolism and sleep homeostasis. Sleep Med Rev 2011;15:123–35.

51. Satoh S, Matsumura H, Suzuki F, et al. Promotion of sleep mediated by the A2a adenosine receptor and possible involvement of this receptor in the sleep induced by prostaglandin D2 in rats. Proc Natl Acad Sci U S A 1996;93:5980–4.

52. Zhang BJ, Huang ZL, Chen JF, et al. Adenosine A2A receptor deficiency attenuates the somnogenic effect of prostaglandin D2 in mice. Acta Pharmacol Sin 2017;38:469–76.

53. Scammell TE, Gerashchenko DY, Mochizuki T, et al. An adenosine A2a agonist increases sleep and induces Fos in ventrolateral preoptic neurons. Neuroscience 2001;107:653–63.

54. Scammell T, Gerashchenko D, Urade Y, et al. Activation of ventrolateral preoptic neurons by the somnogen prostaglandin D2. Proc Natl Acad Sci U S A 1998;95:7754–9.

55. Hong ZY, Huang ZL, Qu WM, et al. An adenosine A receptor agonist induces sleep by increasing GABA release in the tuberomammillary nucleus to inhibit histaminergic systems in rats. J Neurochem 2005;92:1542–9.

56. Sherin JE, Elmquist JK, Torrealba F, et al. Innervation of histaminergic tuberomammillary neurons by GABAergic and galaninergic neurons in the ventrolateral preoptic nucleus of the rat. J Neurosci 1998; 18:4705–21.

57. Sherin JE, Shiromani PJ, McCarley RW, et al. Activation of ventrolateral preoptic neurons during sleep. Science 1996;271:216–9.

58. Saper CB, Scammell TE, Lu J. Hypothalamic regulation of sleep and circadian rhythms. Nature 2005; 437:1257–63.

59. Chu M, Huang ZL, Qu WM, et al. Extracellular histamine level in the frontal cortex is positively correlated with the amount of wakefulness in rats. Neurosci Res 2004;49:417–20.

60. Oishi Y, Huang ZL, Fredholm BB, et al. Adenosine in the tuberomammillary nucleus inhibits the histaminergic system via A1 receptors and promotes non-rapid eye movement sleep. Proc Natl Acad Sci U S A 2008;105:19992–7.

61. Lazarus M, Shen HY, Cherasse Y, et al. Arousal effect of caffeine depends on adenosine A2A receptors in the shell of the nucleus accumbens. J Neurosci 2011;31:10067–75.

62. Huang ZL, Qu WM, Eguchi N, et al. Adenosine A2A, but not A1, receptors mediate the arousal effect of caffeine. Nat Neurosci 2005;8:858–9.

63. Lazarus M, Chen JF, Urade Y, et al. Role of the basal ganglia in the control of sleep and wakefulness. Curr Opin Neurobiol 2013;23(5):780–5.

64. Lazarus M, Huang ZL, Lu J, et al. How do the basal ganglia regulate sleep-wake behavior? Trends Neurosci 2012;35:723–32.

65. Qiu MH, Liu W, Qu WM, et al. The role of nucleus accumbens core/shell in sleep-wake regulation

and their involvement in modafinil-induced arousal. PLoS One 2012;7:e45471.

66. Islam F, Watanabe Y, Morii H, et al. Inhibition of rat brain prostaglandin D synthase by inorganic selenocompounds. Arch Biochem Biophys 1991;289: 161–6.

67. Matsumura H, Takahata R, Hayaishi O. Inhibition of sleep in rats by inorganic selenium compounds, inhibitors of prostaglandin D synthase. Proc Natl Acad Sci U S A 1991;88:9046–50.

68. Qu WM, Huang ZL, Xu XH, et al. Lipocalin-type prostaglandin D synthase produces prostaglandin D2 involved in regulation of physiological sleep. Proc Natl Acad Sci U S A 2006;103:17949–54.

69. Segawa Y, Sato M, Sakai N, et al. Wake-promoting effects of ONO-4127Na, a prostaglandin DP1 receptor antagonist in hypocretin/orexin deficient narcoleptic mice. Neuropharmacology 2016;110: 268–76.

70. Pinzar E, Kanaoka Y, Inui T, et al. Prostaglandin D synthase gene is involved in the regulation of non-rapid eye movement sleep. Proc Natl Acad Sci U S A 2000;97:4903–7.

71. Kaushik MK, Aritake K, Kamauchi S, et al. Prostaglandin D2 is crucial for seizure suppression and postictal sleep. Exp Neurol 2014;253:82–90.

72. Jordan W, Tumani H, Cohrs S, et al. Narcolepsy increased L-PGDS (beta-trace) levels correlate with excessive daytime sleepiness but not with cataplexy. J Neurol 2005;252:1372–8.

73. Chihara Y, Chin K, Aritake K, et al. A urine biomarker for severe obstructive sleep apnoea patients: lipocalintype prostaglandin D synthase. Eur Respir J 2013;42:1563–74.

74. Krueger JM, Majde JA, Obal F Jr. Sleep in host defense. Brain Behav Immun 2003;17:41–7.

75. Krueger JM, Obal F Jr, Fang J, et al. The role of cytokines in physiological sleep regulation. Ann NY Acad Sci 2001;933:211–21.

76. Opp MR. Cytokines and sleep. Sleep Med Rev 2005;9:355–64.

77. Terao A, Matsumura H, Saito M. Interleukin-1 induces slow-wave sleep at the prostaglandin D2-sensitive sleep-promoting zone in the rat brain. J Neurosci 1998;18:6599–607.

78. Zhang BJ, Shao SR, Aritake K, et al. Interleukin-1β induces sleep independent of prostaglandin D2 in rats and mice. Neuroscience 2017;340:258–67.

79. Oishi Y, Yoshida K, Scammell TE, et al. The roles of prostaglandin E2 and D2 in lipopolysaccharide-mediated changes in sleep. Brain Behav Immun 2015;47:172–7.

80. Inui T, Mase M, Shirota R, et al. Lipocalin-type prostaglandin D synthase scavenges biliverdin in the cerebrospinal fluid of patients with aneurysmal subarachnoid hemorrhage. J Cereb Blood Flow Metab 2014;34:1558–67.

81. Mase M, Yamada K, Iwata A, et al. Acute and transient increase of lipocalin-type prostaglandin D synthase (beta-trace) level in cerebrospinal fluid of patients with aneurysmal subarachnoid hemorrhage. Neurosci Lett 1999;270:188–90.

82. Mohri I, Taniike M, Okazaki I, et al. Lipocalin-type prostaglandin D synthase is up-regulated in oligodendrocytes in lysosomal storage diseases and binds gangliosides. J Neurochem 2006;97:641–51.

83. Taniike M, Mohri I, Eguchi N, et al. Perineuronal oligodendrocytes protect against neuronal apoptosis through the production of lipocalin-type prostaglandin D synthase in a genetic demyelinating model. J Neurosci 2002;22:4885–96.

84. Trimarco A, Forese MG, Alfieri V, et al. Prostaglandin D2 synthase/GPR44: a signaling axis in PNS myelination. Nat Neurosci 2014;17(12): 1682–92.

85. Mohri I, Taniike M, Taniguchi H, et al. Prostaglandin D2-mediated microglia/astrocyte interaction enhances astrogliosis and demyelination in twitcher. J Neurosci 2006;26:4383–93.

86. Kagitani-Shimono K, Mohri I, Oda H, et al. Lipocalin-type prostaglandin D synthase (beta-trace) is upregulated in the alphaB-crystallin-positive oligodendrocytes and astrocytes in the chronic multiple sclerosis. Neuropathol Appl Neurobiol 2006;32:64–73.

87. Liu M, Eguchi N, Yamasaki Y, et al. Focal cerebral ischemia/reperfusion injury in mice induces hematopoietic prostaglandin D synthase in microglia and macrophages. Neuroscience 2007;145:520–9.

88. Taniguchi H, Mohri I, Okabe-Arahori H, et al. Prostaglandin D2 protects neonatal mouse brain from hypoxic ischemic injury. J Neurosci 2007;27:4303–12.

89. Mohri I, Kadoyama K, Kanekiyo T, et al. Hematopoietic prostaglandin D synthase and DP1 receptor are selectively upregulated in microglia and astrocytes within senile plaques from human patients and in a mouse model of Alzheimer disease. J Neuropathol Exp Neurol 2007;66:469–80.

90. Redensek A, Rathore KI, Berard JL, et al. Expression and detrimental role of hematopoietic prostaglandin D synthase in spinal cord contusion injury. Glia 2011;59:603–14.

91. Shinozawa T, Urade Y, Maruyama T, et al. Tetranor PGDM analyses for the amyotrophic lateral sclerosis: positive and simple diagnosis and evaluation of drug effect. Biochem Biophys Res Commun 2011;415:539–44.

92. Makino Y, Kondo S, Nishimura Y, et al. Hastatoside and verbenalin are sleep-promoting components in Verbena officinalis. Sleep Biol Rhythm 2009;7:211–7.

93. Omori K, Kagami Y, Yokoyama C, et al. Promotion of non–rapid eye movement sleep in mice after oral administration of ornithine. Sleep Biol Rhythm 2012;10:38–45.

94. Masaki M, Aritake K, Tanaka H, et al. Crocin promotes non-rapid eye movement sleep in mice. Mol Nutr Food Res 2012;56:304–8.

95. Soeda S, Aritake K, Urade Y, et al. Neuroprotective activities of saffron and crocin. Adv Neurobiol 2016;12:275–92.

96. Kawai N, Sakai N, Okuro M, et al. The sleep-promoting and hypothermic effects of glycine are mediated by NMDA receptors in the suprachiasmatic nucleus. Neuropsychopharmacology 2015;40(6):1405–16.

97. Qiu MH, Qu WM, Xu XH, et al. D(1)/D(2) receptor-targeting L-stepholidine, an active ingredient of the Chinese herb Stephonia, induces non-rapid eye movement sleep in mice. Pharmacol Biochem Behav 2009;94:16–23.

98. Qu WM, Yue XF, Sun Y, et al. Honokiol promotes non-rapid eye movement sleep via the benzodiazepine site of the GABAA receptor in mice. Br J Pharmacol 2012;167:587–98.

99. Chen CR, Zhou XZ, Luo YJ, et al. Magnolol, a major bioactive constituent of the bark of Magnolia officinalis, induces sleep via the benzodiazepine site of GABAA receptor in mice. Neuropharmacology 2012;63:1191–9.

100. Cho S, Yoon M, Pae AN, et al. Marine polyphenol phlorotannins promote non-rapid eye movement sleep in mice via the benzodiazepine site of the GABAA receptor. Psychopharmacology (Berl) 2014;231(14):2825–37.

101. Monoi N, Matsuno A, Nagamori Y, et al. Japanese sake yeast supplementation improves the quality of sleep: a double-blind randomised controlled clinical trial. J Sleep Res 2016;25:116–23.

102. Nakamura Y, Midorikawa T, Monoi N, et al. Oral administration of Japanese sake yeast (Saccharomyces cerevisiae sake) promotes non-rapid eye movement sleep in mice via adenosine A2A receptors. J Sleep Res 2016;25:746–53.

103. Cherasse Y, Saito H, Nagata N, et al. Zinc-containing yeast extract promotes nonrapid eye movement sleep in mice. Mol Nutr Food Res 2015;59:2087–93.

104. Saito H, Cherasse Y, Suzuki R, et al. Zinc-rich oysters as well as zinc yeast- and astaxanthin-enriched food improved sleep efficiency and sleep onset in a randomized controlled trial of healthy individuals. Mol Nutr Food Res 2017. [Epub ahead of print].

105. Kaushik MK, Kaul SC, Wadhwa R, et al. Triethylene glycol, an active component of Ashwagandha (Withania somnifera) leaves, is responsible for sleep induction. PLoS One 2017;12:e0172508.

The Immune Basis of Narcolepsy
What Is the Evidence?

Shahrad Taheri, MSc, PhD, FRCP[a,b,*]

KEYWORDS

- Narcolepsy • Autoimmune • Human leukocyte antigen • Influenza

KEY POINTS

- Narcolepsy is a chronic neurological sleep disorder associated with abnormal transitions into rapid eye movement sleep.
- Type 1 narcolepsy, which is associated with cataplexy, appears to be due to a specific destruction of lateral hypothalamic hypocretin neurons.
- Type 1 narcolepsy is closely associated with HLA DQB1*0602. This suggests that an autoimmune process is involved in type 1 narcolepsy.
- An association between influenza H1N1 infection, its vaccination, and narcolepsy has been observed, suggesting an infectious trigger for type 1 narcolepsy and molecular mimicry.
- Definitive evidence regarding pathogenic autoantibodies and/or autoreactive T lymphocytes in narcolepsy is still unavailable.

INTRODUCTION

Narcolepsy is a profound chronic neurologic sleep disorder associated with excessive daytime sleepiness (hypersomnia).[1–4] Narcolepsy is a disorder of abnormal transitions into rapid eye movement (REM) sleep, resulting in other key features, such as cataplexy, sleep paralysis, and hypnagogic hallucinations. Paradoxically, nighttime sleep is disturbed in narcolepsy. Cataplexy, an important feature triggered by emotions such as laughter, is partial or generalized muscle weakness with preserved consciousness. It can be mild, such as drooping of the eyelids and jaw dropping, or severe, resulting in collapse when larger muscles are affected. Cataplexy is seen in only a few other disorders and is thus a distinctive feature of narcolepsy. In the International Classification of Sleep Disorders, third edition (ICSD-3),[5] narcolepsy is subdivided into type 1 (cataplexy present) and type 2 (cataplexy absent). Although it can occur at any age, narcolepsy commonly presents in the second decade of life.[1,6] Narcolepsy results in a significant impact on quality of life, but does not limit lifespan. The diagnosis of narcolepsy is often delayed (as long as 10 years), which adversely affects patients and has hindered efforts to understand its triggers and pathophysiology.

The role of the hypothalamus in the regulation of homeostatic mechanisms is well established. The hypothalamus is also a key regulator of sleep and circadian rhythms. The encephalitis lethargica epidemic (1918–1926),[2] thought to have been triggered by an as yet undetermined viral infection, resulted in individuals who developed postencephalitic Parkinsonism and excessive sleepiness. Those affected with posterior (lateral) hypothalamic and midbrain junction lesion were affected by sleepiness, whereas those whose anterior hypothalamus was affected suffered from insomnia

[a] Department of Medicine, Weill Cornell Medicine, New York, NY 10065, USA; [b] Department of Medicine, Weill Cornell Medicine Qatar, Qatar Foundation–Education City, PO Box 24144, Doha, Qatar
* Department of Medicine, Weill Cornell Medicine Qatar, Qatar Foundation–Education City, PO Box 24144, Doha, Qatar.
E-mail address: staheri@me.com

Sleep Med Clin 12 (2017) 279–287
http://dx.doi.org/10.1016/j.jsmc.2017.03.004

and chorea. These observations not only established a key role for the posterior (lateral) hypothalamus in the maintenance of wakefulness but also demonstrated the possibility of a postinfectious process affecting the hypothalamus and triggering a sleep phenotype. Indeed, postinfectious immune-mediated neurologic disorders are well established, for example, Sydenham chorea associated with rheumatic fever secondary to streptococcal infection, Guillain-Barré syndrome triggered by multiple infectious organisms, and many others.

The important role of the hypothalamus in sleep and narcolepsy is now well established through several human and animal observations. Narcolepsy is associated with a specific dysfunction of hypocretin (orexin) peptide producing neurons whose cell bodies are specifically located in the lateral hypothalamus.[6–10] Hypocretin neurons produce 2 key peptide neurotransmitters: hypocretin-1 and hypocretin-2, derived from the enzymatic cleavage of preprohypocretin.[11–13] Hypocretins act through 2 key 7-transmembrane G-protein–coupled receptors named hypocretin receptor 1 (HCRTR1) and hypocretin receptor 2 (HCRTR2).[6] Lateral hypothalamic hypocretin neurons project throughout the brain suggesting multiple functions, and their dysfunction explains the key features of narcolepsy.[9,14] Postmortem brains from patients with narcolepsy have shown a specific loss of hypocretin neurons, whereas other neurons (melanin concentrating hormone, MCH neurons) whose cell bodies are interspersed with hypocretin neurons in the lateral hypothalamus are preserved.[15,16] Furthermore, hypocretin-1 levels are low or undetectable in patients with type 1 narcolepsy,[17–19] whereas MCH levels are normal,[20] and cerebrospinal fluid (CSF) hypocretin 1 measurement is included in the ICSD-3 diagnostic criteria for type 1 narcolepsy.[5]

An autosomal recessive canine model of narcolepsy has provided important information regarding narcolepsy.[21,22] Genetic canine narcolepsy, with a strong cataplexy phenotype, is associated with several mutations in the HCRTR2 gene resulting in a dysfunctional receptor.[21,23] Human narcolepsy, however, is not a simple genetic disorder and is not associated, except is a rare reported case,[16] with mutations in hypocretin system genes. The presence of the canine genetic model, however, resulted in the early pursuit of genetic associations with narcolepsy. A key discovered association was with the HLA markers.[1,24,25] HLA associations are commonly observed in relation to autoimmune disorders. Proteins colocalizing with hypocretin peptides, such as dynorphin and neuronal activity–regulated pentraxin, have been observed to be absent in the lateral hypothalamus of postmortem brains from those with narcolepsy, suggesting the absence (destruction) of hypocretin neurons.[26] The HLA association with narcolepsy, in combination with the observation that narcolepsy has a peripubertal onset, suggests that hypocretin neuron destruction results from an autoimmune process.[27–31] In the following sections, the current evidence regarding the autoimmune basis of narcolepsy is presented and discussed, with gaps in current knowledge regarding the pathophysiology of narcolepsy highlighted.

NARCOLEPSY AND HUMAN LEUKOCYTE ANTIGEN GENES

The HLA system has a major role in immune function.[1,32] HLA genes are highly polymorphic, and, in humans, map to the short arm of chromosome 6 (6p21.31) and encode glycoproteins. HLA class I and II encoded glycoproteins are involved in antigen processing and presentation to cytotoxic and regulatory T lymphocytes, respectively. HLA class I genes encode an alpha polypeptide chain that combines with a beta-chain (beta$_2$ microglobulin), encoded by a nonpolymorphic gene on chromosome 15, to result in a molecule present on the cell surface of all nucleated cells. HLA class I molecules interact with T-cell receptors on cytotoxic CD8+ cells. HLA class II genes are normally expressed in immune cells (B and T lymphocytes, macrophages and dendritic cells, and thymic epithelial cells). They encode the alpha and beta polypeptide chains of HLA-DR, DQ, and DP. Alpha- and beta-chains form heterodimers on antigen-presenting cells and play a key role in antigen presentation to T lymphocytes (T-helper CD4+ cells) through the T-cell receptor. Activation of helper T cells mobilizes the immune system to protect against foreign antigens.

Given the diversity of the HLA system, a specific nomenclature is used to describe HLA genes and molecules. HLA class I molecules are named HLA-A, HLA-B, and HLA-C. HLA class II molecules are named HLA-DR, HLA-DQ, and HLA-DP. The *A* designation in HLA (eg, HLA DQA1*102) refers to alpha-chain genes, whereas the *B* designation (eg, HLA DQB1*0602) refers to beta-chain genes. The numbers following the * (eg, HLA DQB1*0602) refer to the gene variant. Autoimmune disorders are associated with specific HLA class II genes: type 1 diabetes mellitus (DR3, DR4, DQB1*0302, DQB1*0201, DQB1*0602), rheumatoid arthritis (DR4), seronegative arthritides (B27), multiple sclerosis (DR2, DQB1*0602), celiac disease (DQA1*05, DQB1*02), and pemphigus vulgaris (DRB1*0402).

Autoimmune diseases are thought to be triggered by the environment. They may be triggered by foreign antigens, usually associated with infectious agents, that interact with susceptible HLA class II antigens to mobilize the immune system against self-antigens through the proliferation and/or development of self-reactive T cells and/or through generation of autoantibodies. The autoimmune process may be triggered by an infectious agent that results in molecular mimicry and bystander activation. Molecular mimicry is when foreign antigens from the infectious agent share similar epitopes to normal host molecules. Mimicry may generate autoantibodies and/or self-reactive T cells. Bystander activation can occur when the presentation of the foreign antigen in conjunction with susceptible HLA II antigens triggers pre-primed self-reactive T cells. T-cell and immune-mediated damage of infected cells can spread damage to neighboring healthy cells, resulting in bystander damage. Release of self-peptides from damaged cells, including the differential processing of self-peptides by antigen-presenting cells, may result in activation of the immune system in response to self-antigens (epitope spreading).

Type 1 narcolepsy has a close association with specific HLA alleles.[33] An association between narcolepsy and HLA DR2 and DQ1 was first reported in the Japanese population[24] and subsequently confirmed in European populations,[34,35] but found to be more variable in African Americans.[36] HLA DQB1*0602 (a subtype of DQ1/DQ6), occurring in about 90% of patients, shows consistent association with narcolepsy across all ethnic groups,[33] and its structure appears to be essential for narcolepsy.[37] HLA DQB1*0602 allele occurs with HLA DQA1*102 on a haplotype with HLA DRB1*1501 in the Japanese and Europeans. This association has not been observed in African Americans, whereby HLA DQB1 and HLA DQA1 alleles occur with distinct HLA DRB1 haplotypes (HLA DRB1*1503, HLA DRB1*1501, HLA DRB1*1101, and HLA DRB1*806).[33] Interestingly, HLA DQB1*0602 is in almost complete linkage disequilibrium with HLA DQA1*102, but HLA DQA1*102 alone is not associated with increased narcolepsy risk. It is important to note that although 90% of those with narcolepsy have the HLA DQB1*0602 susceptibility, this allele is common in the general population (12% in Japanese to 38% in African Americans).[33] Also, relatives sharing HLA DQB1*0602 only rarely develop narcolepsy. Thus, HLA alone is not responsible for narcolepsy. HLA DQB1*0602 homozygotes, however, have a 2- to 4-fold greater narcolepsy risk compared with heterozygotes.[38–41] HLA DQB1*0602 homozygotes have been observed to have greater white cell DQB1*0602 mRNA and protein expression.[33] Another observed HLA association is with HLA DQB1*0301 across several ethnic groups. HLA DQB1*0301 predisposition occurs in the face of multiple DQA1 haplotypes. Thus, it appears that the beta-chain plays a greater role in antigen binding and immune engagement. It is of note that HLA DQB1*0601 is protective for narcolepsy. HLA DQB1*0601 has a structure close to HLADQB1*0602, suggesting that small variations in HLA can have significant effects. DQA1*0103-DQB1*603 is associated with lesser protection from narcolepsy. Exploration of the region around HLADQB1*0602 suggests that it is the susceptibility gene rather than other genes close to the HLA DQ region. Furthermore, HLADQB1*0602 has been reported to bind preprohypocretin. Interestingly, HLA DQB1*602 status has been associated with sleepiness and alterations in sleep architecture.

Other narcolepsy-related HLA loci have also been observed. A protective variant of HLA-DQA2 was observed in a genome-wide association study. This variant was strongly linked to HLA DRB1*03-DQB1*02 and HLA DRB1*1301-DQB1*0603. Narcolepsy cases almost never carried a trans-HLA DRB1*1301-DQB1*0603 haplotype. Following the observed potential relationship between upper respiratory infections (eg, influenza A H1N1), a case control study with HLA-DR and HLA-DQ matching, observed protective effects for HLA DPA1*0103-DPB1*0402 and HLA DPA1*0103-DPB1*0401. Other studies have suggested a role for HLA class I (HLA A*1101, HLA B*3503, and HLA B*51:01) susceptibility effects.[42] These alleles point to additional roles for HLA markers in infection-triggered autoimmune disease with previous work reporting changes in HLA associations after the 2009 H1N1 pandemic.[43]

NARCOLEPSY AND NON–HUMAN LEUKOCYTE ANTIGEN IMMUNE GENES

Recent genetic studies have identified a potential contribution of non-HLA immune-related genes to narcolepsy, although the association of polymorphisms in these genes with narcolepsy is significantly weaker (odds ratio, range 1.3–1.8) than the HLA association. The T-lymphocyte cell receptor consists of unique alpha- and beta-chains assembled to recognize a specific antigen. The antigen-presenting cell engages the T-cell receptor through presenting the antigen bound to HLA molecules. A narcolepsy-associated polymorphism (especially rs1154155) in the TRA@ (T-cell receptor alpha) gene locus (chromosome 14q11.2) has been observed.[44] A custom genotyping array

(ImmunoChip) approach, examining immune-related genes, confirmed the importance of TRA@ and identified 2 additional loci: Cathepsin H (CTSH) and tumor necrosis factor (ligand) super-family member 4 (TNFSF4/OX40L).[45,46] Interestingly, CTSH, expressed by antigen-presenting cells, is a cysteine protease important for peptide processing, which occurs as part of antigen presentation. TNFSF4/OX40L is found in antigen-presenting cells and is involved in T-cell regulation.

A single nucleotide polymorphism (rs4804122) has been associated with HLA DQB1*0602 narcolepsy compared with HLA DQB1*0602-positive controls. This polymorphism is downstream on purinergic receptor subtype 2Y11 (P2RY11) gene (chromosome 19p13.2), which has high linkage disequilibrium with PPAN (Peter Pan), P2RY11, EIF3G (Eukaryotic translation initiation factor 3), and DNMT1 (DNA (Cytosine-5-)-Methyltransferase 1) genes. Purinergic signaling plays an important role in immune cell regulation, chemotaxis, proliferation, and apoptosis. DNMT1 is found in immune cells and has a role in T-cell differentiation. DNMT1 gene mutations are associated with narcolepsy, deafness, cerebellar ataxia, and neuropathy.[47] In a further study, the disease-associated EIF3G allele (rs3826784) was associated with increased EIF3G expression.[48] EIF3G expression correlates with expression of PPAN and PRY11, suggesting shared regulatory mechanisms. A Japanese study has identified a role for chemokine receptors (CCR1/CCR3), which plays a role in monocyte migration. A polymorphism (rs3181077) located upstream of CCR1 and CCR3 has been associated with narcolepsy. The expression of CCR1 and CCR3 was observed to be lower in patients with narcolepsy.[49] The above findings suggest the contribution of multiple immune-related genes to narcolepsy and highlight the complexity of narcolepsy. The precise role of these immune-related gene polymorphisms in the pathophysiology of narcolepsy remains to be determined.

NARCOLEPSY, INFECTIONS, AND VACCINES

The encephalitis lethargica epidemic and the fact that several immune-mediated neurologic and autoimmune diseases are triggered by infectious organisms suggest that if narcolepsy is an autoimmune disorder, there may also be an infectious trigger for it. Infectious diseases occur in a seasonal fashion. In narcolepsy, however, given that the onset of disease tends to differ markedly from the time of diagnosis, it is difficult to confirm if there is a seasonal effect.

In a study of 200 patients close to disease onset, it was noted that anti-streptolysin O and anti-DNAse B antibody titers were higher in patients compared with age-matched controls, especially within the first 3 years of disease onset.[50] The investigators suggested several explanations for their findings: (1) streptococcal infection, through molecular mimicry, is directly implicated in narcolepsy; or (2) streptococcal infection enables other factors to trigger narcolepsy, by increasing susceptibility, reactivating the immune system nonspecifically or through superantigens (triggering a widespread nonspecific T-cell activation and massive cytokine release), or increasing blood-brain barrier permeability. In a study from Sweden, a role for streptococcal infection was proposed in those who developed narcolepsy after Pandemrix H1N1 (α-tocopherol containing ASO3-adjuvanated A(H1N1) pandemic vaccine) vaccination.[51] Higher levels of serum antistreptolysin O were found in narcolepsy cases compared with vaccinated controls. Also, interferon-gamma production in whole blood of narcolepsy cases was higher in response to streptococcal antigens. This study suggests a potential role for streptococcal infections in triggering narcolepsy.

The 2009 pandemic of H1N1 influenza infection was noted to be associated with a 3- to 4-fold increased incidence of narcolepsy in Beijing, China. This incidence returned to baseline with the conclusion of the pandemic.[52] In the observations from China, it was suggested that narcolepsy was associated with winter infections.[53] This observation may have been made mainly in China because of the high population density and low vaccination rates. An association between ASO3-adjuvanated A(H1N1) pandemic vaccine and increased incidence of narcolepsy was first observed in Finland and Sweden.[54] A 12.7-fold risk was observed in 4 to 19 year olds within about 8 months after vaccination compared with unvaccinated age-matched controls. The narcolepsy in response to vaccination was associated with the presence of HLADQB1*0602.

Countries where vaccination coverage was high also reported and increased incidence of narcolepsy.[55] Some have argued that the ASO3 adjuvant may be the key contributor, but although ASO3 is likely to enhance the immune response, it is most likely, especially in the context of data from China, that H1N1 is likely to be the culprit.[56,57] However, molecular mimicry of H1N1 with hypocretin peptides has not been clearly demonstrated. It is possible that prior exposure to streptococcal infection may enhance the effect of H1N1 in triggering an autoimmune attack on hypocretin neurons to result in narcolepsy.

NARCOLEPSY AND HUMORAL IMMUNITY

Autoimmune diseases are commonly associated with disease-specific and nonspecific autoantibodies. If narcolepsy is an autoimmune disease, then it would be expected that it would be associated with the presence of autoantibodies against components of hypocretin neurons and/or hypocretin receptors. To date, no confirmed antibodies against the hypocretin system components have been reported. One study used western blots to examine serum immunoreactivity to lateral hypothalamic proteins from brains of dogs, rats, and mice.[27,58] The study also examined the binding to lateral hypothalamic protein of purified immunoglobulin G (IgG) derived from CSF of HLADQB1*0602-positive patients, including those close to disease onset. No binding was observed for serum or CSF. Others have tested a similar hypothesis using immunocytochemistry,[59-61] but again, no convincing evidence of antibodies against lateral hypothalamic neurons that might explain the pathophysiology of narcolepsy has been demonstrated. Although some interesting binding to nonhypocretin neurons has been observed, the binding patterns are not specific to narcolepsy.

Passive transfer of immunoglobulins from patients to animals has also been attempted without any clear evidence for a pathophysiologic role. The lack of observed autoantibodies weakens the case for narcolepsy being an autoimmune disease. However, given that the disease is rarely captured at onset, these antibodies may only be circulating at very low titers beyond the detection of current methods. A small study examined the presence of encephalopathy-related autoantibodies (N-methyl-D-aspartate receptor [NMDAR]) and contactin-associated protein 2 (CASPR2) in children who developed narcolepsy after ASO3-adjuvanated A (H1N1) pandemic vaccination. No positive binding to NMDAR and CASPR2 was observed.[62] There was no evidence of specific antibodies to hypocretin neurons. Several studies have examined antibodies against nonhypocretin targets including the presence of neuron-specific antibodies. One study examined both antibodies against neuronal and nonneuronal antibodies, but although autoantibodies were observed, no single potential autoantibody emerged.

Some patients with Guillain-Barré syndrome have low hypocretin-1 levels in their CSF.[63] Screening for antiganglioside antibodies did not demonstrate a correlation between these antibodies and narcolepsy. Another study noted that those with Pandemrix-associated narcolepsy had higher titers of anti-GM3 antibodies compared with vaccinated nonnarcolepsy controls (14.3% vs 3.5%).[64] Vaccination, by itself, was associated with greater percentage of having antiganglioside antibodies. Interestingly, these antibodies demonstrated a significant association with HLA-DQB1*0602 in both narcolepsy cases and controls. Given that vaccine-associated narcolepsy cases are generally diagnosed earlier, it is possible that antiganglioside antibodies have a role in Pandemrix-associated narcolepsy.

One study has reported cross-reactivity between antibodies from Pandemrix-associated narcolepsy cases for both HCRTR2 and influenza nucleoprotein.[65] These antibodies were specific to Pandemrix vaccination. However, hypocretin neurons do not express HCRTR2 autoreceptors, so it is unlikely that the observed antibodies are directly related to hypocretin neuron destruction.[66] Narcolepsy symptoms have been described with anti-Ma2 paraneoplastic-associated encephalitis. In one case report, neuropathologic examination revealed inflammation and injury of the hypothalamus, with loss of hypocretin neurons. A cytotoxic CD8+ T-cell infiltration was observed.[67] Cytotoxic CD8+ T cells, but not helper CD4+ T cells, have been shown to induce a narcolepsy phenotype in mice expressing hemagglutinin (HA) in hypothalamic hypocretin neurons (HA-hypocretin neo-self-antigen) after transfer of neo-self-antigen–specific T cells.[68]

An association between early onset type 1 narcolepsy and autoantibodies against tribbles homolog 2 (TRIB2), which was found to be enriched in hypocretin neurons, has been reported.[69,70] Anti-TRIB2 antibodies have previously been associated with autoimmune uveitis. Early onset type 1 narcolepsy patients (within 2–3 years of diagnosis) had higher levels of anti-TRIB2 antibodies.[71] Intracerebroventricular (ICV) passive transfer of pooled IgG antibodies against TRIB2 into mice was associated with loss of hypocretin neurons and a narcolepsy phenotype.[72] Anti-TRB2 immunization in rats has been observed to result in decreased hypocretin mRNA and release into CSF.[73]

TRIB2 antibodies fulfill several criteria that suggest a potential causal link:

1. Antibodies are detected in sera from patients with type 1 narcolepsy;
2. The antibodies are detected in those with early onset disease;
3. Reports of improvement of narcolepsy with intravenous immunoglobulin (IVIg) treatment[74-82];
4. Passive transfer of narcolepsy to animals with anti-TRIB2 antibodies;
5. Immunization against TRIB2 was observed to result in alterations in hypocretin production and release.

However, TRIB2 antibodies have not been observed in the CSF or histologically in the vicinity of lateral hypothalamic hypocretin neurons. TRIB2 is widely distributed in the brain, which suggests that anti-TRIB2 antibodies are likely to be insufficient as a cause of narcolepsy. Ataxin-3 mice that lose hypocretin neurons through toxic destruction demonstrate TRIB2 reactivity, suggesting that anti-TRIB2 antibodies are the consequence rather than cause of destruction of hypocretin cells.[73] Observations from ICV passive transfer experiments remain to be replicated, and beneficial effects of IVIg[74,78–80,82] and other treatments that affect the immune system[83] are unconfirmed, and their putative mechanisms undetermined. Although passive transfer of antibodies can confirm pathogenic processes, this may be too simplistic and is generally easier to demonstrate when an antibody has direct pathophysiologic effects, for example, in myasthenia gravis, where the autoantibody binds the acetylcholine receptor. Similarly, oligoclonal bands, observed in multiple sclerosis, are helpful in diagnosis and assessment of disease severity. Oligoclonal bands have not been observed in the CSF of most patients with narcolepsy.[84]

SUMMARY

Although there are is a significant body of evidence pointing to narcolepsy being an autoimmune disorder, the definitive proof has eluded efforts to date. Several researchers have hypothesized how the immune system may be triggered resulting in the autoimmune destruction of hypocretin neurons. Also, a key role for T lymphocytes (both helper and cytotoxic) has been proposed,[85,86] but definitive evidence is lacking. There is no evidence of a systemic or local inflammatory process[87] in narcolepsy. Only one postmortem study has suggested the potential of immune infiltration and gliosis in the hypothalamus in narcolepsy,[15] but all postmortem studies suffer from the fact that they are very distal to disease onset. Common markers of neurodegeneration appear to be lower in narcolepsy.[88] Although narcolepsy occurs in a genetic fashion in dogs, there are also sporadic cases, similar to the human condition. Examination of these sporadic cases could provide important clues. These cases are usually euthanized and are lost to investigation.

The H1N1 pandemic provided an exceptional opportunity to advance the understanding of the pathogenesis of narcolepsy. Understanding the pathogenesis of narcolepsy can open avenues to greater understanding and treatment of other autoimmune disorders. However, the experimental evidence to establish narcolepsy as an autoimmune disease (caused by autoreactive T cells and/or autoantibodies) remains elusive.

REFERENCES

1. Chabas D, Taheri S, Renier C, et al. The genetics of narcolepsy. Annu Rev Genomics Hum Genet 2003; 4:459–83.
2. Mignot E, Taheri S, Nishino S. Sleeping with the hypothalamus: emerging therapeutic targets for sleep disorders. Nat Neurosci 2002;5(Suppl):1071–5.
3. Taheri S. The genetics of sleep disorders. Minerva Med 2004;95(3):203–12.
4. Taheri S, Mignot E. The genetics of sleep disorders. Lancet Neurol 2002;1(4):242–50.
5. American Academy of Sleep Medicine. International classification of sleep disorders. 3rd edition. American Academy of Sleep Medicine; 2014.
6. Taheri S, Zeitzer JM, Mignot E. The role of hypocretins (orexins) in sleep regulation and narcolepsy. Annu Rev Neurosci 2002;25:283–313.
7. Taheri S, Bloom S. Orexins/hypocretins: waking up the scientific world. Clin Endocrinol (Oxf) 2001; 54(4):421–9.
8. Taheri S, Hafizi S. The orexins/hypocretins: hypothalamic peptides linked to sleep and appetite. Psychol Med 2002;32(6):955–8.
9. Taheri S, Mahmoodi M, Opacka-Juffry J, et al. Distribution and quantification of immunoreactive orexin A in rat tissues. FEBS Lett 1999;457(1):157–61.
10. Taheri S, Ward H, Ghatei M, et al. Role of orexins in sleep and arousal mechanisms. Lancet 2000; 355(9206):847.
11. Beuckmann CT, Sinton CM, Williams SC, et al. Expression of a poly-glutamine-ataxin-3 transgene in orexin neurons induces narcolepsy-cataplexy in the rat. J Neurosci 2004;24(18):4469–77.
12. Sakurai T. Orexins and orexin receptors: implication in feeding behavior. Regul Pept 1999;85(1):25–30.
13. Sakurai T, Amemiya A, Ishii M, et al. Orexins and orexin receptors: a family of hypothalamic neuropeptides and G protein-coupled receptors that regulate feeding behavior. Cell 1998;92(4):573–85.
14. Poli F, Pizza F, Mignot E, et al. High prevalence of precocious puberty and obesity in childhood narcolepsy with cataplexy. Sleep 2013;36(2):175–81.
15. Thannickal TC, Moore RY, Nienhuis R, et al. Reduced number of hypocretin neurons in human narcolepsy. Neuron 2000;27(3):469–74.
16. Peyron C, Faraco J, Rogers W, et al. A mutation in a case of early onset narcolepsy and a generalized absence of hypocretin peptides in human narcoleptic brains. Nat Med 2000;6(9):991–7.
17. Mignot E, Lammers GJ, Ripley B, et al. The role of cerebrospinal fluid hypocretin measurement in the

diagnosis of narcolepsy and other hypersomnias. Arch Neurol 2002;59(10):1553–62.

18. Nishino S, Ripley B, Overeem S, et al. Low cerebrospinal fluid hypocretin (Orexin) and altered energy homeostasis in human narcolepsy. Ann Neurol 2001;50(3):381–8.

19. Ripley B, Overeem S, Fujiki N, et al. CSF hypocretin/orexin levels in narcolepsy and other neurological conditions. Neurology 2001;57(12):2253–8.

20. Schrolkamp M, Jennum PJ, Gammeltoft S, et al. Normal morning MCH levels and no association with REM or NREM sleep parameters in narcolepsy type 1 and type 2. J Clin Sleep Med 2016; 13:235–43.

21. Lin L, Faraco J, Li R, et al. The sleep disorder canine narcolepsy is caused by a mutation in the hypocretin (orexin) receptor 2 gene. Cell 1999;98(3):365–76.

22. Mignot EJ. History of narcolepsy at Stanford University. Immunol Res 2014;58(2–3):315–39.

23. Hungs M, Fan J, Lin L, et al. Identification and functional analysis of mutations in the hypocretin (orexin) genes of narcoleptic canines. Genome Res 2001; 11(4):531–9.

24. Juji T, Matsuki K, Tokunaga K, et al. Narcolepsy and HLA in the Japanese. Ann N Y Acad Sci 1988;540: 106–14.

25. Lin L, Hungs M, Mignot E. Narcolepsy and the HLA region. J Neuroimmunol 2001;117(1–2):9–20.

26. Crocker A, Espana RA, Papadopoulou M, et al. Concomitant loss of dynorphin, NARP, and orexin in narcolepsy. Neurology 2005;65(8):1184–8.

27. Taheri S, Paterno J, Mignot E. Narcolepsy and autoimmunity. In: Nishino S, Sakurai T, editors. The orexin/hypocretin system: physiology and pathophysiology. Totowa (NJ): Humana Press; 2006. p. 341–6.

28. Mahlios J, De la Herran-Arita AK, Mignot E. The autoimmune basis of narcolepsy. Curr Opin Neurobiol 2013;23(5):767–73.

29. Overeem S, Black JL 3rd, Lammers GJ. Narcolepsy: immunological aspects. Sleep Med Rev 2008;12(2): 95–107.

30. Langdon N, Lock C, Welsh K, et al. Immune factors in narcolepsy. Sleep 1986;9(1 Pt 2):143–8.

31. Parkes JD, Langdon N, Lock C. Narcolepsy and immunity. Br Med J (clin Res Ed) 1986;292(6517):359–60.

32. Alvaro-Benito M, Morrison E, Wieczorek M, et al. Human leukocyte antigen-DM polymorphisms in autoimmune diseases. Open Biol 2016;6(8):1–22.

33. Taheri S. The genetics of narcolepsy. In: Goswami M, Thorpy MJ, Pandi-Perumal SR, editors. Narcolepsy: a clinical guide. Switzerland: Springer International Publishing; 2016. p. 1–3.

34. Mueller-Eckhardt G, Strohmaier P, Schendel DJ, et al. Possible male segregation distortion of DR2 haplotypes in narcolepsy patients. Hum Immunol 1987;20(3):189–93.

35. Marcadet A, Gebuhrer L, Betuel H, et al. DNA polymorphism related to HLA-DR2 Dw2 in patients with narcolepsy. Immunogenetics 1985;22(6):679–83.

36. Neely S, Rosenberg R, Spire JP, et al. HLA antigens in narcolepsy. Neurology 1987;37(12):1858–60.

37. Siebold C, Hansen BE, Wyer JR, et al. Crystal structure of HLA-DQ0602 that protects against type 1 diabetes and confers strong susceptibility to narcolepsy. Proc Natl Acad Sci U S A 2004; 101(7):1999–2004.

38. Pelin Z, Guilleminault C, Risch N, et al. HLA-DQB1*0602 homozygosity increases relative risk for narcolepsy but not disease severity in two ethnic groups. US Modafinil in Narcolepsy Multicenter Study Group. Tissue Antigens 1998;51(1):96–100.

39. Watson NF, Ton TG, Koepsell TD, et al. Does narcolepsy symptom severity vary according to HLA-DQB1*0602 allele status? Sleep 2010;33(1):29–35.

40. Mignot E, Lin L, Rogers W, et al. Complex HLA-DR and -DQ interactions confer risk of narcolepsy-cataplexy in three ethnic groups. Am J Hum Genet 2001;68(3):686–99.

41. Hong SC, Lin L, Lo B, et al. DQB1*0301 and DQB1*0601 modulate narcolepsy susceptibility in Koreans. Hum Immunol 2007;68(1):59–68.

42. Tafti M, Lammers GJ, Dauvilliers Y, et al. Narcolepsy-associated HLA class I alleles implicate cell-mediated cytotoxicity. Sleep 2016;39(3):581–7.

43. Han F, Faraco J, Dong XS, et al. Genome wide analysis of narcolepsy in China implicates novel immune loci and reveals changes in association prior to versus after the 2009 H1N1 influenza pandemic. PLoS Genet 2013;9(10):e1003880.

44. Hallmayer J, Faraco J, Lin L, et al. Narcolepsy is strongly associated with the T-cell receptor alpha locus. Nat Genet 2009;41(6):708–11.

45. Faraco J, Lin L, Kornum BR, et al. ImmunoChip study implicates antigen presentation to T cells in narcolepsy. PLoS Genet 2013;9(2):e1003270.

46. Han F, Lin L, Li J, et al. TCRA, P2RY11, and CPT1B/CHKB associations in Chinese narcolepsy. Sleep Med 2012;13(3):269–72.

47. Winkelmann J, Lin L, Schormair B, et al. Mutations in DNMT1 cause autosomal dominant cerebellar ataxia, deafness and narcolepsy. Hum Mol Genet 2012;21(10):2205–10.

48. Holm A, Lin L, Faraco J, et al. EIF3G is associated with narcolepsy across ethnicities. Eur J Hum Genet 2015;23(11):1573–80.

49. Toyoda H, Miyagawa T, Koike A, et al. A polymorphism in CCR1/CCR3 is associated with narcolepsy. Brain Behav Immun 2015;49:148–55.

50. Aran A, Lin L, Nevsimalova S, et al. Elevated anti-streptococcal antibodies in patients with recent narcolepsy onset. Sleep 2009;32(8):979–83.

51. Ambati A, Poiret T, Svahn BM, et al. Increased beta-haemolytic group A streptococcal M6 serotype and

streptodornase B-specific cellular immune responses in Swedish narcolepsy cases. J Intern Med 2015; 278(3):264–76.

52. Han F, Lin L, Li J, et al. Decreased incidence of childhood narcolepsy 2 years after the 2009 H1N1 winter flu pandemic. Ann Neurol 2013;73(4):560.

53. Han F, Lin L, Warby SC, et al. Narcolepsy onset is seasonal and increased following the 2009 H1N1 pandemic in China. Ann Neurol 2011;70(3):410–7.

54. Partinen M, Kornum BR, Plazzi G, et al. Narcolepsy as an autoimmune disease: the role of H1N1 infection and vaccination. Lancet Neurol 2014;13(6): 600–13.

55. Ahmed SS, Schur PH, MacDonald NE, et al. Narcolepsy, 2009 A(H1N1) pandemic influenza, and pandemic influenza vaccinations: what is known and unknown about the neurological disorder, the role for autoimmunity, and vaccine adjuvants. J Autoimmun 2014;50:1–11.

56. Jacob L, Leib R, Ollila HM, et al. Comparison of Pandemrix and Arepanrix, two pH1N1 AS03-adjuvanted vaccines differentially associated with narcolepsy development. Brain Behav Immun 2015;47:44–57.

57. Ahmed SS, Steinman L. Mechanistic insights into influenza vaccine-associated narcolepsy. Hum Vaccin Immunother 2016;12(12):3196–201.

58. Taheri S, Kremptez M, Jackson M, et al. Investigation of the autoimmune basis of narcolepsy using western blot analysis of lateral hypothalamus protein extract with serum and cerebrospinal fluid (CSF). Sleep 2003;A285.

59. Overeem S, Verschuuren JJ, Fronczek R, et al. Immunohistochemical screening for autoantibodies against lateral hypothalamic neurons in human narcolepsy. J Neuroimmunol 2006;174(1–2):187–91.

60. Bergman P, Adori C, Vas S, et al. Narcolepsy patients have antibodies that stain distinct cell populations in rat brain and influence sleep patterns. Proc Natl Acad Sci U S A 2014;111(35):E3735–44.

61. van der Heide A, Hegeman-Kleinn IM, Peeters E, et al. Immunohistochemical screening for antibodies in recent onset type 1 narcolepsy and after H1N1 vaccination. J Neuroimmunol 2015;283:58–62.

62. Thebault S, Waters P, Snape MD, et al. Neuronal antibodies in children with or without narcolepsy following H1N1-AS03 vaccination. PLoS One 2015; 10(6):e0129555.

63. Nishino S, Kanbayashi T, Fujiki N, et al. CSF hypocretin levels in Guillain-Barre syndrome and other inflammatory neuropathies. Neurology 2003;61(6): 823–5.

64. Saariaho AH, Vuorela A, Freitag TL, et al. Autoantibodies against ganglioside GM3 are associated with narcolepsy-cataplexy developing after Pandemrix vaccination against 2009 pandemic H1N1 type influenza virus. J Autoimmun 2015;63: 68–75.

65. Ahmed SS, Volkmuth W, Duca J, et al. Antibodies to influenza nucleoprotein cross-react with human hypocretin receptor 2. Sci Transl Med 2015;7(294): 294ra105.

66. Vassalli A, Li S, Tafti M. Comment on "Antibodies to influenza nucleoprotein cross-react with human hypocretin receptor 2". Sci Transl Med 2015;7(314): 314le2.

67. Dauvilliers Y, Bauer J, Rigau V, et al. Hypothalamic immunopathology in anti-Ma-associated diencephalitis with narcolepsy-cataplexy. JAMA Neurol 2013; 70(10):1305–10.

68. Bernard-Valnet R, Yshii L, Queriault C, et al. CD8 T cell-mediated killing of orexinergic neurons induces a narcolepsy-like phenotype in mice. Proc Natl Acad Sci U S A 2016;113(39):10956–61.

69. Cvetkovic-Lopes V, Bayer L, Dorsaz S, et al. Elevated Tribbles homolog 2-specific antibody levels in narcolepsy patients. J Clin Invest 2010; 120(3):713–9.

70. Toyoda H, Tanaka S, Miyagawa T, et al. Anti-Tribbles homolog 2 autoantibodies in Japanese patients with narcolepsy. Sleep 2010;33(7):875–8.

71. Kawashima M, Lin L, Tanaka S, et al. Anti-Tribbles homolog 2 (TRIB2) autoantibodies in narcolepsy are associated with recent onset of cataplexy. Sleep 2010;33(7):869–74.

72. Katzav A, Arango MT, Kivity S, et al. Passive transfer of narcolepsy: anti-TRIB2 autoantibody positive patient IgG causes hypothalamic orexin neuron loss and sleep attacks in mice. J Autoimmun 2013;45: 24–30.

73. Tanaka S, Honda Y, Honda M, et al. Anti-tribbles pseudokinase 2 (TRIB2)-immunization modulates HYPOCRETIN/OREXIN neuronal functions. Sleep 2017;40(1).

74. Lecendreux M, Berthier J, Corny J, et al. Intravenous immunoglobulin therapy in pediatric narcolepsy: a nonrandomized, open-label, controlled, longitudinal observational study. J Clin Sleep Med 2017;13: 441–53.

75. Lecendreux M, Maret S, Bassetti C, et al. Clinical efficacy of high-dose intravenous immunoglobulins near the onset of narcolepsy in a 10-year-old boy. J Sleep Res 2003;12(4):347–8.

76. Dauvilliers Y, Abril B, Mas E, et al. Normalization of hypocretin-1 in narcolepsy after intravenous immunoglobulin treatment. Neurology 2009;73(16): 1333–4.

77. Dauvilliers Y, Carlander B, Rivier F, et al. Successful management of cataplexy with intravenous immunoglobulins at narcolepsy onset. Ann Neurol 2004; 56(6):905–8.

78. Dalakas MC. Role of IVIg in autoimmune, neuroinflammatory and neurodegenerative disorders of the central nervous system: present and future prospects. J Neurol 2006;253(Suppl 5):V25–32.

79. Gadian J, Kirk E, Holliday K, et al. Systematic review of immunoglobulin use in paediatric neurological and neurodevelopmental disorders. Dev Med Child Neurol 2017;59(2):136–44.

80. Knudsen S, Biering-Sorensen B, Kornum BR, et al. Early IVIg treatment has no effect on post-H1N1 narcolepsy phenotype or hypocretin deficiency. Neurology 2012;79(1):102–3.

81. Knudsen S, Mikkelsen JD, Bang B, et al. Intravenous immunoglobulin treatment and screening for hypocretin neuron-specific autoantibodies in recent onset childhood narcolepsy with cataplexy. Neuropediatrics 2010;41(5):217–22.

82. Plazzi G, Poli F, Franceschini C, et al. Intravenous high-dose immunoglobulin treatment in recent onset childhood narcolepsy with cataplexy. J Neurol 2008;255(10):1549–54.

83. Hecht M, Lin L, Kushida CA, et al. Report of a case of immunosuppression with prednisone in an 8-year-old boy with an acute onset of hypocretin-deficiency narcolepsy. Sleep 2003;26(7):809–10.

84. Fredrikson S, Carlander B, Billiard M, et al. CSF immune variables in patients with narcolepsy. Acta Neurol Scand 1990;81(3):253–4.

85. Partinen M, Kornum BR, Plazzi G, et al. Does autoreactivity have a role in narcolepsy? Lancet Neurol 2014;13(11):1072–3.

86. Degn M, Kornum BR. Type 1 narcolepsy: a CD8(+) T cell-mediated disease? Ann N Y Acad Sci 2015;1351:80–8.

87. Kornum BR, Pizza F, Knudsen S, et al. Cerebrospinal fluid cytokine levels in type 1 narcolepsy patients very close to onset. Brain Behav Immun 2015;49:54–8.

88. Jennum PJ, Pedersen LO, Bahl JM, et al. Cerebrospinal fluid biomarkers of neurodegeneration are decreased or normal in narcolepsy. Sleep 2017;40(1).

Genetic Markers of Sleep and Sleepiness

Namni Goel, PhD

KEYWORDS

- Candidate gene • GWAS • Sleepiness • Sleep • Individual differences • Chronotype
- Circadian clock genes • Heritability

KEY POINTS

- The circadian clock interacts with the sleep homeostatic drive in humans.
- Chronotype and sleep parameters show substantial heritability, underscoring their genetic component.
- Candidate gene and genome-wide association (GWA) studies indicate circadian clock genes and noncircadian genes are related to individual differences in chronotype.
- Similarly, candidate gene and GWA studies show circadian clock genes and noncircadian genes are associated with variation in sleep parameters.

Both sleep and wakefulness are modulated by an endogenous biological clock located in the suprachiasmatic nuclei of the anterior hypothalamus. Beyond driving the timing of wake and sleep, the clock modulates waking behavior, as reflected in sleepiness.[1] The daily sleep and wakefulness modulations have been instantiated in the 2-process mathematical model of sleep regulation and its variants.[2–4]

This 2-process model has been applied to the temporal profiles of sleep[3,5] and wakefulness.[6] The model consists of a sleep homeostatic process and a circadian process that interact to determine sleep onset and offset timing.[1,7] The homeostatic process, represented by the drive for sleep, increases during wakefulness (observed when wakefulness is maintained beyond habitual bedtime into the night and subsequent day) and decreases during sleep (represented by recuperation obtained from sleep). When this homeostatic drive increases above a certain threshold, sleep is triggered; when it decreases below a different threshold, wakefulness is invoked.

The circadian process represents daily oscillatory modulation of these threshold levels. The circadian system actively promotes wakefulness more than sleep.[8] The circadian drive for wakefulness can be experienced as spontaneously enhanced alertness in the early evening after a sleepless night. Notably, there are robust individual differences in the sleep homeostatic and circadian processes, underscoring genetic underpinnings.

This article, which focuses on healthy adult sleepers, begins with a discussion of the heritability (h^2) and genetic basis of chronotype, drawing on candidate gene and genome-wide association (GWA) studies. The h^2 of sleep is discussed and candidate gene studies using circadian clock genes to investigate variation in sleep parameters are described. GWA studies of sleep are then reviewed. The article concludes with a discussion of future research areas.

Grant support: Office of Naval Research N00014-11-1-0361, National Aeronautics and Space Administration NNX14AN49G.
Disclosure Statement: The author has nothing to disclose.
Division of Sleep and Chronobiology, Department of Psychiatry, Perelman School of Medicine, University of Pennsylvania, 1017 Blockley Hall, 423 Guardian Drive, Philadelphia, PA 19104-6021, USA
E-mail address: goel@mail.med.upenn.edu

Sleep Med Clin 12 (2017) 289–299
http://dx.doi.org/10.1016/j.jsmc.2017.03.005
1556-407X/17/© 2017 Elsevier Inc. All rights reserved.

GENETICS OF INDIVIDUAL DIFFERENCES IN CIRCADIAN RHYTHMS AND CHRONOTYPE

Healthy adults show interindividual differences in free-running circadian period (tau),[9–15] which shows robust stability within individuals.[12] They also demonstrate interindividual differences in circadian amplitude[16,17] and circadian phase,[10,16–18] partly due to genetic influences.[17]

Chronotype (Morningness-Eveningness)

Chronotype or morningness-eveningness (ie, the tendency to be an early lark or a late owl) is the most frequently measured interindividual variation in circadian rhythmicity. Morning-type and evening-type individuals differ endogenously in the circadian phase of their biological clocks.[16,18]

Self-report questionnaires, such as the Horne-Östberg Morningness-Eveningness Questionnaire[19] and its variants,[20] and the Munich ChronoType Questionnaire,[21,22] are the most commonly used measures of circadian phase preference. Chronotype is a phenotypic aspect of circadian rhythmicity in humans.[1] As predicted from the 2-process model, chronotypes show differences in homeostatic sleep regulation[23–25] and responses to sleep fragmentation in laboratory studies.[26]

Heritability of Chronotype

The fraction of variance in a trait or phenotype explained by genetic influence is the h^2. Twin studies, which allow for assessment of the relative contributions of genetics and environment, demonstrate chronotype has substantial h^2 (.40–.54) across diverse populations.[27–36] Family studies also demonstrate substantial h^2 (.23–.48).[37–39]

Candidate Gene Studies of Chronotype

Most candidate gene studies investigating the genetic basis of chronotype have targeted circadian clock genes. The 3111C allele (single nucleotide polymorphism [SNP] rs1801260) in the Circadian Locomotor Output Cycles Kaput (CLOCK) gene 5'-UTR region has been associated with eveningness and delayed sleep timing[40–42] (but see[13,43–48]) and CLOCK rs11824092[49] has also been linked to chronotype. The variable number tandem repeat (VNTR) polymorphism in the PERIOD3 (PER3) gene (rs57875989) has been linked to chronotype (albeit not consistently[44,50–64]), as have PER3 SNPs rs228697,[65] rs10462020,[66] and rs2640909.[67] The bp2114 G/A G3853 A and 111G polymorphisms of PERIOD2 (PER2)[68–70] have also been associated with

chronotype (but see[43]); however, rs6753456 does not show an association.[71]

Similarly, the PERIOD1 (PER1) T2434C polymorphism has been associated with morning preference.[72] Moreover, rs7221412 near PER1 has been related to activity rhythm timing in 2 independent cohorts: activity timing was delayed by 67 minutes in GG versus AA homozygotes and GG individuals died about 7 hours later than AA/AG individuals.[73]

SNPs rs922270, rs11824092, and rs1481892 of the Aryl Hydrocarbon Receptor Nuclear Translocator-like 2 (ARNTL2) gene[49,66] and the Nuclear Receptor Subfamily 1 Group D Member 1 (NR1D1) gene encoding for nuclear receptor REV-ERBα[74] have been associated with chronotype, whereas the G-protein B3 subunit (GNβ3) gene 825 C/T SNP,[48] the Timeless (TIM) gene A2634G SNP,[75] and the Melanopsin (OPN4) gene Ile394Thr SNP[76] all failed to show such an association.

Genome-Wide Association Studies of Chronotype

Both h^2 and candidate gene studies of chronotype successfully laid the groundwork for GWA studies, which are comprehensive and unbiased approaches to identify genes and genomic variants associated with a phenotype, trait, or disease, using population samples. Different alleles (risk variants) are characterized by the frequency of their occurrence, spanning from rare (frequency <1%) to common (frequency >5%). These are associated with a range of effects, from small (increased risk by a factor of 0.1) to large (increased risk by a factor of >100) on a given phenotype, trait, or disease.

The first GWAS of chronotype capitalized on personalized genetic platforms, using 89,283 individuals from the 23andMe database.[77] This study found 15 genetic variants associated with morningness, including 7 near well-established circadian genes: PER2, PER3, Regulator of G-Protein Signaling 16 (RGS16), Vasoactive Intestinal Peptide (VIP), Hypocretin Receptor 2 (HCRTR2), Ras Related Dexamethasone Induced 1 (RASD1), and F-Box and Leucine-Rich Repeat Protein 3 (FBXL3) (**Table 1**).

Using 100,420 individuals from the UK Biobank cohort, Lane and colleagues[78] identified 12 significant and 1 suggestive genetic loci associated with chronotype, including variants near 4 circadian genes: PER2, RGS16, F-Box and Leucine-Rich Repeat Protein 13 (FBXL13), and Aph-1 Homolog A, Gamma Secretase Subunit (APH1A). Notably, 8 of the 15 previously reported gene loci[77] were replicated, and all 15 showed a consistent directional effect (see **Table 1**).

Table 1
Circadian and noncircadian genes associated with self-reported chronotype from genome-wide association studies

SNP or Marker	Gene	Chromosome	Reference
rs12736689, rs1144566, rs516134	RGS16	1	Hu et al,[77] 2016; Lane et al,[78] 2016; Jones et al,[79] 2016
rs55694368, rs35333999, rs75804782	PER2	2	Hu et al,[77] 2016; Lane et al,[78] 2016; Jones et al,[79] 2016
rs11121022	PER3	1	Hu et al,[77] 2016
rs9479402	VIP	6	Hu et al,[77] 2016
rs35833281, rs76899638	HCRTR2	6	Hu et al,[77] 2016; Jones et al,[79] 2016
rs11545787	RASD1	17	Hu et al,[77] 2016
rs9565309	FBXL3	13	Hu et al,[77] 2016
rs10493596, rs76681500, rs11162296	AK5	1	Hu et al,[77] 2016; Lane et al,[78] 2016; Jones et al,[79] 2016
rs34714364, rs10157197	APH1A	1	Hu et al,[77] 2016; Lane et al,[78] 2016
rs1595824	PLCL1	2	Hu et al,[77] 2016
rs3972456, rs372229746	FBXL13	7	Hu et al,[77] 2016; Lane et al,[78] 2016
rs2948276	DLX5	7	Hu et al,[77] 2016
rs6582618	ALG10B	12	Hu et al,[77] 2016
rs12927162	TOX3	16	Hu et al,[77] 2016
rs12965577	NOL4	18	Hu et al,[77] 2016
rs141175086	LINC01128	1	Lane et al,[78] 2016
rs2050122	HTR6	1	Lane et al,[78] 2016; Jones et al,[79] 2016
rs11895698	ASB1	2	Lane et al,[78] 2016
rs11708779, rs12635074	ERC2	3	Lane et al,[78] 2016; Jones et al,[79] 2016
rs148750727	FAT1	4	Lane et al,[78] 2016
rs17311976	ADCY8	8	Lane et al,[78] 2016
rs542675489	RNF10	12	Lane et al,[78] 2016
rs4821940	TNRC6B	22	Lane et al,[78] 2016
rs10157197	PRPF3	1	Jones et al,[79] 2016
rs372229746	ORAI2	7	Jones et al,[79] 2016
rs77641763	EXD3	9	Jones et al,[79] 2016
rs9961653	RAX	18	Jones et al,[79] 2016
rs70944707	FKBP1B	2	Jones et al,[79] 2016
rs72720396	CALB1	1	Jones et al,[79] 2016
rs12140153	INADL	1	Jones et al,[79] 2016
rs1075265	PSME4	2	Jones et al,[79] 2016
rs4821940	SGSM3	22	Jones et al,[79] 2016
rs192534763	UNC5D	8	Jones et al,[79] 2016

A third GWAS[79] using 128,266 individuals from the UK Biobank cohort found 16 variants associated with chronotype, including 2 near circadian genes RGS16 and PER2; both were detected in prior GWAS (see **Table 1**).[77,78] The investigators replicated their results using the Biobank and 23andMe[77] datasets: 13 signals remained significant, with 11 in the same direction as in the 23andMe dataset. Thus, all 3 GWAS found associations of circadian and noncircadian genetic variants with self-rated chronotype (see **Table 1**).

GENETICS OF INDIVIDUAL DIFFERENCES IN NORMAL SLEEP

Sleep is a highly complex trait involving many genes and their interactions with environmental factors. Both self-rated sleep measures and electroencephalogram (EEG) sleep show substantial h^2.

Heritability of Self-Rated and Electroencephalogram Sleep

Sleep quality shows substantial h^2 (.31–.49) in twin studies.[31,32,80–83] Twin studies also show sleep duration has substantial h^2 (.27–.44).[30,31,80,81,83–88] Similarly, family studies demonstrate substantial h^2 in sleep duration (.13–.26).[37,89] Daytime sleepiness assessed in twin studies show substantial h^2 (.37–.48).[31,81,90–94] Similarly, family studies demonstrate substantial h^2 in daytime sleepiness (.17).[38]

Twin studies indicate a strong genetic basis underlying objective sleep, including sleep duration, onset, quality, and homeostasis.[31,36,95–98] The sleep EEG power spectrum also shows strong h^2 (h^2 = .50–.96) and consistency across nights within individuals but differences among individuals.[31,98–100] Nonrapid eye movement (NREM) and rapid eye movement (REM) sleep also show trait-like features.[36,101–107] REM sleep microstructure features are heritable.[108,109] Waking EEG patterns are also strongly heritable (h^2 = .76–.89).[97,98]

Candidate Gene Studies of Sleep

The h^2 of sleep parameters underscores the role of genetics in these measures. Many candidate gene studies investigating the genetic basis of sleep in not sleep-deprived conditions have targeted circadian clock genes; these are reviewed alphabetically by clock gene name in this section. Studies in noncircadian genes and in response to sleep deprivation are reviewed elsewhere.[110]

ARNTL

Parsons and colleagues[66] found a polymorphism (rs922270) in *ARNTL2* was associated with sleep latency and quality. The rs3816358 SNP (T allele) in *ARNTL* also was associated with later actigraphic sleep onset time.[111]

BHLHE41/DEC2

In 2 adults, a point mutation in the *BHLHE41/DEC2* gene was associated with a short sleep duration phenotype (average of 6.25 hours vs 8.06 hours of self-reported sleep), characterized by an earlier nonworkday habitual sleep offset time, with normal onset time.[112]

CLOCK

Allebrandt and colleagues[113] reported an association between 2 uncorrelated, common *CLOCK* genetic variants (rs12649507 and rs11932595) and sleep duration in 2 independent European populations from South Tyrol (n = 283) and

Estonia (n = 1011). Another group failed to replicate either of these associations using 3 independent cohorts.[114] Vanderlind and colleagues[115] found rs11932595 was associated with sleep quality but not with actigraphic sleep measures.

DBP

Parsons and colleagues[66] found the rs3848543 polymorphism in *D site of albumin promoter (albumin D-box) binding protein* (*DBP*) was significantly associated with sleep latency.

GNβ3

The rs5443 polymorphism in *GNβ3* was significantly associated with global sleep quality and duration.[66] In addition, the rs1047776A and rs2238114C alleles in *GNβ3* were significantly associated with more actigraphic wake after sleep onset.[111]

MTNR1B

Chang and colleagues[71] reported that a rare genetic variant (rs7942988) in *Melatonin Receptor 1B* (*MTNR1B*) was associated with longer REM sleep latency, with minor allele carriers showing an average of 65 minutes longer latency from sleep onset to REM sleep compared with noncarriers.

NPAS2

Evans and colleagues[111] found the rs3768984 SNP (C allele) in *Neuronal PAS Domain Protein 2* (*NPAS2*) was associated with later actigraphic wake onset time.

OPN4

Lee and colleagues[76] investigated the role of Ile394Thr SNP in *OPN4* in self-rated sleep-wake timing: during weekdays, bedtime, waketime, and sleep midpoint were significantly later for *C/C* subjects than for *T/T* and *T/C* subjects. Similarly, during weekends, bedtime and sleep midpoints were significantly later for *C/C* subjects than for *T* allele carriers.

PER2

A rare polymorphism (rs2304672) in *PER2* was significantly related to sleep duration and quality.[66] In another study, *PER2* rs6753456 was associated with 20 minutes less slow-wave sleep in carriers of the minor allele than in noncarriers and with reduced EEG power density in the delta range (0.25–1.0 Hz) during NREM sleep and less slow-wave activity (0.75–4.5 Hz) in the early part of the sleep episode.[71]

Genome-Wide Association Studies of Sleep

Candidate gene studies have detected several potential loci underlying sleep parameters, some which lack replication. Recent GWAS have examined phenotypic-genotypic interactions in healthy sleepers, and have uncovered numerous associations of circadian and noncircadian genetic variants with self-rated sleep duration and timing, sleepiness, sleep latency and quality, and with actigraphic sleep measures (**Table 2**).

Self-rated sleep duration and sleep timing

Using 749 subjects from the Sleep Heart Health Study, linkage analysis revealed sleep duration

was related to genes such as Casein Kinase 2 Alpha 2 (CSNK2A2) and Myosin VIIA and Rab Interacting Protein (MYRIP).[116] Furthermore, a nonsynonymous-coding SNP in Neuropeptide S Receptor 1 (NPSR1) and an SNP in Opioid Binding Protein/Cell Adhesion Molecule-Like (OPCML) were identified as a putative mediators of habitual bedtime.[116]

Another GWAS found an association between an intronic variant (rs11046205) in the Adenosine

Table 2
Circadian and noncircadian genes associated with sleep parameters from genome-wide association studies

SNP or Marker	Gene	Chromosome	Reference
rs1380703, rs17190618	VRK2	2	Jones et al,[79] 2016
rs17601612, rs11214607	DRD2	11	Cade et al,[89] 2016
rs28168	CSNK2A2	16	Gottlieb et al,[116] 2007
rs6599077, rs10492604	MYRIP	3	Gottlieb et al,[116] 2007
rs1940013	OPCML	11	Gottlieb et al,[116] 2007
rs2218488	EYA1	8	Gottlieb et al,[116] 2007
rs324981	NPSR1	7	Gottlieb et al,[116] 2007
rs1823068	PDE4D	5	Gottlieb et al,[116] 2007
rs11046205, rs11046211, rs11046209, rs2544443	ABCC9	12	Allebrandt et al,[117] 2013; Parsons et al,[118] 2013; Scheinfeldt et al,[121] 2015
rs13092077	KCNAB1	3	Allebrandt et al,[117] 2013
rs2697804, rs2245601	CHRND	2	Allebrandt et al,[117] 2013
rs9911832	RNF157	17	Allebrandt et al,[117] 2013
rs16929277, rs7304986, rs7316184, rs7301906, rs16929275, rs16929276, rs16929278, rs2051990	CACNA1C	12	Parsons et al,[118] 2013; Byrne et al,[122] 2013
rs10914351	PTPRU	1	Ollila et al,[119] 2014
rs1037079	PCDH7-CENTD1	4	Ollila et al,[119] 2014
rs2031573	KLF6	10	Ollila et al,[119] 2014
rs62158211, rs1191685	PAX8	2	Jones et al,[79] 2016; Gottlieb et al,[120] 2015
rs4587207	IER3, FLOT1	6	Gottlieb et al,[120] 2015
rs7233717	FBXO15	18	Scheinfeldt et al,[121] 2015
rs17122013	SORCS1	10	Scheinfeldt et al,[121] 2015
rs41463746	ELOVL2	6	Scheinfeldt et al,[121] 2015
rs41348446	ARNTL	11	Scheinfeldt et al,[121] 2015
rs1412611	NFATC2	20	Scheinfeldt et al,[121] 2015
rs2256551	ATP9A	20	Scheinfeldt et al,[121] 2015
rs9900428, rs9907432, rs7211029	RBFOX3	17	Amin et al,[123] 2016
rs75842709	UFL1	6	Spada et al,[124] 2016
chr9:864201:D	DMRT1	9	Spada et al,[124] 2016
rs74448913	CSNK2A1	20	Spada et al,[124] 2016
rs2919869	SMYD1	2	Spada et al,[124] 2016
rs12069385, rs12441664	ZMYM4	1	Spada et al,[124] 2016

Triphosphate-binding Cassette, Sub-family C Member 9 (ABCC9) gene and sleep duration in 7 European populations (n = 4251 subjects).[117] An independent group replicated this association.[118]

Using a Finnish sample (n = 1941), Ollila and colleagues[119] did not detect any significant genome-wide signals for sleep duration, although 31 SNPs showed suggestive associations. Three of these SNPs were nominally associated with sleep duration in a replication sample (n = 6834): rs10914351 near Protein Tyrosine Phosphatase, Receptor Type U (PTPRU), rs1037079 in Proto-cadherin 7-Centaurin, Delta 1 (PCDH7-CENTD1), and rs2031573 in Krueppel-like Factor 6 (KLF6). SNPs rs2031573 and rs1037079 were also associated with higher KLF6 and PCDH7 expression levels, suggesting they may affect sleep duration regulation via gene expression.

A GWAS using 18 population-based European cohorts (n = 47,180)[120] found 2 novel genome-wide significant loci associated with sleep duration: 1 was located in an intergenic region (rs1191685) upstream from Paired Box Gene 8 (PAX8), and the second was located in an intergenic region (rs4587207) upstream of Immediate Early Response 3 (IER3), Flotillin-1 (FLOT1), and Long Intergenic NonProtein Coding RNA 243 (LINC00243). The rs1191685 association was replicated in 4771 African Americans. This study also failed to replicate a previous association of the ABCC9 gene with sleep duration.[117] Jones and colleagues[79] found associations of sleep duration with rs62158211 in PAX8 and rs1380703 and rs17190618 in Vaccinia Related Kinase 2 (VRK2).

Using data from the Coriell Personalized Medicine Collaborative (n = 4401), Scheinfeldt and colleagues[121] found several genes linked to sleep duration, including ABCC9, ARNTL, F-Box Protein 15 (FBXO15), Sortilin Related VPS10 Domain Containing Receptor 1 (SORCS1), and ELOVL Fatty Acid Elongase 2 (ELOVL2). Cade and colleagues[89] conducted meta-analyses of genetic associations with sleep duration using 7 Candidate Gene Association Resource cohorts of more than 25,000 individuals of African, Asian, European, and Hispanic ancestry. They found Dopamine D2 Receptor (DRD2) SNPs rs17601612 and rs11214607 were associated with sleep duration.

Self-rated sleepiness, sleep quality and latency
One SNP located in an intron of cyclic adenosine monophosphate-specific 3′,5′-cyclic Phosphodiesterase 4D (PDE4D) and 1 SNP located in EYA Transcriptional Coactivator and Phosphatase 1 (EYA1) have been identified as mediators of subjective sleepiness.[116]

Using an Australian sample (n = 2323), Byrne and colleagues[122] failed to detect any genome-wide significant signals for sleep habits. However, they found 7 SNPs in the third intron of Calcium Voltage-Gated Channel Subunit Alpha1 C (CACNA1C) that were suggestively associated with sleep latency and another CACNA1C variant (rs7304986) that was suggestively associated with sleep quality. A replication study using the G1219 British sample found CACNA1C variant rs16929277 was significantly associated with sleep latency and quality.[118] In a sample of 4242 individuals from 7 European cohorts, sleep latency was associated with 3 highly correlated variants (rs9900428, rs9907432, and rs7211029) in RNA-binding Protein Fox-1 Homolog 3 (RBFOX3); notably, this finding was replicated.[123]

Actigraphic sleep measures
In the only GWA using actigraphy to measure sleep, Spada and colleagues[124] found UFM1 Specific Ligase 1 (UFL1) was associated with sleep efficiency on weekdays, and Doublesex and Mab-3 Related Transcription Factor 1 (DMRT1) and Casein Kinase 2 Alpha 1 (CSNK2A1) were associated with sleep latency. They also found SET and MYND Domain Containing 1 (SMYD1) was related to sleep offset, and Zinc Finger MYM-Type Containing 4 (ZMYM4) was related to sleep duration and onset.

SUMMARY AND FUTURE DIRECTIONS

Numerous circadian and noncircadian genetic polymorphisms underlie interindividual differences in chronotype and sleep parameters. As predicted by the 2-process model of the circadian clock interacting with the sleep homeostat, findings from recent candidate gene and GWA studies show substantial overlap in the genes influencing sleep and chronotype.

Replication in independent samples is needed to determine whether results are genuine and are not due to chance, particularly because many of the candidate gene studies, especially those in laboratory settings, have been conducted in smaller samples. Moreover, both candidate gene and GWA studies should also be replicated in different ethnic and racial groups to increase the generalizability of the findings, given significant admixture in groups such as African Americans. GWAS using physiologic sleep and circadian measures as outcomes, rather than self-rated measures, are also needed to assess individual biological differences; however, these will likely require pooling of data across a large number of laboratories, given the expense, time, and effort required for such rigorous studies.

GWAS have notable advantages and disadvantages.[125] They generate large amounts of genetic data and are well-powered to detect common variants associated with a trait such as chronotype or sleep duration. However, they fail to account for all of the h^2 associated with a trait; they rarely detect the causal variants linking heredity genotypes to trait phenotypes (ie, epigenomics); and they can produce high false-negative rates due to the stringent statistical cutoff points required for multiple testing corrections.[125] Alternatively, SNPs provide specific pathways and underlying mechanisms but are limited and intensive for eliciting genotype-phenotype relationships. Therefore, a crucial next step is the utilization of genomics, epigenetics, and transcriptomics, along with bioinformatics and specific phenotyping, to better understand mechanisms and pathways related to sleep and circadian parameters in humans.

REFERENCES

1. Goel N, Basner M, Dinges DF. Phenotyping of neurobehavioral vulnerability to circadian phase during sleep loss. Methods Enzymol 2015;552:285–308.

2. Achermann P, Dijk DJ, Brunner DP, et al. A model of human sleep homeostasis based on EEG slow-wave activity; quantitative comparison of data and simulations. Brain Res Bull 1993;31:97–113.

3. Borbély AA. A two process model of sleep regulation. Hum Neurobiol 1982;1:195–204.

4. Mallis MM, Mejdal S, Nguyen TT, et al. Summary of the key features of seven biomathematical models of human fatigue and performance. Aviat Space Environ Med 2004;75:A4–14.

5. Daan S, Beersma DGM, Borbély AA. Timing of human sleep: recovery process gated by a circadian pacemaker. Am J Physiol 1984;246:R161–78.

6. Achermann P, Borbély AA. Simulation of daytime vigilance by the additive interaction of a homeostatic and a circadian process. Biol Cybern 1994; 71:115–21.

7. Khalsa SBS, Jewett ME, Duffy JF, et al. The timing of the human circadian clock is accurately represented by the core body temperature rhythm following phase shifts to a three-cycle light stimulus near the critical zone. J Biol Rhythms 2000;15:524–30.

8. Edgar DM, Dement WC, Fuller CA. Effect of SCN lesions on sleep in squirrel monkeys: evidence for opponent processes in sleep-wake regulation. J Neurosci 1993;13:1065–79.

9. Czeisler CA, Duffy JF, Shanahan TL, et al. Stability, precision, and near-24-hour period of the human circadian pacemaker. Science 1999;284:2177–81.

10. Smith MR, Burgess HJ, Fogg LF, et al. Racial differences in the human endogenous circadian period. PLoS One 2009;4:e6014.

11. Lázár AS, Santhi N, Hasan S, et al. Circadian period and the timing of melatonin onset in men and women: predictors of sleep during the weekend and in the laboratory. J Sleep Res 2013;22:155–9.

12. Hasan S, Santhi N, Lázár AS, et al. Assessment of circadian rhythms in humans: comparison of real-time fibroblast reporter imaging with plasma melatonin. FASEB J 2012;26:2414–23.

13. Chang AM, Buch AM, Bradstreet DS, et al. Human diurnal preference and circadian rhythmicity are not associated with the CLOCK 3111C/T gene polymorphism. J Biol Rhythms 2011;26:276–9.

14. Eastman CI, Molina TA, Dziepak ME, et al. Blacks (African Americans) have shorter free-running circadian periods than whites (Caucasian Americans). Chronobiol Int 2012;29:1072–7.

15. Eastman CI, Suh C, Tomaka VA, et al. Circadian rhythm phase shifts and endogenous free-running circadian period differ between African-Americans and European-Americans. Sci Rep 2015;5:8381.

16. Baehr EK, Revelle W, Eastman CI. Individual differences in the phase and amplitude of the human circadian temperature rhythm: with an emphasis on morningness-eveningness. J Sleep Res 2000; 9:117–27.

17. Burgess HJ, Fogg LF. Individual differences in the amount and timing of salivary melatonin secretion. PLoS One 2008;3:e3055.

18. Kerkhof GA, Van Dongen HPA. Morning-type and evening-type individuals differ in the phase position of their endogenous circadian oscillator. Neurosci Lett 1996;218:153–6.

19. Horne JA, Östberg O. A self-assessment questionnaire to determine morningness–eveningness in human circadian rhythms. Int J Chronobiol 1976; 4:97–110.

20. Smith CS, Reilly D, Midkiff K. Evaluation of three circadian rhythm questionnaires with suggestions for an improved measure of morningness. J Appl Psychol 1989;74:728–38.

21. Roenneberg T, Wirz-Justice A, Merrow M. Life between clocks: daily temporal patterns of human chronotypes. J Biol Rhythms 2003;18:80–90.

22. Roenneberg T, Kuehnle T, Juda M, et al. Epidemiology of the human circadian clock. Sleep Med Rev 2007;11:429–38.

23. Mongrain V, Carrier J, Dumont M. Chronotype and sex effects on sleep architecture and quantitative sleep EEG in healthy young adults. Sleep 2005; 28:819–27.

24. Mongrain V, Carrier J, Dumont M. Difference in sleep regulation between morning and evening circadian types as indexed by antero-posterior analyses of the sleep EEG. Eur J Neurosci 2006;23: 497–504.

25. Mongrain V, Carrier J, Paquet J, et al. Morning and evening-type differences in slow waves during

NREM sleep reveal both trait and state-dependent phenotypes. PLoS One 2011;6:e22679.

26. Mongrain V, Dumont M. Increased homeostatic response to behavioral sleep fragmentation in morning types compared to evening types. Sleep 2007; 30:773–80.

27. Hur YM. Stability of genetic influence on morningness-eveningness: a cross-sectional examination of South Korean twins from preadolescence to young adulthood. J Sleep Res 2007;16: 17–23.

28. Hur YM, Bouchard TJ Jr, Lykken DT. Genetic and environmental influence on morningness–eveningness. Pers Indiv Differ 1998;25:917–25.

29. Vink JM, Groot AS, Kerkhof GA, et al. Genetic analysis of morningness and eveningness. Chronobiol Int 2001;18:809–22.

30. Watson NF, Buchwald D, Noonan C, et al. Is circadian type associated with sleep duration in twins? Sleep Biol Rhythms 2012;10:61–8.

31. Barclay NL, Gregory AM. Quantitative genetic research on sleep: a review of normal sleep, sleep disturbances and associated emotional, behavioural, and health-related difficulties. Sleep Med Rev 2013;17:29–40.

32. Barclay NL, Eley TC, Buysse DJ, et al. Diurnal preference and sleep quality: same genes? A study of young adult twins. Chronobiol Int 2010;27:278–96.

33. Barclay NL, Watson NF, Buchwald D, et al. Moderation of genetic and environmental influences on diurnal preference by age in adult twins. Chronobiol Int 2014;31:222–31.

34. Koskenvuo M, Hublin C, Partinen M, et al. Heritability of diurnal type: a nationwide study of 8753 adult twin pairs. J Sleep Res 2007;16:156–62.

35. Toomey R, Panizzon MS, Kremen WS, et al. A twin-study of genetic contributions to morningness-eveningness and depression. Chronobiol Int 2015; 32:303–9.

36. Kuna ST, Maislin G, Pack FM, et al. Heritability of performance deficit accumulation during acute sleep deprivation in twins. Sleep 2012;35:1223–33.

37. Klei L, Reitz P, Miller M, et al. Heritability of morningness-eveningness and self-report sleep measures in a family-based sample of 521 hutterites. Chronobiol Int 2005;22:1041–54.

38. Evans DS, Snitker S, Wu SH, et al. Habitual sleep/wake patterns in the Old Order Amish: heritability and association with non-genetic factors. Sleep 2011;34:661–9.

39. von Schantz M, Taporoski TP, Horimoto AR, et al. Distribution and heritability of diurnal preference (chronotype) in a rural Brazilian family-based cohort, the Baependi study. Sci Rep 2015;5:9214.

40. Katzenberg D, Young T, Finn L, et al. A CLOCK polymorphism associated with human diurnal preference. Sleep 1998;21:569–76.

41. Mishima K, Tozawa T, Satoh K, et al. The 3111T/C polymorphism of hClock is associated with evening preference and delayed sleep timing in a Japanese population sample. Am J Med Genet B Neuropsychiatr Genet 2005;133:101–4.

42. Garaulet M, Sánchez-Moreno C, Smith CE, et al. Ghrelin, sleep reduction and evening preference: relationships to CLOCK 3111 T/C SNP and weight loss. PLoS One 2011;6:e17435.

43. Choub A, Mancuso M, Coppedè F, et al. Clock T3111C and Per2 C111G SNPs do not influence circadian rhythmicity in healthy Italian population. Neurol Sci 2011;32:89–93.

44. Barclay NL, Eley TC, Mill J, et al. Sleep quality and diurnal preference in a sample of young adults: associations with 5HTTLPR, PER3, and CLOCK 3111. Am J Med Genet B Neuropsychiatr Genet 2011; 156B:681–90.

45. Robilliard DL, Archer SN, Arendt J, et al. The 3111 Clock gene polymorphism is not associated with sleep and circadian rhythmicity in phenotypically characterized human subjects. J Sleep Res 2002; 11:305–12.

46. Iwase T, Kajimura N, Uchiyama M, et al. Mutation screening of the human Clock gene in circadian rhythm sleep disorders. Psychiatry Res 2002;109: 121–8.

47. Pedrazzoli M, Louzada FM, Pereira DS, et al. Clock polymorphisms and circadian rhythms phenotypes in a sample of the Brazilian population. Chronobiol Int 2007;24:1–8.

48. Lee HJ, Paik JW, Kang SG, et al. Allelic variants interaction of CLOCK gene and G-protein beta3 subunit gene with diurnal preference. Chronobiol Int 2007;24:589–97.

49. Dmitrzak-Węglarz M, Pawlak J, Wiłkość M, et al. Chronotype and sleep quality as a subphenotype in association studies of clock genes in mood disorders. Acta Neurobiol Exp 2016;76:32–42.

50. Archer SN, Robilliard DL, Skene DJ, et al. A length polymorphism in the circadian clock gene PER3 is linked to delayed sleep phase syndrome and extreme diurnal preference. Sleep 2003;26:413–5.

51. Pereira DS, Tufik S, Louzada FM, et al. Association of the length polymorphism in the human PER3 gene with the delayed sleep-phase syndrome: does latitude have an influence upon it? Sleep 2005;28:29–32.

52. Jones KH, Ellis J, von Schantz M, et al. Age-related change in the association between a polymorphism in the PER3 gene and preferred timing of sleep and waking activities. J Sleep Res 2007;16: 12–6.

53. Ebisawa T, Uchiyama M, Kajimura N, et al. Association of structural polymorphisms in the human period3 gene with delayed sleep phase syndrome. EMBO Rep 2001;2:342–6.

54. Viola AU, Archer SN, James LM, et al. PER3 polymorphism predicts sleep structure and waking performance. Curr Biol 2007;17:613–8.

55. Groeger JA, Viola AU, Lo JC, et al. Early morning executive functioning during sleep deprivation is compromised by a PERIOD3 polymorphism. Sleep 2008;31:1159–67.

56. Lázár AS, Slak A, Lo JC, et al. Sleep, diurnal preference, health, and psychological well-being: a prospective single-allelic-variation study. Chronobiol Int 2012;29:131–46.

57. Osland TM, Bjorvatn BR, Steen VM, et al. Association study of a variable-number tandem repeat polymorphism in the clock gene PERIOD3 and chronotype in Norwegian university students. Chronobiol Int 2011;28:764–70.

58. Voinescu BI, Coogan AN. A variable-number tandem repeat polymorphism in PER3 is not associated with chronotype in a population with self-reported sleep problems. Sleep Biol Rhythms 2012;10:23–6.

59. Goel N, Banks S, Mignot E, et al. PER3 polymorphism predicts cumulative sleep homeostatic but not neurobehavioral changes to chronic partial sleep deprivation. PLoS One 2009;4:e5874.

60. Perea CS, Niño CL, López-León S, et al. Study of a functional polymorphism in the PER3 gene and diurnal preference in a Colombian sample. Open Neurol J 2014;8:7–10.

61. Kunorozva L, Stephenson KJ, Rae DE, et al. Chronotype and PERIOD3 variable number tandem repeat polymorphism in individual sports athletes. Chronobiol Int 2012;29:1004–10.

62. Ellis J, von Schantz M, Jones KH, et al. Association between specific diurnal preference questionnaire items and PER3 VNTR genotype. Chronobiol Int 2009;26:464–73.

63. An HJ, Zhou CX, Geng P, et al. Influence of Per3 genotypes on circadian rhythmicity in flight cadets after militarized management. Int J Clin Exp Pathol 2014;7:6980–4.

64. An H, Zhu Z, Zhou C, et al. Chronotype and a PERIOD3 variable number tandem repeat polymorphism in Han Chinese pilots. Int J Clin Exp Med 2014;7:3770–6.

65. Hida A, Kitamura S, Katayose Y, et al. Screening of clock gene polymorphisms demonstrates association of a PER3 polymorphism with morningness-eveningness preference and circadian rhythm sleep disorder. Sci Rep 2014;4:6309.

66. Parsons MJ, Lester KJ, Barclay NL, et al. Polymorphisms in the circadian expressed genes PER3 and ARNTL2 are associated with diurnal preference and GNβ3 with sleep measures. J Sleep Res 2014;23:595–604.

67. Ojeda DA, Perea CS, Niño CL, et al. A novel association of two non-synonymous polymorphisms in PER2 and PER3 genes with specific diurnal preference subscales. Neurosci Lett 2013;553:52–6.

68. Carpen JD, Archer SN, Skene DJ, et al. A single-nucleotide polymorphism in the 5'-untranslated region of the hPER2 gene is associated with diurnal preference. J Sleep Res 2005;14:293–7.

69. Lee HJ, Kim L, Kang SG, et al. PER2 variation is associated with diurnal preference in a Korean young population. Behav Genet 2011;41:273–7.

70. Matsuo M, Shiino Y, Yamada N, et al. A novel SNP in hPer2 associates with diurnal preference in a healthy population. Sleep Biol Rhythms 2007;5:141–5.

71. Chang AM, Bjonnes AC, Aeschbach D, et al. Circadian gene variants influence sleep and the sleep electroencephalogram in humans. Chronobiol Int 2016;33:561–73.

72. Carpen JD, von Schantz M, Smits M, et al. A silent polymorphism in the PER1 gene associates with extreme diurnal preference in humans. J Hum Genet 2006;51:1122–5.

73. Lim AS, Chang AM, Shulman JM, et al. A common polymorphism near PER1 and the timing of human behavioral rhythms. Ann Neurol 2012;72:324–34.

74. Kang JI, Park CI, Namkoong K, et al. Associations between polymorphisms in the NR1D1 gene encoding for nuclear receptor REV-ERBα and circadian typologies. Chronobiol Int 2015;32:568–72.

75. Pedrazzoli M, Ling L, Finn L, et al. A polymorphism in the human timeless gene is not associated with diurnal preferences in normal adults. Sleep Res Online 2000;3:73–6.

76. Lee SI, Hida A, Kitamura S, et al. Association between the melanopsin gene polymorphism OPN4*Ile394Thr and sleep/wake timing in Japanese university students. J Physiol Anthropol 2014;33:9.

77. Hu Y, Shmygelska A, Tran D, et al. GWAS of 89,283 individuals identifies genetic variants associated with self-reporting of being a morning person. Nat Commun 2016;7:10448.

78. Lane JM, Vlasac I, Anderson SG, et al. Genome-wide association analysis identifies novel loci for chronotype in 100,420 individuals from the UK Biobank. Nat Commun 2016;7:10889.

79. Jones SE, Tyrrell J, Wood AR, et al. Genome-wide association analyses in >128,266 individuals identifies new morningness and sleep duration loci. PLoS Genet 2016;12:e1006125.

80. Partinen M, Kaprio J, Koskenvuo M, et al. Genetic and environmental determination of human sleep. Sleep 1983;6:179–85.

81. Heath AC, Kendler KS, Eaves LJ, et al. Evidence for genetic influences on sleep disturbance and sleep pattern in twins. Sleep 1990;13:318–35.

82. Barclay NL, Eley TC, Buysse DJ, et al. Genetic and environmental influences on different components of the 'Pittsburgh Sleep Quality Index' and their overlap. Sleep 2010;33:659–68.

83. Genderson MR, Rana BK, Panizzon MS, et al. Genetic and environmental influences on sleep quality in middle-aged men: a twin study. J Sleep Res 2013;22:519–26.

84. Watson NF, Buchwald D, Vitiello MV, et al. A twin study of sleep duration and body mass index. J Clin Sleep Med 2010;6:11–7.

85. Watson NF, Harden KP, Buchwald D, et al. Sleep duration and body mass index in twins: a gene-environment interaction. Sleep 2012;35:597–603.

86. De Castro JM. The influence of heredity on self-reported sleep patterns in free-living humans. Physiol Behav 2002;76:479–86.

87. Liu R, Liu X, Arguelles LM, et al. A population-based twin study on sleep duration and body composition. Obesity (Silver Spring) 2012;20:192–9.

88. Hublin C, Partinen M, Koskenvuo M, et al. Genetic factors in evolution of sleep length–a longitudinal twin study in Finnish adults. J Sleep Res 2013;22:513–8.

89. Cade BE, Gottlieb DJ, Lauderdale DS, et al. Common variants in DRD2 are associated with sleep duration: the CARe consortium. Hum Mol Genet 2016;25:167–79.

90. Carmelli D, Bliwise DL, Swan GE, et al. Genetic factors in self-reported snoring and excessive daytime sleepiness: a twin study. Am J Respir Crit Care Med 2001;164:949–52.

91. Carmelli D, Bliwise DL, Swan GE, et al. A genetic analysis of the epworth sleepiness scale in 1560 world war II male veteran twins in the NAS-NRC twin registry. J Sleep Res 2001;10:53–8.

92. Watson NF, Goldberg J, Arguelles L, et al. Genetic and environmental influences on insomnia, daytime sleepiness, and obesity in twins. Sleep 2006;29:645–9.

93. Desai AV, Cherkas LF, Spector TD, et al. Genetic influences in self-reported symptoms of obstructive sleep apnoea and restless legs: a twin study. Twin Res 2004;7:589–95.

94. Lessov-Schlaggar CN, Bliwise DL, Krasnow RE, et al. Genetic association of daytime sleepiness and depressive symptoms in elderly men. Sleep 2008;31:1111–7.

95. Dauvilliers Y, Maret S, Tafti M. Genetics of normal and pathological sleep in humans. Sleep Med Rev 2005;9:91–100.

96. Tafti M, Maret S, Dauvilliers Y. Genes for normal sleep and sleep disorders. Ann Med 2005;37:580–9.

97. Tafti M. Genetic aspects of normal and disturbed sleep. Sleep Med 2009;10:S17–21.

98. Landolt HP. Genotype-dependent differences in sleep, vigilance, and response to stimulants. Curr Pharm Des 2008;14:3396–407.

99. Ambrosius U, Lietzenmaier S, Wehrle R, et al. Heritability of sleep electroencephalogram. Biol Psychiatry 2008;64:344–8.

100. De Gennaro L, Marzano C, Fratello F, et al. The electroencephalographic fingerprint of sleep is genetically determined: a twin study. Ann Neurol 2008;64:455–60.

101. Werth E, Achermann P, Dijk DJ, et al. Spindle frequency activity in the sleep EEG: individual differences and topographic distribution. Electroencephalogr Clin Neurophysiol 1997;103:535–42.

102. Tan X, Campbell IG, Palagini L, et al. High inter-night reliability of computer-measured NREM delta, sigma, and beta: biological implications. Biol Psychiatry 2000;48:1010–9.

103. Finelli LA, Achermann P, Borbely AA. Individual 'fingerprints' in human sleep EEG topography. Neuropsychopharmacology 2001;25:S57–62.

104. De Gennaro L, Ferrara M, Vecchio F, et al. An electroencephalographic fingerprint of human sleep. Neuroimage 2005;26:114–22.

105. Tucker AM, Dinges DF, Van Dongen HP. Trait interindividual differences in the sleep physiology of healthy young adults. J Sleep Res 2007;16:170–80.

106. Buckelmuller J, Landolt HP, Stassen HH, et al. Trait-like individual differences in the human sleep electroencephalogram. Neuroscience 2006;138:351–6.

107. Andretic R, Franken P, Tafti M. Genetics of sleep. Annu Rev Genet 2008;42:361–88.

108. Adamczyk M, Ambrosius U, Lietzenmaier S, et al. Genetics of rapid eye movement sleep in humans. Transl Psychiatry 2015;5:e598.

109. Adamczyk M, Genzel L, Dresler M, et al. Automatic sleep spindle detection and genetic influence estimation using continuous wavelet transform. Front Hum Neurosci 2015;9:624.

110. Goel N. Genetics in sleep medicine. Rev Sleep Med, in press.

111. Evans DS, Parimi N, Nievergelt CM, et al. Common genetic variants in ARNTL and NPAS2 and at chromosome 12p13 are associated with objectively measured sleep traits in the elderly. Sleep 2013;36:431–6.

112. He Y, Jones CR, Fujiki N, et al. The transcriptional repressor DEC2 regulates sleep length in mammals. Science 2009;325:866–70.

113. Allebrandt KV, Teder-Laving M, Akyol M, et al. CLOCK gene variants associate with sleep duration in two independent populations. Biol Psychiatry 2010;67:1040–7.

114. Lane JM, Tare A, Cade BE, et al. Common variants in CLOCK are not associated with measures of sleep duration in people of European ancestry from the sleep heart health study. Biol Psychiatry 2013;74:e33–5.

115. Vanderlind WM, Beevers CG, Sherman SM, et al. Sleep and sadness: exploring the relation among sleep, cognitive control, and depressive symptoms in young adults. Sleep Med 2014;15:144–9.

116. Gottlieb DJ, O'Connor GT, Wilk JB. Genome-wide association of sleep and circadian phenotypes. BMC Med Genet 2007;8:S9.

117. Allebrandt KV, Amin N, Müller-Myhsok B, et al. A K(ATP) channel gene effect on sleep duration: from genome-wide association studies to function in Drosophila. Mol Psychiatry 2013;18:122–32.

118. Parsons MJ, Lester KJ, Barclay NL, et al. Replication of genome-wide association studies (GWAS) loci for sleep in the British G1219 cohort. Am J Med Genet B Neuropsychiatr Genet 2013;162B:431–8.

119. Ollila HM, Kettunen J, Pietiläinen O, et al. Genome-wide association study of sleep duration in the Finnish population. J Sleep Res 2014;23:609–18.

120. Gottlieb DJ, Hek K, Chen TH, et al. Novel loci associated with usual sleep duration: the CHARGE Consortium Genome-Wide Association Study. Mol Psychiatry 2015;20:1232–9.

121. Scheinfeldt LB, Gharani N, Kasper RS, et al. Using the Coriell Personalized Medicine Collaborative Data to conduct a genome-wide association study of sleep duration. Am J Med Genet B Neuropsychiatr Genet 2015;168:697–705.

122. Byrne EM, Gehrman PR, Medland SE, et al. A genome-wide association study of sleep habits and insomnia. Am J Med Genet B Neuropsychiatr Genet 2013;162B:439–51.

123. Amin N, Allebrandt KV, van der Spek A, et al. Genetic variants in RBFOX3 are associated with sleep latency. Eur J Hum Genet 2016;24:1488–95.

124. Spada J, Scholz M, Kirsten H, et al. Genome-wide association analysis of actigraphic sleep phenotypes in the LIFE Adult Study. J Sleep Res 2016;25:690–701.

125. Parsons MJ. On the genetics of sleep disorders: genome-wide association studies and beyond. Adv Genomics Genet 2015;5:293–303.

Evaluation of the Sleepy Patient: Differential Diagnosis

 CrossMark

Renee Monderer, MD*, Imran M. Ahmed, MD, Michael Thorpy, MD

KEYWORDS

- Excessive daytime sleepiness • Hypersomnolence • Evaluation • Sleep disorders

KEY POINTS

- Excessive daytime sleepiness is defined as the inability to maintain wakefulness during waking hours, resulting in unintended lapses into sleep. It is important to distinguish sleepiness from fatigue.
- The evaluation of a sleep patient begins with a careful clinical assessment that includes a detailed sleep history, medical and psychiatric history, a review of medications, as well as a social and family history.
- Physical examination should include a general medical examination with careful attention to the upper airway and the neurological examination.
- Appropriate objective testing with a polysomnogram and a multiple sleep latency test if needed will help confirm the diagnosis and direct the appropriate treatment plan.

INTRODUCTION

Excessive daytime sleepiness (EDS) is defined as the inability to maintain wakefulness during waking hours, resulting in unintended lapses into sleep.[1] Patients often describe their sleepiness using vague terms such as tired, fatigue, or lack of energy. It is important to distinguish sleepiness from fatigue. Fatigue is a physical or psychological feeling that may occur in a variety of other disorders, such as depression or Parkinson disease.[2,3] Unlike sleepiness, fatigued patients do not fall asleep when sedentary, such as while watching television or reading. This distinction is important because sleepiness indicates the presence of a sleep disorder or a problem with nighttime sleep. In a study of 190 obstructive sleep apnea (OSA) patients, approximately 47% used the term sleepiness to describe their symptoms. In contrast, 62% reported a lack of energy, 61% described themselves as feeling tiredness, and 57% used the term fatigue. When these patients were asked to select the most prominent symptom, only about

22% chose sleepiness, whereas more than 40% chose lack of energy.[4]

Patients may or may not be aware of their sleepiness before falling asleep, but it often significantly affects quality of life. EDS has many implications, including increased risk of injury at work or home, decreased alertness, car accidents, and lower productivity overall. EDS may also lead to heightened tension with family, friends, and co-workers, who may attribute the patient's symptoms to laziness or poor work ethic.

Driving while sleepy is perhaps the most worrisome behavior associated with EDS. This may take the form of dozing at a red light, while in stop-and-go traffic, or while traveling at higher speeds on a highway. Approximately 52% of drivers have driven while drowsy, with 50% reporting doing so within the last month.[5] Sleepiness while driving should be considered a medical emergency, and immediate evaluation and treatment should be initiated.[6,7]

Sleepiness can manifest in many different forms. For some patients, sleepiness is associated

Sleep-Wake Disorders Center, Department of Neurology, Montefiore Medical Center, Albert Einstein College of Medicine, 111 East 210th Street, Bronx, NY 10467, USA
* Corresponding author.
E-mail address: rmondere@montefiore.org

Sleep Med Clin 12 (2017) 301–312
http://dx.doi.org/10.1016/j.jsmc.2017.03.006
1556-407X/17/© 2017 Elsevier Inc. All rights reserved.

with more hours of sleep per day without feeling refreshed. For others, naps can be refreshing but sleepiness recurs. Children can paradoxically present with symptoms of hyperactivity or poor attention.

Many of the sleep disorders listed in the International Classifications of Sleep Disorders, 3rd edition (ICSD-3) can present with excessive sleepiness (**Box 1**). These disorders result in daytime sleepiness either because of shortened sleep time, fragmentation of the major sleep period, or central nervous system (CNS) dysfunction. Several studies of patients with OSA have demonstrated a significant correlation between the total number of arousals on a polysomnogram with the severity of sleepiness.[8–10] Other disorders, such as narcolepsy type 1 (with cataplexy) or type 2 (without cataplexy), idiopathic hypersomnia, or Kleine-Levin syndrome, are caused by a suspected CNS abnormality.[11–14] In contrast, insufficient sleep syndrome is caused by patients sleeping less than their biologic sleep requirement. Sleepiness in shift work disorder often results from insufficient sleep time because patients cannot sleep on their hours off due to noise, family, or social obligations. Medications, alcohol, substance abuse, and certain medical, neurologic, and psychiatric disorders can cause excessive sleepiness either by disturbing CNS sleep-wake mechanisms or by fragmenting the major sleep period (**Box 2**).

Box 1
Common sleep disorders associated with excessive daytime somnolence

1. Hypersomnia due to medical or psychiatric disorder or drug or substance
2. Narcolepsy type 1 or 2
3. Idiopathic hypersomnia
4. Kleine-Levin syndrome
5. Insufficient sleep syndrome (sleep deprivation)
6. OSA
7. Central sleep apnea
8. Shift work disorder
9. Delayed sleep phase type
10. Advanced sleep phase type
11. Long sleeper
12. Periodic limb movement disorder
13. Hypersomnia due to a medical disorder
14. Hypersomnia due to a medication or substance

Box 2
Common medical and psychiatric disorders that can cause excessive sleepiness

Brain tumors

Strokes

Head trauma

Seizures

Congestive heart failure

Bronchial asthma

Endocrine abnormalities (eg, excessive growth hormone, hypothyroidism, diabetes mellitus)

Chronic renal insufficiency

Infectious diseases (eg, human immunodeficiency virus, CNS Lyme disease)

Metabolic or infectious encephalopathies

Fibromyalgia

Chronic fatigue syndrome

Schizophrenia

Mood (depressive) disorders

Seasonal affective disorder

Conversion disorder

Factitious disorder

Malingering

Drug intoxication or withdrawal

Approximately 14% of the population report EDS at least a few days per week.[15] The prevalence seems to be higher among subjects age 65 years and older, ranging from 15% to 20%.[16,17] Although exact statistics are not known, the most common causes of daytime sleepiness are insufficient sleep syndrome, shift work disorder, and OSA. Central causes of daytime sleepiness, such as narcolepsy and idiopathic hypersomnia, are less prevalent but important to screen for as well.[15,18]

A systematic approach to the sleepy patient is needed to be able to distinguish between the many causes of daytime sleepiness. A thorough sleep history from the patient and, preferably, the patient's bed partner or caregiver, is needed. In addition, past medical, psychiatric history, surgical history, family history, physical examination, and appropriate laboratory tests are needed to form a complete differential diagnosis.

SLEEP EVALUATION

A thorough sleep evaluation begins with taking a careful history to determine the chief complaint; a detailed sleep history; and a medical, psychiatric, social, and family history. This should be followed by a focused physical examination; an appropriate sleep questionnaire; possible laboratory testing; and, if necessary, a sleep study.

History

As previously discussed, many patients with excessive sleepiness do not report sleepiness but rather describe their symptoms as fatigue, tiredness, lethargy, moodiness, or difficulty concentrating. If sleepiness is present, it is important to determine how that sleepiness affects daily activities. Many patients will report difficulty staying awake at work or completing tasks at home. Others will report negative effects on education, recreation, or personal relationships.[7] Discerning the effect that sleepiness has on a person's quality of life helps guide the evaluation and treatment to alleviate those symptoms.

Occasionally, patients, such as those with Parkinson disease or Alzheimer dementia, may not be aware of their sleepiness. It is helpful to have a bed partner or caretaker present to determine whether patients are unaware of episodes of falling asleep.[19]

To determine the severity of sleepiness, it is important to identify those situations in which a person experiences sleepiness. Mild sleepiness will manifest as falling asleep when sedentary and inactive, such as while watching television or reading. Moderate sleepiness is present when patients fall asleep during activities that require some attention, for instance during a meeting for work. Severe sleepiness is defined as sleepiness occurring during active situations, such as while driving.[20] The Epworth Sleepiness Scale (ESS) is an important tool that addresses the likelihood of falling asleep in these and other daily situations (Fig. 1). The patient reports on a score from

The Epworth Sleepiness Scale (ESS) has 8 routine daytime situations that you rate on a scale from 0 to 3, based on your likelihood of dozing off or falling asleep in each situation. Write the number that corresponds with your answer for each situation in the "My score" box. Then add up your score, and share the results with your doctor.

SITUATION	Would Never Doze Nunca se Queda Dormido (a)	Slight Chance Of Dozing Posibilidad minina de Dormirse	Moderate Chance of Dozing Posibilidad Moderada de Dormirse	High Chance Of Dozing Major Posibilidad de Dormirse
Sitting and reading *Sentando(a) y leyendo*	0	1	2	3
Watching television *Mirando television*	0	1	2	3
Sitting inactive in a public place-for example, a theater or meeting *Sentado,(a) sin hacer nada en un lugar public por ejemplo, en el cine o en una reunion.*	0	1	2	3
As a passenger in a car for an hour without a break *Como un pasajero en un carro for una hora sin ningun descanso.*	0	1	2	3
Lying down to rest in the afternoon when circumstances permit *Recostado (a) en la tarde para descansar cuando sea permitido.*	0	1	2	3
Sitting and talking to someone *Setando (a) hablando con alguien*	0	1	2	3
Sitting quietly after lunch without alcohol *Setando (a) en silencio despues del almuerzo sin haber tomado alcohol*	0	1	2	3
In a car, while stopped for a few minutes in traffic *En un carro detenido mientras espera por el trafico.*	0	1	2	3
	TOTAL SCORE:			

Fig. 1. Epworth sleepiness scale.

0 to 3 the chance of dozing in 8 typical daytime activities. A score of 10 or more is considered significant daytime sleepiness, and above 15 is considered severe daytime sleepiness.

To discern if sleepiness while driving is present, it is important to inquire whether a person is using techniques such as rolling down the windows, turning up the volume on the radio, or talking to a passenger to keep themselves awake. Additionally, drivers should be asked about near-miss accidents to determine the level of sleepiness while driving. Sleepy near-miss accidents may be precursors to driving accidents.[21]

Sleep history

Obtaining a sleep history is essential to identifying a sleep disorder. Symptoms during the 24-hour cycle, rather than only those that occur at night, should be evaluated. The sleep history consists of the patient's bedtime, the length of time it takes to fall asleep, wake time, number of awakenings, naps, periods of dozing off, and any additional time spent in bed awake. It is often helpful to obtain a sleep log over a 2-week period to determine if there is sufficient amount of sleep per night or whether a circadian rhythm disorder, such as advanced or delayed sleep phase disorder, is present (**Fig. 2**). A person with delayed sleep phase may report sleepiness on awakening in the morning, whereas a person with advanced sleep phase may complain of sleepiness in the evening hours. A sleep log may help a shift

worker recognize lost sleep and formulate a strategy for how to obtain more hours of sleep. The sleep log can also help identify behaviors that disrupt the major sleep period and lead to daytime sleepiness.

Other sleep features

The diagnosis of a primary sleep disorder causing EDS needs to be considered. Sleep disorders such as narcolepsy, OSA, recurrent hypersomnia, insufficient sleep time, and circadian rhythm disorders can often be determined by the patient's history.

Obstructive sleep apnea

The presence of snoring, episodes of choking or gasping for air, or witnessed apnea may be reported by the patient or bed partner and often indicate sleep-related breathing disorders. Occasionally, only snoring is reported because the patient is unaware that she or he has trouble breathing while asleep. Additional signs of sleep apnea include awakening with a dry mouth, nasal congestion, nighttime cough, nocturnal enuresis, and morning headaches. It is helpful to have a bed partner present to identify variations in the quality of snoring, because apnea may present as episodes of loud snoring that alternate with quiet episodes of pauses in breathing.[22] The presence of a bed partner can also be helpful in identifying the deleterious effects of snoring on interpersonal relationships, a possibility that is

SLEEP DIARY

Fatigue Rating Scale	0 extremely fatigued	25 moderately fatigued	50 mildly fatigued	75 somewhat fatigued	100 very energetic

COMPLETE AT NIGHT in reference to today　　　　　　　　COMPLETE IN MORNING in reference to night before

Day and Date	Unusual daytime stressors	Fatigue rating (use rating scale on top of page)	Naps (time & length)	Exercise (Y/N, time of day and how long)	Caffeine (note type and time) Cigarettes	Sleep meds or alcohol (name & dose)	Time you went to bed and turned out the lights	How long it took you to fall asleep for the first time	Number of times you woke falling asleep	How long you were awake in total after falling asleep	Time you finally woke up	Time you finally got out of bed
.												
Mon. 9/14	Pain/ Stress	68	2–4 pm	No	Coffee, 8oz at noon	Ambien 10mg	12:00	60 min.	3	60 min.	6:30	8:00

Fig. 2. Sleep diary.

often a key motivating factor in seeking out a sleep evaluation.

Obesity is an established risk factor for sleep apnea. The weight and height of each patient should be documented, as well as any weight changes over the past few years or attempts at weight loss.[23]

Menopause, independent of age and body mass index, is also a risk factor for sleep apnea.[24] Determining if a woman is premenopausal or postmenopausal can help determine if she is at risk for sleep apnea.

Narcolepsy

Daytime sleepiness is the hallmark of narcolepsy. Cataplexy, characterized by sudden loss of muscle tone brought on by emotions, is pathognomonic for narcolepsy. Additional features, such as hypnogogic hallucinations and sleep paralysis, can also help establish a diagnosis of narcolepsy; however, neither is specific to narcolepsy and both can be seen in disorders of sleep fragmentation.[25,26] Narcolepsy patients often report fragmented sleep and automatic behaviors. A detailed history of excessive, frequent, and bizarre dreams, as well as out-of-body experiences, delusional or lucid dreams, and dreams in naps can be consistent with a diagnosis of narcolepsy. A diagnosis of narcolepsy without cataplexy (narcolepsy type 2) is appropriate when EDS is present with rapid eye movement (REM) phenomenology (hypnogogic hallucinations and sleep paralysis) but without cataplexy.

Idiopathic hypersomnia

EDS without the presence of REM phenomena, such as cataplexy and hypnagogic hallucinations, that has persisted for more than 3 months may indicate idiopathic hypersomnia if all other causes of hypersomnia have been ruled out by polysomnography. This is often a diagnosis of exclusion.

Kleine-Levin syndrome

A history of relapsing and remitting episodes of sleepiness that occur at least once a year, lasting 2 days to 4 weeks, and that are associated with cognitive and behavioral disturbances, might suggest Kleine-Levin Syndrome. Normal levels of alertness, behavior, and cognition are present in between episodes.

Circadian rhythm disorders

Obtaining a detailed sleep history, as well as a sleep log, can help diagnose circadian rhythm disorders. Sleepiness in these disorders is caused by a misalignment between the endogenous circadian clock and the schedules imposed by society. In shift work disorder it is essential to determine the patient's work schedule. Rotating shifts that alternate schedules every few weeks can make patients particularly vulnerable to work-related injuries resulting from sleepiness.[27] Night shifts are usually the most disruptive to circadian rhythms; however, early morning shifts, especially when traveling to work is involved, can also present a problem and result in excessive sleepiness.

Other sleep disorders

It is important to differentiate fatigue and lack of energy from daytime sleepiness in insomnia patients. Insomnia patients do not generally report a propensity to fall asleep when sedentary. If EDS is present in the setting of insomnia, a suspicion for an underlying sleep disorder, such as sleep apnea, should be raised.[28]

Although restless leg syndrome (RLS) and periodic limb movement disorder are not a common cause of EDS, an inquiry into the presence of unpleasant sensations in the legs, an urge to move the limbs, or jerking of the legs in bed should be done.

Medical History

A comprehensive medical history should be performed with particular focus on cardiovascular, cerebrovascular, and nasopharyngeal disease. Hypertension, type II diabetes, ischemic heart disease, heart failure, atrial fibrillation, and pulmonary hypertension have all been linked to OSA.[29–36] Congestive heart failure is also a risk factor for central sleep apnea.[37] Sleep apnea and stroke have also been linked in a bidirectional manner, with sleep apnea, increasing the risk for stroke and the incidence of sleep apnea being increased following a stroke.[38–41]

Chronic nasal congestion is associated with fragmented sleep and sleep-disordered breathing.[42,43] It is helpful to inquire about the presence of nasal allergies, postnasal drip, sinus disease, and rhinitis. Additionally, any prior history of adenoid or tonsil surgery or upper airway surgery should be documented.

The association of sleep and pain is bidirectional.[44] Pain syndromes, such as neuropathy or arthritis, can fragment sleep, leading to daytime sleepiness.[45,46] Conversely, newer studies have shown that disrupted sleep can reliably predict new occurrence and worsening of chronic pain.[47,48]

Metabolic disorders, such as thyroid dysfunction or diabetes, can cause EDS and should be inquired about in a medical history.[49–51]

Many prescription medications can cause either daytime sleepiness or impair nighttime sleep.[52]

Pain medications, such as opioids, have been linked with an increase in sleep-disordered breathing.[53,54] Methadone has been linked to an increase in both central sleep apnea and OSA.[55,56]

Psychiatric History

It is prudent to inquire about mood disorders, such as depression or bipolar disorder, because these disorders can manifest as excessive sleepiness. Sleepiness can be due to a psychiatric condition, psychiatric medications, or a comorbid sleep disorder. Prolonged nocturnal sleep or EDS can be a presenting symptom in atypical depression or some bipolar depression.[57,58] Nocturnal panic attacks, which can present as part of an anxiety disorder, can cause fragmented nocturnal sleep and result in daytime sleepiness.[59]

Tricyclic antidepressants, antipsychotic medications, benzodiazepines, and certain serotonin reuptake inhibitors can lead to daytime sleepiness.[60,61] Additionally, many mood stabilizing medications can lead to weight gain, which is a risk factor for OSA.[62]

Social and Family History

The social history should focus on any personal stressors that may disrupt nighttime sleep. The frequency and timing of exercise should also be determined because it can also have an effect on nighttime sleep.[63]

Caffeine consumption should be inquired about because of its disruptive effects on sleep.[64] Furthermore, excessive caffeine consumption can indicate a need to self-medicate to combat daytime sleepiness.

Smoking tobacco, both during consumption and withdrawal, has been associated with fragmented sleep. Additionally, it may be a risk factor for sleep-disordered breathing.[65,66]

Alcohol decreases sleep latency and consolidates sleep in the first part of the night, but it disrupts the second half of sleep.[67,68] Alcoholics, both during binge drinking and withdrawal, experience excessive sleepiness, insomnia, and fragmented nighttime sleep.[69,70] Illicit drugs, such as cocaine, methylenedioxymethamphetamine (ecstasy), and ketamine, can also cause severe sleep disruption both during consumption and withdrawal.[71,72]

A family history is found in many sleep disorders, such as narcolepsy, RLS, and OSA with or without obesity, and should be inquired about.[1]

Physical Examination

The physical examination should include an evaluation of the nose, throat, neck, heart, lungs, abdomen, extremities, and neurologic system. Vital signs, including blood pressure, heart rate, weight, height, body mass index, and neck circumference, should be collected. Evaluation of the upper airway should focus on size and shape of the soft palate, tongue, uvula, airway, pharyngeal tissue, and tongue. Nasal examination should look for the presence of a deviated nasal septum and/or turbinate hypertrophy. The cervicofacial angle should be examined for possible retrognathia or micrognathia, both of which can be associated with OSA.[73,74] A patient can be referred to an otolaryngologist for upper airway endoscopy to establish the location and severity of obstruction in the nasopharynx and/or oropharynx. Thyroid size should be determined because enlargement can obstruct the upper airway.[75,76] For a patient suspected of having narcolepsy and cataplexy, observing the patients face during the interview may reveal facial muscle weakness or twitching during emotion that can indicate cataplexy.

A neurologic examination should be performed to look for secondary causes of narcolepsy, idiopathic hypersomnia, and RLS. Additionally, a neurologic examination to evaluate the possibility of Parkinson disease or a previous stroke can help with differentiating causes of excessive sleepiness. A vascular examination, including assessing for distal pulses and for the presence of peripheral edema, is also helpful in ruling out secondary causes of leg symptoms that disturb sleep.

Sleep Questionnaires

Sleep questionnaires can be valuable tools for obtaining information regarding sleep complaints, sleep pattern, sleep hygiene, and medical and social history. The ESS is widely used to assess the degree of daytime sleepiness (see **Fig. 1**). Other sleep questionnaires that can be useful in assessing sleepiness include the Stanford Sleepiness Scale, the Pittsburgh Sleep Quality Index, the Ullanlinna Narcolepsy Scale, or the Karolinska Sleepiness Scale. The Swiss Narcolepsy Scale can be helpful to detect cataplexy. When positive, it is consistent with a diagnosis of narcolepsy type 1 (**Box 3**).

A sleep log kept over a 2-week period that documents time of sleep onset, awakenings during the night, wake time, naps, and other sleep-related habits can be helpful in monitoring sleep patterns and determining what factors are contributing to daytime sleepiness.

Blood and Urine Tests

Screening blood work is usually done by the primary care physician before referral to the sleep

Box 3
Swiss narcolepsy scale

1. How often are you unable to fall asleep?

   a. Never

   b. Rarely (less than once a month)

   c. Sometimes (1–3 times a month)

   d. Often (1–2 times a week)

   e. Almost always

2. How often do you feel bad or not well rested in the morning?

   a. Never

   b. Rarely (less than once a month)

   c. Sometimes (1–3 times a month)

   d. Often (1–2 times a week)

   e. Almost always

3. How often do you take a nap during the day?

   a. Never

   b. I would like to but cannot

   c. 1 to 2 times a week

   d. 3 to 5 times a week

   e. Almost daily

4. How often have you experienced weak knees or buckling of the knees during emotions like laughing, happiness, or anger?

   a. Never

   b. Rarely (less than once a month)

   c. Sometimes (1–3 times a month)

   d. Often (1–2 times a week)

   e. Almost always

5. How often have you experienced sagging of the jaw during emotions like laughing, happiness, or anger?

   a. Never

   b. Rarely (less than once a month)

   c. Sometimes (1–3 times a month)

   d. Often (1–2 times a week)

   e. Almost always

Each question (Q) is weighted by a positive or negative factor, with the score calculated using the following equation: $(6 \times Q1 + 9 \times Q2 - 5 \times Q3 - 11 \times Q4 - 13 \times Q5 + 20)$.[101,102] Interpretation: A Swiss Narcolepsy Scale (SNS) score less than 0 is suggestive of narcolepsy with cataplexy.[101,102] Validation: In patients with narcolepsy with cataplexy, an SNS score less than 0 was shown to have a sensitivity of 96% and specificity of 98%.[102]

physician for EDS. If signs of thyroid dysfunction are present, the patient should be sent for thyroid function tests. However, this is not recommended routinely unless the patient is in a high-risk group for the development of hypothyroidism, such as women over age 60 years.[77,78]

Blood work should be done as part of the evaluation of patients with RLS. These tests should include a complete blood count, chemistry panel, iron studies, and serum ferritin levels. An iron saturation below 16% or a serum ferritin below 50 µg/L indicates a need for iron supplementation.[79]

Serum and urine drug screening can be an important part of the evaluation for EDS. Recent studies suggest that use of opioids, cannabis, and/or amphetamines can mimic the findings of idiopathic hypersomnia and/or narcolepsy on a multiple sleep latency test (MSLT).[80,81] In these studies, substance use was not reported on initial interview and most physicians did not suspect drug use.[80] Undetected drug or substance abuse could lead to over-diagnosing central causes of hypersomnia and inappropriate treatment. A genetic blood test for the HLA antigen HLA-DQB1*0602 can be helpful in the diagnosis of narcolepsy because it is nearly 100% positive in narcolepsy type 1.

Polysomnography

Polysomnography is an objective measure of sleep that is indicated in evaluating a patient with EDS, unless a circadian rhythm disorder or insufficient sleep disorder is suspected by history. The amount of sleep, percentage of time in each sleep stage, sleep fragmentation, as well as the possible cause of sleep fragmentation is recorded. Causes of sleep fragmentation on polysomnography include respiratory events, such as apneas or hypopneas; abnormal movements in sleep, such as periodic limb movements; and/or other disruptive behaviors, such as parasomnias or epileptiform activity.

An overnight attended polysomnogram in the sleep laboratory monitors sleep parameters and stages via electroencephalogram (EEG), body movements via electromyography (EMG) applied to the lower limbs and chin, eye movement to differentiate sleep stages via electrooculogram, and cardiac tracing via electrocardiogram (EKG). Respiratory parameters are measured with respiratory effort belts that monitor movement of the chest and abdomen, airflow and air pressure sensors applied to the nose and mouth, and oxygen saturation using an infrared oximeter. Other sensors that can be placed when appropriate are upper-extremity EMG to record arm movements, sensors to record end-tidal carbon dioxide concentration, body position, snoring sounds, or gastroesophageal pH. The information is stored digitally on a computer that is later analyzed. Recording speed is typically at 15 mm per second, but this can be adjusted when needed, such as when epileptiform activity is suspected.[82]

The attended polysomnogram is invaluable in providing the information needed to elucidate most causes of sleep fragmentation and resultant daytime sleepiness. An unattended ambulatory polysomnogram done at the patient's home can be used when there is a high suspicion for OSA as the cause of daytime sleepiness.[83–85] However, technical difficulties associated with an unattended recording often limit its value. Additionally, other causes of daytime sleepiness can be missed on home polysomnogram because it routinely only monitors respiratory parameters and EKG without capturing sleep stages and awakenings via EEG.

An in-laboratory, attended, polysomnography is needed in the diagnosing of parasomnias, such as REM sleep behavior disorder; abnormal movements in sleep, such as periodic limb movements; and central causes of sleepiness, such as narcolepsy. Video monitoring, extra EEG leads, and additional EMG leads on the arms are needed to capture abnormal activity in sleep and to help differentiate parasomnias from epileptic disorders.[86] In-laboratory polysomnography can also help confirm the presence of narcolepsy by documenting a short REM latency and by ruling out other causes of sleepiness on the polysomnogram, such as OSA. When narcolepsy is suspected, the polysomnogram is followed by a MSLT. A diagnosis of narcolepsy can be made when the MSLT demonstrates 2 or more sleep-onset REM periods (SOREMPs) with a mean sleep latency of 8 minutes or less.[1] The presence of a SOREMP within 15 minutes on a polysomnogram is highly suggestive of narcolepsy and can count as 1 of the 2 required for a diagnosis of narcolepsy[1]

Polysomnography is not indicated in the diagnosis of insomnia, unless a second sleep disorder is suspected. If EDS, defined as the tendency to fall asleep in the daytime, is present in a patient with insomnia, then a second sleep disorder, such as OSA, should be considered. Older patients with OSA often present with symptoms of insomnia because of their disturbed nighttime sleep. Often these patients report symptoms of insomnia as well as EDS, and a polysomnogram should be done.[87]

Multiple Sleep Latency Test

The MSLT is used to document the degree of daytime sleepiness. It is performed 2 hours after waking from an overnight polysomnogram and consists of 4 or 5 naps, each 2 hours apart. Twenty minutes are allotted to achieve sleep, and the average time to fall asleep on each of the naps is documented. Additionally, the presence of REM sleep in the daytime naps is also documented. Multiple studies have determined that a mean sleep latency of 11.1 minutes or greater with 1 episode of REM sleep is normal for the general population.[88–94] Narcolepsy is suspected when there is a mean sleep latency of less than 8 minutes and 2 SOREMPs, 1 of which may be seen during the preceding night's polysomnogram.[1] Idiopathic hypersomnia patients have a similar mean sleep latency without the presence of REM sleep in daytime naps.[1] Studies of shift workers have documented an average mean sleep latency of less than 5 minutes, which indicates severe sleepiness.[95,96]

Maintenance of Wakefulness Test

The maintenance of wakefulness test (MWT) is used to measure the ability to stay awake. It consists of 4 40-minute intervals in which a patient is asked to sit still and not engage in any stimulating activities. It is often used to measure the effects of alerting medication on daytime functioning. Additionally, it can be used to assess a person's ability to remain awake during work as a commercial driver, a pilot, or other occupations. The Federal Aviation Administration requires an annual MWT to determine the fitness for work in pilots (www.faa.gov). Some employers use the MWT to document response to continuous positive airway pressure in OSA patients.

Performance Testing

Research studies often use performance tests, such as the psychomotor vigilance test (PVT), to assess the behavioral consequences of EDS. The PVT measures reaction time to tasks with high stimulus density to measure attention and performance. Reliable performance changes have been demonstrated on the PVT even with moderate levels of sleepiness due to sleep deprivation.[97] Memory and executive functioning can also be assessed using various cognitive assessment tests when needed.[98]

The Oxford Sleepiness Resistance Test (OSLER) is an alternative test that combines elements of the MWT and psychomotor testing. The OSLER tracks continuing behavioral responses to the activation of a light turning on. A failure to respond to 7 consecutive presentations suggests sleep onset. Multiple studies have shown the OSLER to be a reliable tool for determining a patient's ability to stay awake and vigilant.[99,100]

Electroencephalogram

The EEG is used to investigate possible seizures and to differentiate seizures from other abnormal activity in sleep, such as parasomnias. If seizures are suspected, extra EEG leads are placed in addition to the standard number of leads used for a routine polysomnogram. If epileptiform activity is captured, a more detailed seizure work up should be done.

Neuroimaging

Neuroimaging is needed when an underlying neurologic disorder is being considered as a cause of daytime sleepiness. It can be used to rule out structural lesions in the brainstem that may cause sleepiness. It is usually not required in narcolepsy but may be indicated in patients with idiopathic hypersomnia and patients with REM sleep behavior disorder.

Other Studies

EMG and nerve conduction studies may be used when underlying neuropathy is a possible cause of symptoms of RLS. Upper airway endoscopy can be used in patients with OSA to determine the location of obstruction and guide possible intervention. Pulmonary function tests can be used when an underlying respiratory disorder is suspected in patients with sleep-related breathing disorders. An EKG or echocardiogram is needed when underlying ischemic heart disease or congestive heart failure is suspected, such as in patients with central sleep apnea.

SUMMARY

This article outlines the approach to a patient presenting with excessive sleepiness. The evaluation begins with a careful clinical assessment that includes a detailed sleep history, medical, psychiatric, medications, and social and family history. Physical examination should include a general medical examination, as well as an examination of the upper airway and a neurologic examination. A sleep log can often be very helpful. The patient's history and physical examination will often reveal the suspected cause of daytime sleepiness. Appropriate objective testing with a polysomnogram and possibly an MSLT will help confirm the diagnosis and direct the appropriate treatment plan.

REFERENCES

1. ICSD-3. International classification of sleep disorders. 3rd edition. Chicago: American Academy of Sleep Medicine; 2014.
2. Neu D, Linkowski P, le Bon O. Clinical complaints of daytime sleepiness and fatigue: how to distinguish and treat them, especially when they become 'excessive' or 'chronic'? Acta Neurol Belg 2010; 110(1):15–25.
3. Chaudhuri KR. Nocturnal symptom complex in PD and its management. Neurology 2003;61(6 Suppl 3):S17–23.
4. Chervin RD. Sleepiness, fatigue, tiredness, and lack of energy in obstructive sleep apnea. Chest 2000;118(2):372–9.
5. Gradisar M, Wolfson AR, Harvey AG, et al. The sleep and technology use of Americans: findings from the National Sleep Foundation's 2011 Sleep in America poll. J Clin Sleep Med 2013;9(12):1291–9.
6. Thorpy M. Current concepts in the etiology, diagnosis and treatment of narcolepsy. Sleep Med 2001;2(1):5–17.
7. Broughton R, Ghanem Q, Hishikawa Y, et al. Life effects of narcolepsy in 180 patients from North America, Asia and Europe compared to matched controls. Can J Neurol Sci 1981;8(4):299–304.
8. Stepanski E, Lamphere J, Badia P, et al. Sleep fragmentation and daytime sleepiness. Sleep 1984; 7(1):18–26.
9. McKenna JT, Tartar JL, Ward CP, et al. Sleep fragmentation elevates behavioral, electrographic and neurochemical measures of sleepiness. Neuroscience 2007;146(4):1462–73.
10. Oksenberg A, Arons E, Nasser K, et al. Severe obstructive sleep apnea: sleepy versus non sleepy patients. Laryngoscope 2010;120(3):643–8.
11. Frenette E, Kushida CA. Primary hypersomnias of central origin. Semin Neurol 2009;29(4):354–67.
12. Bove A, Culebras A, Moore JT, et al. Relationship between sleep spindles and hypersomnia. Sleep 1994;17(5):449–55.
13. Sforza E, Gaudreau H, Petit D, et al. Homeostatic sleep regulation in patients with idiopathic hypersomnia. Clin Neurophysiol 2000;111(2): 277–82.
14. Nishino S, Kanbayashi T. Symptomatic narcolepsy, cataplexy and hypersomnia, and their implications in the hypothalamic hypocretin/orexin system. Sleep Med Rev 2005;9(4):269–310.
15. Swanson LM, Arned JT, Rosekind MR, et al. Sleep disorders and work performance: findings from the 2008 National Sleep Foundation Sleep in America poll. J Sleep Res 2011;20(3):487–94.
16. Enright P, Newman A, Wahl P, et al. Prevalence and correlates of snoring and observes apneas in 5,201 older adults. Sleep 1996;19:531–8.

17. Whitney C, Enright P, Newman A, et al. Correlates of daytime sleepiness in 4578 elderly persons: the Cardiovascular Health Study. Sleep 1998;21: 27–36.

18. Ohayon M. Epidemiology of excessive sleepiness. In: Thorpy M, Billiard M, editors. Sleepiness causes, consequences and treatment. New York: Cambridge University Press; 2011. p. 3–13.

19. Merino-Andreu M, Arnulf I, Konofal E, et al. Unawareness of naps in Parkinson disease and in disorders with excessive daytime sleepiness. Neurology 2003;60(9):1553–4.

20. Sleep-related breathing disorders in adults: recommendations for syndrome definition and measurement techniques in clinical research. The Report of an American Academy of Sleep Medicine Task Force. Sleep 1999;22(5):667–89.

21. Powell N, Schechtman K, Riley R, et al. Sleepy driver near-misses may predict accident risks. Sleep 2007;30(3):331–42.

22. Takegami M, Hayashino Y, Chin K, et al. Simple four-variable screening tool for identification of patients with sleep-disordered breathing. Sleep 2009; 32(7):939–48.

23. Tuomilehto H, Seppä J, Uusitupa M. Obesity and obstructive sleep apnea–clinical significance of weight loss. Sleep Med Rev 2013;17(5):321–9.

24. Young T, Peppard P, Gottlieb D. The epidemiology of obstructive sleep apnea: a population health perspective. Am J Respir Crit Care Med 2002; 165:1217–39.

25. Sharpless BA, Barber JP. Lifetime prevalence rates of sleep paralysis: a systematic review. Sleep Med Rev 2011;15(5):311–5.

26. Ohayon MM, Priest RG, Caulet M, et al. Hypnagogic and hypnopompic hallucinations: pathological phenomena? Br J Psychiatry 1996;169(4):459–67.

27. Wong I, Smith P, Mustard C, et al. For better or worse? Changing shift schedules and the risk of work injury among men and women. Scand J Work Environ Health 2014;40(6):621–30.

28. Fung C, Martin J, Dzierzewski J, et al. Prevalence and symptoms of occult sleep disordered breathing among older veterans with insomnia. J Clin Sleep Med 2013;9(11):1173–8.

29. Wang Y, Li C, Feng L, et al. Prevalence of hypertension and circadian blood pressure variations in patients with obstructive sleep apnoea-hypopnoea syndrome. J Int Med Res 2014;42(3): 773–80.

30. Herrscher TE, Akre H, Overland B, et al. High prevalence of sleep apnea in heart failure outpatients: even in patients with preserved systolic function. J Card Fail 2011;17:420–5.

31. Levy P, Ryan S, Oldenburg O, et al. Sleep apnoea and the heart. Eur Respir Rev 2013;22(129): 333–52.

32. Bradley TD, Floras JS. Obstructive sleep apnoea and its cardiovascular consequences. Lancet 2009;373(9657):82–93.

33. Dumitrascu R, Tiede H, Eckermann J, et al. Sleep apnea in precapillary pulmonary hypertension. Sleep Med 2013;14:247–51.

34. Reichmuth KJ, Austin D, Skatrud JB, et al. Association of sleep apnea and type II diabetes: a population-based study. Am J Respir Crit Care Med 2005;172(12):1590–5.

35. Botros N, Concato J, Mohsenin V, et al. Obstructive sleep apnea as a risk factor for type 2 diabetes. Am J Med 2009;122(12):1122–7.

36. Gami AS, Hodge DO, Herges RM, et al. Obstructive sleep apnea, obesity, and the risk of incident atrial fibrillation. J Am Coll Cardiol 2007;49(5):565–71.

37. Garcia-Touchard A, Somers VK, Olson LJ, et al. Central sleep apnea: implications for congestive heart failure. Chest 2008;133:1495–504.

38. Redline S, Yenokyan G, Gottlieb DJ, et al. Obstructive sleep apnea-hypopnea and incident stroke: the sleep heart health study. Am J Respir Crit Care Med 2010;182:269–77.

39. Yaggi HK, Concato J, Kernan WN, et al. Obstructive sleep apnea as a risk factor for stroke and death. N Engl J Med 2005;353:2034–41.

40. Broadley SA, Jorgensen L, Cheek A, et al. Early investigation and treatment of obstructive sleep apnea after stroke. J Clin Neurosci 2007;14(4): 328–33.

41. Noradina AT, Hamidon BB, Roslan H, et al. Risk factors for developing sleep-disordered breathing in patients with recent ischaemic stroke. Singapore Med J 2006;47(5):392–9.

42. Lunn M, Craig T. Rhinitis and sleep. Sleep Med Rev 2011;15(5):293–9.

43. Sardana N, Craig TJ. Congestion and sleep impairment in allergic rhinitis. Asian Pac J Allergy Immunol 2011;29(4):297–306.

44. Finan P, Goodin B, Smith M. The association of sleep and pain: an update and a path forward. J Pain 2013;14(12):1539–52.

45. Allen KD, Renner JB, Devellis B, et al. Osteoarthritis and sleep: the Johnston county osteoarthritis project. J Rheumatol 2008;35(6):1102–7.

46. Palermo TM, Kiska R. Subjective sleep disturbances in adolescents with chronic pain: relationship to daily functioning and quality of life. J Pain 2005;6(3):201–7.

47. Odegard S, Sand T, Engstrom M, et al. The long-term effect of insomnia on primary headaches: a prospective population-based cohort study (HUNT-2 and HUNT-3) headache. Headache 2011;51:570–80.

48. Mork PJ, Nilsen TI. Sleep problems and risk of fibromyalgia: longitudinal data on an adult female population in Norway. Arthritis Rheum 2012;64:281–4.

49. Misiolek M, Marek B, Namyslowski G, et al. Sleep apnea syndrome and snoring in patients with hypothyroidism with relation to overweight. J Physiol Pharmacol 2007;58(Suppl 1):77–85.

50. Chasens ER, Umlauf MG, Weaver TE. Sleepiness, physical activity, and functional outcomes in veterans with type 2 diabetes. Appl Nurs Res 2009;22(3): 176–82.

51. Saaresranta T, Irjala K, Aittokallio T, et al. Sleep quality, daytime sleepiness and fasting insulin levels in women with chronic obstructive pulmonary disease. Respir Med 2005;99(7):856–63.

52. Obermeyer WH, Benca RM. Effects of drugs on sleep. Neurol Clin 1996;14(4):827–40.

53. Morasco B, O'Hearn D, Turk D, et al. Associations between prescription opioid use and sleep impairment among veterans with chronic pain. Pain Med 2014;15(11):1902–10.

54. Cheatle MD, Webster LR. Opioid therapy and sleep disorders: risks and mitigation strategies. Pain Med 2015;16(Suppl 1):S22–6.

55. Wang D, Teichtahl H, Drummer O. Central sleep apnea in stable methadone maintenance treatment patients. Chest 2005;128(3):1348–56.

56. Sharkey K, Kurth M, Anderson B. Obstructive sleep apnea is more common than central sleep apnea in methadone maintenance patients with subjective sleep complaints. Drug Alcohol Depend 2010; 108(1–2):77–83.

57. Posternak MA, Zimmerman M. Symptoms of atypical depression. Psychiatry Res 2001;104(2):175–81.

58. Mitchell PB, Wilhelm K, Parker G, et al. The clinical features of bipolar depression: a comparison with matched major depressive disorder patients. J Clin Psychiatry 2001;62(3):212–6.

59. Vgontzas AN, Bixler EO, Kales A, et al. Differences in nocturnal and daytime sleep between primary and psychiatric hypersomnia: diagnostic and treatment implications. Psychosom Med 2000;62(2): 220–6.

60. Wichniak A, Wierzbicka A, Jernajczyk W. Sleep and antidepressant treatment. Curr Pharm Des 2012; 18(36):5802–17.

61. Waters F, Faulkner D, Naik N, et al. Effects of polypharmacy on sleep in psychiatric inpatients. Schizophr Res 2012;139(1–3):225–8.

62. Rishi MA, Shetty M, Wolff A, et al. Atypical antipsychotic medications are independently associated with severe obstructive sleep apnea. Clin Neuropharmacol 2010;33(3):109–13.

63. Youngstedt SD, Kline CE. Epidemiology of exercise and sleep. Sleep Biol Rhythms 2006;4(3): 215–21.

64. Drake C, Roehrs T, Shambroom J, et al. Caffeine effects on sleep taken 0, 3, or 6 hours before going to bed. J Clin Sleep Med 2013;9(11): 1195–2000.

65. Deleanu OC, Pocora D, Mihălcuţă S, et al. Influence of smoking on sleep and obstructive sleep apnea syndrome. Pneumologia 2016;65(1):28–35.

66. Balaguer C, Palou A, Alonso-Fernández A. Smoking and sleep disorders. Arch Bronconeumol 2009;45(9):449–58.

67. Thakkar MM, Sharma R, Sahota P. Alcohol disrupts sleep homeostasis. Alcohol 2015;49(4):299–310.

68. Ebrahim IO, Shapiro CM, Williams AJ, et al. Alcohol and sleep I: effects on normal sleep. Alcohol Clin Exp Res 2013;37(4):539–49.

69. Colrain IM, Turlington S, Baker FC. Impact of alcoholism on sleep architecture and EEG power spectra in men and women. Sleep 2009;32:1341–52.

70. Brower KJ, Perron BE. Sleep disturbance as a universal risk factor for relapse in addictions to psychoactive substances. Med Hypotheses 2010;74: 928–33.

71. Schierenbeck T, Riemann D, Berger M, et al. Effect of illicit recreational drugs upon sleep: cocaine, ecstasy and marijuana. Sleep Med Rev 2008;12(5): 381–9.

72. Tang J, Liao Y, He H, et al. Sleeping problems in Chinese illicit drug dependent subjects. BMC Psychiatry 2015;15:28.

73. Lowe AA, Fleetham JA, Adachi S, et al. Cephalometric and computed tomographic predictors of obstructive sleep apnea severity. Am J Orthod Dentofacial Orthop 1995;107(6):589–95.

74. Johns FR, Strollo PJ Jr, Buckley M, et al. The influence of craniofacial structure on obstructive sleep apnea in young adults. J Oral Maxillofac Surg 1998;56(5):596–602.

75. Lin WN, Lee LA, Wang CC, et al. Obstructive sleep apnea syndrome in an adolescent girl with hypertrophic lingual thyroid. Pediatr Pulmonol 2009; 44(1):93–5.

76. Barnes TW, Olsen KD, Morgenthaler TI. Obstructive lingual thyroid causing sleep apnea: a case report and review of the literature. Sleep Med 2004;5(6):605–7.

77. Mickelson SA, Lian T, Rosenthal L. Thyroid testing and thyroid hormone replacement in patients with sleep disordered breathing. Ear Nose Throat J 1999;78(10):768–71, 774-5.

78. Winkelman JW, Goldman H, Piscatelli N, et al. Are thyroid function tests necessary in patients with suspected sleep apnea? Sleep 1996;19(10):790–3.

79. Kryger MH, Otake K, Foerster J. Low body stores of iron and restless legs syndrome: a correctable cause of insomnia in adolescents and teenagers. Sleep 2002;3(2):127–32.

80. Kosky CA, Bonakis A, Yogendran A, et al. Urine toxicology in adults evaluated for a central hypersomnia and how the results modify the Physician's diagnosis. J Clin Sleep Med 2016;12(11): 1499–505.

81. Dzodzomenyo S, Stolfi A, Splaingard D, et al. Urine toxicology screen in multiple sleep latency test: the correlation of positive tetrahydrocannabinol, drug negative patients, and narcolepsy. J Clin Sleep Med 2015;11(2):93–9.

82. Berry RB, Gamaldo CE, Harding SM, et al. AASM Scoring Manual Version 2.2 Updates: new chapters for scoring infant sleep staging and home sleep apnea testing. J Clin Sleep Med 2015;11(11):1253–4.

83. Garg N, Rolle AJ, Lee TA, et al. Home-based diagnosis of obstructive sleep apnea in an urban population. J Clin Sleep Med 2014;10(8):879–85.

84. Dawson A, Loving RT, Gordon RM, et al. Type III home sleep testing versus pulse oximetry: is the respiratory disturbance index better than the oxygen desaturation index to predict the apnoea-hypopnoea index measured during laboratory polysomnography? BMJ Open 2015;5(6): e007956.

85. Tedeschi E, Carratù P, Damiani MF, et al. Home unattended portable monitoring and automatic CPAP titration in patients with high risk for moderate to severe obstructive sleep apnea. Respir Care 2013; 58(7):1178–83.

86. Aldrich M, Jahnke B. Diagnostic value of video-EEG polysomnography. Neurology 1991;41: 1060–6.

87. Littner M, Hirshkowitz M, Kramer M, et al. Practice parameters for using polysomnography to evaluate insomnia: an update. Sleep 2003;26(6):754–60.

88. Levine B, Roehrs T, Zorick F, et al. Daytime sleepiness in young adults. Sleep 1988;11(1): 39–46.

89. Johns MW. Sensitivity and specificity of the multiple latency test (MSLT), the maintenance of wakefulness test and the Epworth sleepiness scale: failure of the MSLT as a gold standard. J Sleep Res 2000; 9(1):5–11.

90. Bliwise DL, Carskadon MA, Seidel WF, et al. MSLT-defined sleepiness and neuropsychological test performance do not correlate in the elderly. Neurobiol Aging 1991;12(5):463–8.

91. Steinberg R, Schonberg C, Weess HG, et al. The validity of the multiple sleep latency test. J Sleep Res 1996;5(Suppl 1):220.

92. Hartse KM, Zorick F, Sicklesteel J, et al. Nap recordings in the diagnosis of daytime somnolence. J Sleep Res 1979;8:190.

93. Van den Hoed J, Kraemer H, Guilleminault C, et al. Disorders of excessive daytime somnolence: polygraphic and clinical data for 100 patients. Sleep 1981;4(1):23–37.

94. Carskadon MA, Dement WC, Mitler MM, et al. Guidelines for the multiple sleep latency test (MSLT): standard measure of sleepiness. Sleep 1986;9(4):519–24.

95. Roehrs T, Roth T. Multiple sleep latency test: technical aspects of normal values. J Clin Neuropsychol 1992;9:63–7.

96. Czeisler CA, Walsh JK, Roth T, et al. Modafinil for excessive sleepiness associated with shift-work sleep disorder. N Engl J Med 2005;353: 476–86.

97. Lim J, Dinges DF. Sleep deprivation and vigilant attention. Ann N Y Acad Sci 2008;1129:305–22.

98. Dubois B, Slachevsky A, Litvan I, et al. The FAB:a frontal assessment battery at bedside. Neurology 2000;55(11):1621–6.

99. Mazza S, Pepin JL, Deschaux C, et al. Analysis of error profiles occurring during the OSLER test: a sensitive means of detecting fluctuation in vigilance in patients with obstructive sleep apnea syndrome. Am J Respir Crit Care Med 2002;166(4): 474–8.

100. Priest B, Brichard C, Aubert G, et al. Microsleep during a simplified maintenance of wakefulness test. A validation study of the OSLER test. Am J Respir Crit Care Med 2001;163(7):1619–25.

101. Bassetti CL. Spectrum of narcolepsy. In: Baumann CR, Bassetti CL, Scammell TE, editors. Narcolepsy: pathophysiology, diagnosis, and treatment. New York: Springer Science+Business Media; 2011. p. 309–19.

102. Sturzenegger C, Bassetti CL. The clinical spectrum of narcolepsy with cataplexy: a reappraisal. J Sleep Res 2004;13(4):395–406.

Subjective and Objective Assessment of Hypersomnolence

Brian James Murray, MD, FRCPC, D,ABSM

KEYWORDS

- Sleepiness • Hypersomnia • Multiple sleep latency test • Maintenance of wakefulness test
- Epworth Sleepiness Scale • Subjective sleepiness • Objective sleepiness

KEY POINTS

- Subjective measures of sleepiness are prone to bias.
- Objective measures of sleepiness should be used where possible.
- The multiple sleep latency test (MSLT) is most appropriate for assessment of narcolepsy.
- The maintenance of wakefulness test (MWT) has better conceptual validity for safety assessments.
- Better tests are needed and under development.

INTRODUCTION

Sleep is important for general health. Lack of sleep and sleep disorders are associated with several psychological[1,2] and medical complications.[3–5] Impaired alertness can lead to accidents.[6] Recent studies have suggested that the financial impact of sleep loss is dramatic in society.[7] Sleepiness can be operationalized in terms of the inability to remain awake for various activities. Lack of sleep itself does not correlate with sleepiness[8] because genetic differences and underlying sleep disorders can affect propensity to sleepiness, and circadian factors[9] can significantly influence moment-to-moment alertness. Subjective report of daytime sleepiness is composed of several characteristic components, including perceived sleepiness and the tendency to fall asleep in passive and active situations.[10]

Appropriate selection of a subjective or objective scale for the assessment of sleepiness should take into account several factors. No test is perfect, but careful consideration of the goals of a tool can help identify techniques that may be able to address particular clinical needs.[11]

Considerations include whether a tool is for clinical or research purposes; whether a tool is for assessment of a trait, such as a diagnosis, or a state, such as current alertness; the practicality of an assessment; and implications of an assessment, such as the commonly queried clinical assessment of driving safety. Repeatability of the assessment, such as assessing circadian variations in alertness or assessing the response to therapies over time, is also a consideration. This article outlines some of the most common instruments and suggests situations where particular tools may be most appropriate.

Ontogeny

Sleep needs change over the course of a life span. The National Sleep Foundation recently published guidelines for suggested sleep times across various age ranges. School-aged children were suggested as requiring 9 hours to 11 hours and young adults 7 hours to 9 hours.[12] Because most of the assessment tools have been developed for adults, special consideration for groups such as children need to be made.

Disclosures: Dr B.J. Murray has written for UpToDate.
Neurology and Sleep Medicine, Sunnybrook Health Sciences Centre, University of Toronto, Room M1-600, 2075 Bayview Avenue, Toronto, Ontario M4N 3M5, Canada
E-mail address: brian.murray@sunnybrook.ca

Sleep Med Clin 12 (2017) 313–322
http://dx.doi.org/10.1016/j.jsmc.2017.03.007
1556-407X/17/© 2017 Elsevier Inc. All rights reserved.

sleep.theclinics.com

Shift Work

Separate consideration should also be made for patients who adopt atypical sleep patterns, such as sleep during the light period. Patients who engage in shift work have sleepiness for a variety of reasons. There are natural periods of vulnerability[13] throughout the day and participants with shift work often become progressively sleep deprived. One problem in interpreting sleepiness in this context is that studies routinely used for the assessment of sleepiness, such as the MSLT, are not standardized at alternate times of day.

PATIENT EVALUATION OVERVIEW

The clinical assessment of patients often starts with subjective assessments. Objective neurophysiologic assessments are subsequently arranged if appropriate.

SUBJECTIVE ASSESSMENT

To understand the clinical presentation of patients with sleepiness, it is important to understand the motivation for the visit. Sometimes sleepiness is identified as a separate issue in the investigation of a clinical problem, such as investigation for obstructive sleep apnea. Frequently in hypersomnia there is a concern about safety. Rarely there are concerns about drug-seeking behaviors in patients looking for stimulant therapy. It is important to interview others familiar with a patient. Family and friends may be more likely to report excessive daytime sleepiness than the patient. Some patients may lack insight into the degree of their sleepiness and under-report the problem. It is not uncommon for patients with daytime sleepiness to deny difficulties but family members bring them to medical attention because they may fall asleep in traffic, for example. In other situations, patients may fall asleep in inappropriate social situations. In children, poor school performance is sometimes a trigger for assessment.

Sleep Log

Patients should keep track of bedtimes and rise times on a calendar and track degree of sleepiness. This can lead to insights, such as individuals reporting excessive sleepiness throughout the week suddenly becoming less sleepy on the weekend, where sleep extended due to increased sleep opportunity might be seen.

Interpretation of sleepiness at any given time point should also consider the effects of medication administration as well as common substances, such as caffeine, which are known to alter alertness.[14]

Epworth Sleepiness Scale

The Epworth Sleepiness Scale (ESS) is a commonly administered scale where subjects indicate how likely they would be to fall asleep or doze in 8 common situations, such as watching television.[15] This scale asks a patient to reflect over a period of time rather than assessing sleepiness at any specific point in time and yields a score from 0 to 24 (least–highest likelihood of falling asleep). This is, therefore, more of a trait measure, although it can clearly be influenced by treatments. One American study looked at a group of persons renewing their driver's licenses in the general population and found a mean score of 7.5, with 26.2% of the populations having a score of 10 of higher, which has typically been used as a cutoff to identify sleepiness.[16] A German study of 9710 people noted 23% of the sample had a score greater than 10.[17] A systematic review of the ESS revealed that this instrument could be used for research group assessments but was not recommended for individual-level comparisons.[18] Although the total score is commonly used, some items are of clinical concern, such as falling asleep while sitting and talking to someone, presumably suggesting a significant degree of impairment.

Barcelona Sleepiness Index

Based on focus groups in patients with sleep-disordered breathing, a set of items was generated and assessed against objective measures, such as the Sustained Attention to Response Task (SART), MWT, and MSLT. Two items on this interviewer-administered scale, ranging from 0 to 6, produced the highest predictive value for the MWT and were sensitive to treatment changes with continuous positive airway pressure.[19] This is, therefore, a simple instrument that can be used for a common clinical problem but validation is required in English.

Observation and Interview Based Diurnal Sleepiness Inventory

The recently developed Observation and Interview Based Diurnal Sleepiness Inventory is a 3-item instrument tested in elderly subjects that was able to quickly screen for daytime sleepiness among elderly patients with obstructive sleep apnea but has so far only been assessed against another subjective scale—the ESS.[20] Again this is more of a trait measure.

Stanford Sleepiness Scale

Other scales are more focused on clinical state. The Stanford Sleepiness Scale (SSS) addresses sleepiness at any given moment in time and ranges over 7 descriptions, from "feeling active, vital, alert, wide awake" to "almost in reverie, cannot stay awake, sleep onset appears imminent." The scale was developed in 5 students over the course of several days and after sleep deprivation[21] but has been extensively used. Psychometric properties of this scale have suggested that descriptors at each level of the scale are not equivalent and that the test does not assess a unidimensional construct. Furthermore, studies comparing the SSS to MSLT and pupillographic assessment of sleepiness suggest that the SSS does not correlate well with physiologic measures of sleepiness.[22]

Karolinska Sleepiness Scale

The Karolinska Sleepiness Scale is a 9-point scale ranging from "extremely alert" to "extremely sleepy, fighting sleep" based on subjective assessment of drowsiness at a given point in time.[23] The scale has been noted to correlate with physiologic variables, such as electroencephalography (EEG) and the psychomotor vigilance task, suggesting high validity at specific time points.[24] Some investigators have adapted this scale to assess longer more trait-like periods of time, such as shift work.[25]

Sleepiness-Wakefulness Inability and Fatigue Test

Another scale called the Sleepiness-Wakefulness Inability and Fatigue Test[26] has been developed to focus less on the tendency to fall asleep and more on the inability to maintain wakefulness and capture associated tiredness. This 12-item scale was assessed in several hundred patients with a variety of sleep disorders, including sleep apnea specifically, was reliable and valid, and had a better discriminant ability than the ESS with factors specific to driving.

Time of Day Sleepiness Scale

Because there are variations in the circadian tendency to be alert, this new scale, The Time of Day Sleepiness Scale, addresses sleepiness in light of circadian variation.[27] The scale takes approximately 5 minutes to complete and assesses sleepiness across morning, afternoon, and evening. There is a need to have further normative data across other times of day, particularly for shift workers.

Pittsburgh Sleep Quality Index

Many general psychiatric or psychological scales, such as the Profile of Mood States,[28] have subscales components that reflect fatigue or sleepiness and could be used if already collected but

were not specifically designed with sleepiness as a focus. The Pittsburgh Sleep Quality Index is commonly used for self-reported general sleep characteristics and reflects a broader set of sleep pathologies aside from alertness, such as insomnia.[29] Nonetheless, a component of the scale, daytime dysfunction, can reflect daytime alertness and may correlate with alertness measures.

Leeds Sleep Evaluation Questionnaire

Similarly, the Leeds Sleep Evaluation Questionnaire is a 10-item linear analog scale based on questions across several domains of sleep. Three questions can be extracted from this tool reflect alertness[30] and have been geared toward the assessment of psychoactive drug responses.[31] This scale may be helpful for assessing treatment responses within an individual and has been widely used in pharmacologic studies.

Pediatric Scales

Several pediatric scales have been developed given the specific needs of this population. The ESS is most directed toward adults and, therefore, children may not commonly experience all 8 clinical situations. An extensive evidence-based review of pediatric sleep measures has recently been published.[32] One scale that focused on alertness was well- established with respect to evidence base—the Pediatric Daytime Sleepiness Scale. This is an 8-item self-report scale developed for 11 to 15 years olds that assesses sleepiness, such as how often individuals fall asleep or get drowsy during classes, and has excellent psychometric properties.[33] Importantly, the scale also correlates with academic performance. Other scales include a modified ESS with pediatric appropriate clinical scenarios[34] and the Cleveland Adolescent Sleepiness Questionnaire, which is a 16-item scale developed for ages 11 years to 17 years[35] and includes items, such as "I feel sleepy when I ride in a bus to a school event like a field trip or sports game."

Problems with Subjective Measures

Patients with subjective sleepiness may not be aware of the degree of their impairment. There can be a disconnect between subjective ratings of sleepiness, such as the ESS, and objective measures, such as the MSLT.[36] Some participants may be prone to underestimate their sleepiness to preserve driving privileges. Others may be prone to exaggerate their symptoms if they are seeking stimulant medications. As such, interpretation of subjective scales is probably best done when a clinician can gauge the reliability of the participant and the participant's insight into the problem. Tracking changes on subjective scales may be more useful than using absolute values for establishing a diagnosis, for example. Some individuals may be nonverbal or unable to participate in daily activities that are assessed in many subjective scales. There may also be language or cultural differences in the scales necessitating that validation be done for specific patient populations. Given some of these concerns, objective scales are frequently essential.

OBJECTIVE MEASURES
Clinical Observation

Clinical impression of sleepiness might be evident from the initial presentation. Observing patients in a waiting room can sometimes identify napping during daytime hours. Patients may have yawning or eyelid drooping or even manifest slow roving eye movements during an interview. Sleepiness can be observed in meetings with a drop in neck muscle tone and quick postural correction.

Clinical Neurophysiology

Often, when sleepiness is of medical concern, objective information should be collected in the form of several standardized neurophysiologic tests. Some recent developments in objective assessment of alertness have been outlined.[37] Polysomnography does not provide for measurement of sleepiness, but limited information may be available in an overnight study. For example, prolonged sleep-onset latency is not typically expected in a patient with narcolepsy. Perhaps the most important feature of polysomnography is ensuring that underlying sleep disorders are not present, such as obstructive sleep apnea. Polysomnography is also required prior to the

MSLT to ensure adequate sleep time has been obtained.

Practice parameters have been published for the use of the MSLT and MWT.[38] The tests are widely used but have problems in interpretation outside the laboratory setting.[39,40] Standardization of the tests and appropriate use help in their interpretation but some investigators have noted that normative values remain limited, particularly for the MWT, and that these tests are limited in terms of their implications in the real world.[41] Although these tests are not perfect, they are the best standardized tests currently available and provide useful objective information, particularly when there is a clear clinical question.[42] All clinical decisions require an appropriate clinical context and these tests should not be seen as absolute without appropriate interpretation. The selection of the appropriate test depends on several factors. See **Table 1** for some considerations in test selection.

Multiple Sleep Latency Test

The MSLT is predominantly a test for narcolepsy. Patients have 4 to 5 nap opportunities of 20 minutes' duration spaced 2 hours apart throughout the day, for example 09:00, 11:00, 13:00, 15:00, and 17:00. A fifth nap is often added if there is 1 sleep-onset rapid eye movement (REM) period (SOREMP) in the first 4 naps to help establish a neurophysiologic diagnosis of narcolepsy. The study is done in darkness in a comfortable bed at an acceptable temperature. Patients are instructed to try to fall asleep. If patients fall asleep, they are allowed to sleep for further 15 minutes to see if they enter REM sleep. Sleep latency on this test can suggest a degree of sleep propensity, for example, the ability to willingly initiate asleep. If a patient achieves REM sleep on 2 of the naps or at

Table 1
Considerations in neurophysiological assessment of sleepiness

	Multiple Sleep Latency Test	Maintenance of Wakefulness Test
General goal of the test	Assesses the ability to fall asleep	Assesses the ability to remain awake
Preceding polysomnography	Required	Not required
Narcolepsy diagnosis	Useful in the diagnosis of narcolepsy	
Assessment of safety		Better conceptual validity
Stimulant-seeking behaviors	Less prone to exaggerating abnormalities—although toxicology screen should be obtained	Highly prone to motivation and may be problematic in interpretation
Medications	Formally interpreted off medications	Can be used to assess response to alerting medications

least 1 nap and falls into REM early on the preceding night's polysomnography, this study can also help support a diagnosis of narcolepsy. Patients are supposed to remain awake between naps but sleepy patients commonly do not, although this does not seem to significantly affect the eventual diagnosis.[43]

Patients must have routine sleep in the week prior to the recording, and the preceding night's polysomnogram ensures that at least 6 hours of good-quality sleep has been recorded for appropriate interpretation. The polysomnogram ensures that certain common intrinsic sleep disorders, such as sleep apnea, are not contributing to daytime sleepiness. Psychoactive medications should be held for several weeks prior to the study. This can be problematic in some participants with, for example, significant psychiatric conditions.

Normative values have been published.[44,45] Subtle differences in test interpretation can provide different interpretations. For example, sleep onset, as defined by the first epoch of stage N1, can suggest diagnostic differences in different disorders compared with a definition of sleep onset constituting consecutive epochs of N1 or another stage of sleep.[46]

It is problematic to use the MSLT in the general population without some pretest probability of an abnormality. One study looked at the prevalence and correlates of SOREMPs in a large community-based sleep group.[47] The study looked at 556 predominantly white participants and noted that there was sleep latency less than 8 minutes and 2 or more SOREMPs in approximately 6% of men and 1% of women. In men, SOREMPs were increased in shift workers and individuals with suggestions of sleep restriction. Another study looking at cross-sectional and longitudinal studies of sleep in the general community noted, in a sample of 1725 polysomnography/MSLT participants, including approximately half who had repeated the test, that the prevalence of a mean sleep latency less than 8 minutes was 22%. A sleep latency less than 8 minutes and 2 or more SOREMPs was noted in 3.4% of the population. The study also noted that the value of the MSLT was significantly altered by shift work and sleep deprivation.[48]

In the context of the repeated MSLTs, there can be variations, particularly with respect to sleepiness.[43] One recent study commented on problems in the test–retest reliability of the MSLT in patients with narcolepsy without cataplexy and idiopathic hypersomnia. Of 36 individuals tested approximately 4 years apart, the mean sleep latency on the first and second tests were 5.5 minutes and 7.3 minutes, respectively, with no significant correlation. Change in diagnosis occurred in 53% of patients, predominantly via change in the mean sleep latency. As such, the investigators concluded the MSLT demonstrates poor test-retest reliability for diagnostic purposes in a clinical population of patients with central nervous system hypersomnia.[49] The diagnosis of narcolepsy can also be aided by a clinical history of cataplexy, HLA typing, or low cerebrospinal fluid orexin/hypocretin levels. Again, no one sleep tool should be used independent of the clinical interpretation.

Practice parameters for use of the MSLT in children have recently been published.[50] This publication notes concerns about the technical capacity for the study and problems with limited age-adjusted normative values. Diagnostic criteria are not available for patients under age 6.[51] It was also noted that patients in early pubertal stages or earlier were less likely to fall asleep than older adolescents. Some clinicians have consequently used 30-minute nap opportunities to have a higher chance of detecting SOREMPs but this has not been validated in large samples. There are also concerns in children with napping behaviors because it is hard to standardize and interpret in the context of the MSLT where adults are typically asked to remain awake between tests. Toxicology screens are required even in children, given that they may have habits unknown to their parents or there may be features of Munchausen syndrome by proxy.

Although the MSLT and MWT are frequently used for the assessment of driving safety, there is a paucity of evidence linking the predictive abilities of these tests. One recent important study looked at MSLT values and 10-year crash rate with records from a Department of Motor Vehicles.[52] In this study of 618 participants who were recruited using random digit dialing, 3 MSLT groups were identified: excessively sleepy, moderately sleepy, and alert. The accident rates for the groups were 59.4%, 52.5%, and 47.3%, respectively. The investigators concluded that the MSLT was predictive of an increased risk of documented automotive crashes. Perhaps this effect would have even been more significant had they assessed the MWT.

Maintenance of Wakefulness Test

The MWT has more conceptual validity for assessing the ability to resist sleep in the day. This could be helpful for patients where safety is a concern.

In this test, patients have 20-minute to 40-minute sessions that are spread 2 hours apart throughout the day for typically 4 sessions, for example, 09:00, 11:00, 13:00, and 15:00. Patients sit in a comfortable chair in a dimly lit room of comfortable temperature and attempt to maintain alertness. Participants are specifically instructed to stay awake as long as possible. They are not allowed to vocalize or make excessive movements. Patients can demonstrate abnormalities on the MWT in a variety of sleep conditions, such as the upper airway resistance syndrome.[53] Normative values have been published[45,54] although there is some controversy about what constitutes a normal MWT. Some experts have noted that with appropriate motivation, patients remain awake longer and clinicians consider no sleep on this test or a value of 40 minutes to be normal.

The 40-minute test is recommended over shorter duration assessments, because this is more sensitive for picking up sleepiness. In 1 study of patients using the MWT for driving safety, participants were instructed that if they failed the test, their driver's license would be revoked.[55] In 39 patients with severe obstructive sleep apnea with a respiratory disturbance index over 40, 48.7% fell asleep. On a 20-minute test, only 7% of patients with severe sleep apnea fell asleep once. The investigators concluded that the MWT for 40 minutes' duration was superior to the 20-minute test for detecting difficulties in remaining alert. One study noted differences in a driving simulator when drivers had a mean sleep latency under 34 minutes,[56] and other studies have noted differences in driving abilities based on level of impairment in several conditions.[57]

Deeper analysis of physiologic data may provide more information than is seen on visual inspection. For example, digital signal interpretation with Fourier analysis is a simple consideration to extract hidden information in an EEG that may be a better marker of sleepiness.[58] Again, definition of sleep onset may be a factor in conditions where there is instability of sleep onset.

Ambulatory Electroencephalogram

Devices that track EEG over prolonged periods of time can also help detect lapses in attention. Consumer purchasable portable EEG headbands are available. Automated computerized scoring of large volumes of data helps facilitate monitoring over prolonged periods.

Actigraphy

There has been rapid development in the use of consumer technologies to track sleep-wake behaviors. Common devices for assessing fitness include activity trackers, which can suggest sleep in the context of absence of movement. Although this relation is not perfect, it can estimate sleep and periods of inactivity in the day that may also reflect a tendency toward sleepiness. Current protocols for assessment of actigraphy in daytime napping are limited,[59] but the tool can be helpful for unobtrusively tracking sleep-wake activity over long periods of time.

Psychomotor Vigilance Test

Several devices track performance metrics to help infer inattention or drowsiness. One commercially available device for assessing state alertness is the psychomotor vigilance task.[60] This paradigm measures reaction time typically over the course of 10 minutes with 2-second to 10-second variable stimulus presentation rates. The reaction time to these signals is recorded and this reaction time can correlate with sleepiness. Perhaps more importantly, lapses are identified that are periods of nonresponse to the target stimulus. A nonresponse of greater than 500 milliseconds has traditionally been reported in the literature, although this is somewhat arbitrary. The lack of response to the stimulus likely represents the first movement of the sleep switch from alert to asleep and implicates a change in brain activation patterns.[61] This device can be used in clinical settings easily, requires little training, and has virtually no learning curve. As such, the test can be repeated multiple times throughout the day for longer duration assessments. The test is sensitive to sleep deprivation as well as circadian variations in alertness.

Oxford Sleep Resistance Test

The Oxford Sleep Resistance Test is another commercially available device available based on a task where subjects are asked to press a switch in response to a light.[62] This is a behavioral variant of the MWT but has the advantage of simplified administration compared with the MWT in that EEG is not required. Sleep latencies on this tool correlate well with the MWT.[63] This assessment has sensitivity of 85% and specificity of 94% in the detection of 3 seconds of sleep.[64] The test was also comparable to a shorter reaction time task presented by visual or auditory means and demonstrated an improvement with treatment of sleep apnea.[65]

Sustained Attention to Response Task

Another variation on this theme is the simple neuropsychological test, the SART, which involves inhibiting response to 1/9 of 225 target stimuli. The test has been assessed in conjunction with the MSLT in patients with narcolepsy and controls and was noted to have good sensitivity and specificity for predicting a mean sleep latency of 5 minutes[66] but did not correlate with the MSLT or

ESS. The test has been used to assess treatment responses in pharmacologic treatment of narcolepsy.[67] The task is short and easy to administer, which provides advantages over conventional neurophysiologic assessments and has been tested in a variety of patient groups.[68]

Eyelid Movement

One of the most common features of drowsiness is eyelid closure. Eyelid closure can be detected with new technologies given advances in computing power and new devices. A variety of eyelid closure characteristics, such as the velocity of closure and duration of eye closure, can be analyzed to assess real-time drowsiness.[69] One recent study used an infrared modified glasses frame to track sleepiness in nurses doing shift work and was able to demonstrate inattention in a naturalistic setting— the drive home from work.[70]

Eye Movements

Roving eye movements are also a feature of sleepiness and can be monitored with ambulatory recordings to assess momentary sleepiness. One study of 8 subjects looked at continuous EEG and electrooculogram recordings to detect slow eye movements; these were most readily detected when subjects reported significant sleepiness.[23]

Pupillography

Another eye tool to track sleepiness is pupillography—measurements of pupil size and variability in size changes. These are best detected in the dark where there is maximal pupillary dilation. Pupillary size oscillations have been used to track level of arousal in medical personnel, although this requires a dark room and specialized equipment currently.[71] One study compared pupillometric studies to the MSLT and noted correlation in some measures but pointed out concerns that need to be addressed before using this as a screening tool.[72]

Driving Simulators

Several driving simulators have been tested as an operationalization of sleepiness and with some conceptual validity for interpretation of a common clinical problem.[73] Unfortunately, there is no standard device because they are often developed for a variety of other driving safety considerations, and they may be large and expensive for better lifelike assessments. Medications may contribute to sleepiness and with deviation of road position is a likely marker for lapses in attention with incipient sleep.[74] Monotonous driving conditions showed correlations with the MSLT and subjective sleepiness as assessed by the SSS and a visual analog scale in normal individuals after sleep deprivation.[75]

FUTURE DIRECTIONS

Again, the increase in wearable technologies should help identify better tools to track variations in alertness. Eye movement tracking characteristics are of interest given the prominence of ptosis and slow-moving eye movements with drowsiness. Measures of gait stability have been used to assess alertness.[76] Auditory evoked potentials have been found to change under conditions of sleepiness[77] and could even be incorporated in devices that record EEG. A few studies have noted changes in autonomic function, such as heart rate variability monitoring that correlated with lapses on the psychomotor vigilance task in normal persons undergoing sleep deprivation conditions,[78,79] suggesting that even less conspicuous recording devices, such as cardiac monitors, could track information over time and eventually even provide real-time feedback to individuals about their safety.

SUMMARY

Given the clinical significance of sleepiness, having ways to track sleepiness is important for clinicians and patients. Subjective scales have some advantages in terms of ease of administration and expense but are prone to bias and have to be interpreted with this potential confound. The use of subjective scales can be helpful when a patient has insight into the degree of the problem and is reporting openly. When there are concerns about reliability of reporting and when there are significant implications of abnormal test results, a reliance on objective measures may be needed. Although the MSLT and MWT have problems, they continue to be used as the best standardized tests to date. Refinements of objective scales are required. Many reaction time–type tasks provide objective information and are easy to use. Further standardization of these tests in clinical scenarios is warranted. Newer devices will provide accurate real world measurement of alertness and may even be adapted to provide real-time feedback. Combinations of physiologic measures may also provide further information.[80] Often, subjective scales and objective scales should be used together in a multicomponent assessment of sleepiness.[81]

REFERENCES

1. Winokur A. The relationship between sleep disturbances and psychiatric disorders: introduction and overview. Psychiatr Clin North Am 2015;38(4):603–14.

2. Pilcher JJ, Huffcutt AI. Effects of sleep deprivation on performance: a meta-analysis. Sleep 1996; 19(4):318–26.

3. Badran M, Yassin BA, Fox N, et al. Epidemiology of sleep disturbances and cardiovascular consequences. Can J Cardiol 2015;31(7):873–9.

4. Newman AB, Spiekerman CF, Enright P, et al. Daytime sleepiness predicts mortality and cardiovascular disease in older adults. The Cardiovascular Health Study Research Group. J Am Geriatr Soc 2000;48(2):115–23.

5. Al Lawati NM, Patel SR, Ayas NT. Epidemiology, risk factors, and consequences of obstructive sleep apnea and short sleep duration. Prog Cardiovasc Dis 2009;51(4):285–93.

6. American Academy of Sleep Medicine Board of Directors, Watson NF, Morgenthaler T, et al. Confronting drowsy driving: the American Academy of sleep medicine perspective. J Clin Sleep Med 2015;11(11):1335–6.

7. Hafner M, Stepanek M, Taylor J, et al. Why sleep matters — the economic costs of insufficient sleep: a cross-country comparative analysis. Santa Monica (CA): RAND Corporation; 2016.

8. Czeisler CA. Impact of sleepiness and sleep deficiency on public health–utility of biomarkers. J Clin Sleep Med 2011;7(5 Suppl):S6–8.

9. Mitler MM, Miller JC. Methods of testing for sleepiness [corrected]. Behav Med 1996;21(4):171–83.

10. Kim H, Young T. Subjective daytime sleepiness: dimensions and correlates in the general population. Sleep 2005;28(5):625–34.

11. Carskadon MA. Evaluation of excessive daytime sleepiness. Neurophysiol Clin 1993;23(1):91–100.

12. Watson NF, Badr MS, Belenky G, et al. Recommended amount of sleep for a healthy adult: a joint consensus statement of the American Academy of sleep medicine and sleep research society. Sleep 2015;38(6):843–4.

13. Akerstedt T, Wright KP Jr. Sleep loss and fatigue in shift work and shift work disorder. Sleep Med Clin 2009;4(2):257–71.

14. Roehrs T, Roth T. Caffeine: sleep and daytime sleepiness. Sleep Med Rev 2008;12(2):153–62.

15. Johns MW. A new method for measuring daytime sleepiness: the Epworth sleepiness scale. Sleep 1991;14(6):540–5.

16. Benbadis SR, Perry MC, Sundstad LS, et al. Prevalence of daytime sleepiness in a population of drivers. Neurology 1999;52(1):209–10.

17. Sander C, Hegerl U, Wirkner K, et al. Normative values of the Epworth Sleepiness Scale (ESS), derived from a large German sample. Sleep Breath 2016;20(4):1337–45.

18. Kendzerska TB, Smith PM, Brignardello-Petersen R, et al. Evaluation of the measurement properties of the Epworth sleepiness scale: a systematic review. Sleep Med Rev 2014;18(4):321–31.

19. Guaita M, Salamero M, Vilaseca I, et al. The barcelona sleepiness Index: a new instrument to assess excessive daytime sleepiness in sleep disordered breathing. J Clin Sleep Med 2015;11(11):1289–98.

20. Onen F, Lalanne C, Pak VM, et al. A three-item instrument for measuring daytime sleepiness: the observation and interview based diurnal sleepiness inventory (ODSI). J Clin Sleep Med 2016;12(4):505–12.

21. Hoddes E, Zarcone V, Smythe H, et al. Quantification of sleepiness: a new approach. Psychophysiology 1973;10(4):431–6.

22. Danker-Hopfe H, Kraemer S, Dorn H, et al. Time-of-day variations in different measures of sleepiness (MSLT, pupillography, and SSS) and their interrelations. Psychophysiology 2001;38(5):828–35.

23. Akerstedt T, Gillberg M. Subjective and objective sleepiness in the active individual. Int J Neurosci 1990;52(1–2):29–37.

24. Kaida K, Takahashi M, Akerstedt T, et al. Validation of the Karolinska sleepiness scale against performance and EEG variables. Clin Neurophysiol 2006; 117(7):1574–81.

25. Geiger Brown J, Wieroney M, Blair L, et al. Measuring subjective sleepiness at work in hospital nurses: validation of a modified delivery format of the Karolinska Sleepiness Scale. Sleep Breath 2014;18(4):731–9.

26. Sangal RB. Evaluating sleepiness-related daytime function by querying wakefulness inability and fatigue: sleepiness-Wakefulness Inability and Fatigue Test (SWIFT). J Clin Sleep Med 2012;8(6):701–11.

27. Dolan DC, Taylor DJ, Okonkwo R, et al. The Time of Day Sleepiness Scale to assess differential levels of sleepiness across the day. J Psychosom Res 2009; 67(2):127–33.

28. McNair DM, Lorr M, Droppelman LF. Manual for the profile of mood states. San Diego (CA): Educational and Industrial Testing Service; 1971. p. 27.

29. Buysse DJ, Reynolds CF 3rd, Monk TH, et al. The Pittsburgh Sleep Quality Index: a new instrument for psychiatric practice and research. Psychiatry Res 1989;28(2):193–213.

30. Parrott AC, Hindmarch I. Factor analysis of a sleep evaluation questionnaire. Psychol Med 1978;8(2): 325–9.

31. Zisapel N, Laudon M. Subjective assessment of the effects of CNS-active drugs on sleep by the Leeds sleep evaluation questionnaire: a review. Hum Psychopharmacol 2003;18(1):1–20.

32. Lewandowski AS, Toliver-Sokol M, Palermo TM. Evidence-based review of subjective pediatric sleep measures. J Pediatr Psychol 2011;36(7):780–93.

33. Drake C, Nickel C, Burduvali E, et al. The pediatric daytime sleepiness scale (PDSS): sleep habits and

school outcomes in middle-school children. Sleep 2003;26(4):455–8.

34. Melendres MC, Lutz JM, Rubin ED, et al. Daytime sleepiness and hyperactivity in children with suspected sleep-disordered breathing. Pediatrics 2004;114(3):768–75.

35. Spilsbury JC, Drotar D, Rosen CL, et al. The Cleveland adolescent sleepiness questionnaire: a new measure to assess excessive daytime sleepiness in adolescents. J Clin Sleep Med 2007;3(6): 603–12.

36. Benbadis SR, Mascha E, Perry MC, et al. Association between the Epworth sleepiness scale and the multiple sleep latency test in a clinical population. Ann Intern Med 1999;130(4 Pt 1):289–92.

37. Coelho FM, Narayansingh M, Murray BJ. Testing sleepiness and vigilance in the sleep laboratory. Curr Opin Pulm Med 2011;17(6):406–11.

38. Littner MR, Kushida C, Wise M, et al. Practice parameters for clinical use of the multiple sleep latency test and the maintenance of wakefulness test. Sleep 2005;28(1):113–21.

39. Lammers GJ, van Dijk JG. The multiple sleep latency test: a paradoxical test? Clin Neurol Neurosurg 1992;94(Suppl):S108–10.

40. Bonnet MH. ACNS clinical controversy: MSLT and MWT have limited clinical utility. J Clin Neurophysiol 2006;23(1):50–8.

41. Sullivan SS, Kushida CA. Multiple sleep latency test and maintenance of wakefulness test. Chest 2008; 134(4):854–61.

42. Wise MS. Objective measures of sleepiness and wakefulness: application to the real world? J Clin Neurophysiol 2006;23(1):39–49.

43. Kasravi N, Legault G, Jewell D, et al. Minimal impact of inadvertent sleep between naps on the MSLT and MWT. J Clin Neurophysiol 2007;24(4):363–5.

44. Roehrs T, Roth T. Multiple Sleep Latency Test: technical aspects and normal values. J Clin Neurophysiol 1992;9(1):63–7.

45. Arand D, Bonnet M, Hurwitz T, et al. The clinical use of the MSLT and MWT. Sleep 2005;28(1):123–44.

46. Pizza F, Vandi S, Detto S, et al. Different sleep onset criteria at the multiple sleep latency test (MSLT): an additional marker to differentiate central nervous system (CNS) hypersomnias. J Sleep Res 2011; 20(1 Pt 2):250–6.

47. Mignot E, Lin L, Finn L, et al. Correlates of sleep-onset REM periods during the multiple sleep latency test in community adults. Brain 2006;129(Pt 6): 1609–23.

48. Goldbart A, Peppard P, Finn L, et al. Narcolepsy and predictors of positive MSLTs in the Wisconsin sleep cohort. Sleep 2014;37(6):1043–51.

49. Trotti LM, Staab BA, Rye DB. Test-retest reliability of the multiple sleep latency test in narcolepsy without cataplexy and idiopathic hypersomnia. J Clin Sleep Med 2013;9(8):789–95.

50. Aurora RN, Lamm CI, Zak RS, et al. Practice parameters for the non-respiratory indications for polysomnography and multiple sleep latency testing for children. Sleep 2012;35(11):1467–73.

51. Nevsimalova S. The diagnosis and treatment of pediatric narcolepsy. Curr Neurol Neurosci Rep 2014; 14(8):469.

52. Drake C, Roehrs T, Breslau N, et al. The 10-year risk of verified motor vehicle crashes in relation to physiologic sleepiness. Sleep 2010;33(6):745–52.

53. Powers CR, Frey WC. Maintenance of wakefulness test in military personnel with upper airway resistance syndrome and mild to moderate obstructive sleep apnea. Sleep Breath 2009;13(3):253–8.

54. Doghramji K, Mitler MM, Sangal RB, et al. A normative study of the maintenance of wakefulness test (MWT). Electroencephalogr Clin Neurophysiol 1997;103(5): 554–62.

55. Arzi L, Shreter R, El-Ad B, et al. Forty- versus 20-minute trials of the maintenance of wakefulness test regimen for licensing of drivers. J Clin Sleep Med 2009;5(1):57–62.

56. Philip P, Sagaspe P, Taillard J, et al. Maintenance of Wakefulness Test, obstructive sleep apnea syndrome, and driving risk. Ann Neurol 2008;64(4):410–6.

57. Philip P, Chaufton C, Taillard J, et al. Maintenance of Wakefulness Test scores and driving performance in sleep disorder patients and controls. Int J Psychophysiol 2013;89(2):195–202.

58. Gast H, Schindler K, Rummel C, et al. EEG correlation and power during maintenance of wakefulness test after sleep-deprivation. Clin Neurophysiol 2011;122(10):2025–31.

59. Martin JL, Hakim AD. Wrist actigraphy. Chest 2011; 139(6):1514–27.

60. Dinges DF, Pack F, Williams K, et al. Cumulative sleepiness, mood disturbance, and psychomotor vigilance performance decrements during a week of sleep restricted to 4-5 hours per night. Sleep 1997;20(4):267–77.

61. Drummond SP, Bischoff-Grethe A, Dinges DF, et al. The neural basis of the psychomotor vigilance task. Sleep 2005;28(9):1059–68.

62. Bennett LS, Stradling JR, Davies RJ. A behavioural test to assess daytime sleepiness in obstructive sleep apnoea. J Sleep Res 1997;6(2):142–5.

63. Krieger AC, Ayappa I, Norman RG, et al. Comparison of the maintenance of wakefulness test (MWT) to a modified behavioral test (OSLER) in the evaluation of daytime sleepiness. J Sleep Res 2004;13(4):407–11.

64. Priest B, Brichard C, Aubert G, et al. Microsleep during a simplified maintenance of wakefulness test. A validation study of the OSLER test. Am J Respir Crit Care Med 2001;163(7):1619–25.

65. Alakuijala A, Maasilta P, Bachour A. The oxford sleep resistance test (OSLER) and the multiple unprepared reaction time test (MURT) detect vigilance modifications in sleep apnea patients. J Clin Sleep Med 2014;10(10):1075–82.

66. Fronczek R, Middelkoop HA, van Dijk JG, et al. Focusing on vigilance instead of sleepiness in the assessment of narcolepsy: high sensitivity of the Sustained Attention to Response Task (SART). Sleep 2006;29(2):187–91.

67. van der Heide A, van Schie MK, Lammers GJ, et al. Comparing treatment effect measurements in narcolepsy: the sustained attention to response task, Epworth sleepiness scale and maintenance of wakefulness test. Sleep 2015;38(7):1051–8.

68. Van Schie MK, Thijs RD, Fronczek R, et al. Sustained attention to response task (SART) shows impaired vigilance in a spectrum of disorders of excessive daytime sleepiness. J Sleep Res 2012;21(4):390–5.

69. Wilkinson VE, Jackson ML, Westlake J, et al. The accuracy of eyelid movement parameters for drowsiness detection. J Clin Sleep Med 2013;9(12):1315–24.

70. Ftouni S, Sletten TL, Howard M, et al. Objective and subjective measures of sleepiness, and their associations with on-road driving events in shift workers. J Sleep Res 2013;22(1):58–69.

71. Wilhelm BJ, Widmann A, Durst W, et al. Objective and quantitative analysis of daytime sleepiness in physicians after night duties. Int J Psychophysiol 2009;72(3):307–13.

72. Yamamoto K, Kobayashi F, Hori R, et al. Association between pupillometric sleepiness measures and sleep latency derived by MSLT in clinically sleepy patients. Environ Health Prev Med 2013;18(5):361–7.

73. George CF. Driving simulators in clinical practice. Sleep Med Rev 2003;7(4):311–20.

74. Rapoport MJ, Lanctot KL, Streiner DL, et al. Benzodiazepine use and driving: a meta-analysis. J Clin Psychiatry 2009;70(5):663–73.

75. Pizza F, Contardi S, Mostacci B, et al. A driving simulation task: correlations with Multiple Sleep Latency Test. Brain Res Bull 2004;63(5):423–6.

76. Forsman P, Wallin A, Tietavainen A, et al. Posturographic sleepiness monitoring. J Sleep Res 2007; 16(3):259–61.

77. Dorokhov VB, Verbitskaya YS, Lavrova TP. Auditory evoked potentials and impairments to psychomotor activity evoked by falling asleep. Neurosci Behav Physiol 2010;40(4):411–9.

78. Chua EC, Tan WQ, Yeo SC, et al. Heart rate variability can be used to estimate sleepiness-related decrements in psychomotor vigilance during total sleep deprivation. Sleep 2012;35(3):325–34.

79. Henelius A, Sallinen M, Huotilainen M, et al. Heart rate variability for evaluating vigilant attention in partial chronic sleep restriction. Sleep 2014;37(7):1257–67.

80. Borghini G, Astolfi L, Vecchiato G, et al. Measuring neurophysiological signals in aircraft pilots and car drivers for the assessment of mental workload, fatigue and drowsiness. Neurosci Biobehav Rev 2014; 44:58–75.

81. Mathis J, Hess CW. Sleepiness and vigilance tests. Swiss Med Wkly 2009;139(15–16):214–9.

Sleepiness in Narcolepsy

Jun Zhang, MD[a], Fang Han, MD[b],*

KEYWORDS

- Excessive daytime sleepiness • Narcolepsy • Cataplexy • Multiple sleep latency test • Stimulant

KEY POINTS

- Excessive daytime sleepiness (EDS) is usually the first and the most disabling symptom in narcolepsy. Understanding the clinical characteristic of EDS in narcolepsy leads to an early diagnosis.
- EDS in narcolepsy varies in different aspects, such as onset age, severity, and clinical characteristics.
- The diagnosis of narcolepsy is based on the clarifying of EDS through history and polysomnography (PSG) followed by the multiple sleep latency test (MSLT). Cerebrospinal fluid (CSF) orexin measurement is helpful to classify type 1 and type 2 narcolepsy.
- The therapeutic goal is to optimize control of EDS through wake-promoting medications and nonpharmacological treatments.

INTRODUCTION

EDS, or hypersomnia, defined as the inability to stay awake and alert during the major waking episodes of the day, resulting in unintended lapses into drowsiness or sleep,[1] and has been well recognized by medical professionals and the public. The problem is common; it is estimated to affect up 9% of the general population[2] and 15% to 30% of patients suffering from sleep disorders. EDS is one of the most common complaints of patients seeking help in sleep clinics. EDS has critical implications for human productivity and safety, because EDS can result in reduced quality of life, impaired mood and cognitive function, and increased risk for motor vehicle accidents. The diagnosis and treatment of sleep disorders with EDS were major triggers of the development of modern sleep medicine. Factors influencing sleep quality and/or quantity may cause EDS. Narcolepsy represents the best understood hypersomnia, due in large part to the elucidation of the role of hypocretin (orexins) in the pathophysiology of animals and human narcolepsy cataplexy decades ago.[3–6] According to the *International Classification of Sleep Disorders, Third Edition (ICSD-3)*, narcolepsy is classified as type 1 and type 2. Specifically, type 1 narcolepsy became defined as either documented low CSF hypocretin-1, even if it does not manifest cataplexy or clear cataplexy and a positive MSLT; cases without cataplexy but with a positive MSLT were called type 2 narcolepsy.

EPIDEMIOLOGY OF EXCESSIVE DAYTIME SLEEPINESS AND NARCOLEPSY

Narcolepsy affects 0.03% to 0.16% of the general population in various ethnic groups.[7–10] The prevalence of narcolepsy with cataplexy falls between 25 and 50 per 100,000 people.[11] Little is known about the epidemiology of type 2 narcolepsy. Two groups independently examined the population prevalence of a positive MSLT result with mean sleep latencies less than or equal to 8 minutes plus greater than or equal to 2 sleep-onset rapid eye movement (REM) periods (SOREMPs). In 1 sample of 539 subjects, 2.5% of subjects met MSLT criteria for narcolepsy.[12] A separate cohort study of 556 subjects found a surprisingly

Disclosure Statement: No conflict of interest declared.
a Department of Neurology, Peking University People's Hospital, 11, Xi Zhi Men Nan Da Jie, Xi Chen Qu, Beijing 100044, China; b Department of Respiratory Medicine, Peking University People's Hospital, 11, Xi Zhi Men Nan Da Jie, Xi Chen Qu, Beijing 100044, China
* Corresponding author.
E-mail address: hanfang1@hotmail.com

high prevalence of positive MSLTs; 4.1% men and 0.4% women met the criteria for narcolepsy and subjective sleepiness (Epworth Sleepiness Scale [ESS] score >10).[13]

Most cases of human narcolepsy are sporadic. Up to 5% are familial cases, and the risk of a first-degree relative developing narcolepsy cataplexy is 1% to 2%, which is 10 times to 40 times higher than in the general population.[14] Higher prevalence of EDS was found in relatives of patients with narcolepsy. In 1 study, including 378 parents of children with type 1 narcolepsy-cataplexy, MSLT testing found that 27% of parents had MSL less than or equal to 8 minutes; further analysis indicated 0.8% of parents have hypocretin deficiency with cataplexy and 2.4% parents are without cataplexy but with MSLT results consistent with narcolepsy, although a large portion of subjects did not report subjective daytime sleepiness or other ancillary symptoms (Yan H and Han F, unpublished data, 2017).

EXCESSIVE DAYTIME SLEEPINESS AS THE CARDINAL SYMPTOM OF NARCOLEPSY

EDS, cataplexy, sleep paralysis, and hypnagogic hallucinations are the classic tetrad of symptoms for narcolepsy. Only approximately one-third of patients, however, have all 4 of these symptoms on initial evaluation in a sleep laboratory.[15] EDS and cataplexy are considered the 2 primary symptoms of narcolepsy. Cataplexy typically presents as an abrupt and reversible decrease or loss of muscle tone usually elicited by strong emotions and is the only truly specific feature of narcolepsy, but it occurs in only 65% to 75% of individuals with confirmed narcolepsy and may improve or even completely disappear during the disease course.[10,16,17] It presents as the first symptom in less than 10% of the patients and appears usually months to years after the onset of EDS. In contrast, presence of objective EDS is considered the cardinal diagnostic criterion for narcolepsy; 100% of the narcoleptic subjects present with chronic sleepiness, and it often abates with time but never phases out completely. Clinically, type 1 and type 2 narcolepsy do not differ qualitatively and qualitatively in regard to daytime sleepiness. In a Japanese series, the mean ESS (14.9 ± 3.5) in 62 patients with type 2 was similar to the mean ESS (14.6 ± 3.7) of 52 patients with type 1 narcolepsy.[18] A similar finding was observed in a French series (ESS 19 ± 3.3 in 54 patients with type 1 vs 17.5 ± 2.7 in 46 patients with type 2).[19] In summary, EDS is often the most frequent cause for consultation in sleep clinics and the first clue to the diagnosis of narcolepsy type 1 and type 2.

Given the average diagnostic delay of more than 10 years,[15] understanding the clinical characteristic of EDS in narcolepsy leads an early diagnosis of the disorder.

PRESENTATIONS OF EXCESSIVE DAYTIME SLEEPINESS IN NARCOLEPSY
Onset of Excessive Daytime Sleepiness in Narcolepsy

EDS and irresistible sleep episodes are usually the first and the most disabling symptoms in patients with narcolepsy. Narcolepsy onset is variable and may appear as either progressive or sudden. A majority of the narcoleptic patients begin to show symptoms, mostly sleepiness, in the second decade of life, with a bimodal distribution, including a large peak around puberty and a smaller peak between 35 years and 45 years.[20] This was confirmed in a US white population and a European Narcolepsy Network study,[21] with mean EDS onset age at 22.7 years old. Emerging evidences indicates that narcolepsy and EDS symptom onset seems different across various ethnic populations. EDS occurred in an earlier age in Chinese narcoleptics.[22] Childhood narcolepsy cases were first reported in a group of Northern Chinese[23] and confirmed in a follow-up study.[22] In a series of 2000 narcolepsy–cataplexy patients seen over 15 years in the same sleep laboratory, two-thirds had onset of symptoms at age 8.5 years, more than 15% with onset prior to 6 years. A major onset peak at approximately 10 years old to 11 years old was observed in Southern Han Chinese,[24,25] and childhood narcoleptics were often seen in Taiwan,[26] a place with mixed Chinese population from both South China and North China. Childhood narcolepsy is considered rare in whites, however. Only in recent years has the number of childhood diagnosis of narcolepsy increased, probably due to the higher disease awareness in the context of the possible association with H1N1 pandemic and vaccination.[27,28] Further comparison between patients in 2 large databases from Beijing University and Stanford University also revealed that age of onset for EDS was younger in Chinese patients versus whites, 2.5 years younger in children less than 18 years, and 6.7 years younger in all patients.[22]

Clinical Characteristics of Excessive Daytime Sleepiness in Narcolepsy

EDS in narcolepsy generally presents as a background of baseline sleepiness that easily leads to sleep episodes of a strong, sometimes overwhelming, desire for sleep not only under conducive circumstances, such as monotonous, sedentary activities like watching television, reading, and attending a meeting or in high temperature environment, but also in unusual situations like eating, walking, talking, bicycle riding, or driving. Sleepiness also aggravates after a heavy meal. Sleep attacks that present as sudden onset of sleepiness without a prodromal warning are often accompanied by microsleep episodes where a patient blanks out. These unconscious microsleep episodes or memory lapses can become more frequent as a patient makes desperate efforts to fight against the urge to sleep. The patient may then continue his or her activity in a semiconscious manner, such as writing incoherent phrases in a letter and even gestural, deambulatory, or speech automatisms. In addition to the sleep episodes, EDS in some patients may manifest as lack of energy, chronic tiredness or fatigue, a low level of alertness with poor concentration, and error-prone performance in school or at work; however, they often go to sleep in several minutes while a passenger in a car. Physicians erroneously think that sleep attacks are unique to narcolepsy or that EDS without sleep attacks cannot be due to narcolepsy.

Daytime sleepiness occurs daily; the frequency shows wide interpersonal variation and generally repeats several times every day. Sleep episodes happen more often in the morning and less frequently in the afternoon. Patients may keep alert the whole afternoon after a noon nap. The episode duration can vary from a few seconds to more than an hour depending on environmental factors. Narcolepsy patients generally do not spend a greater portion of their time asleep across the 24 hours of a day compared with people who do not have narcolepsy. In children narcoleptics, continuous sleep can last for more than 15 hours per day up to the symptom onset, then may switch gradually to a typical episode pattern in several months. EDS and irresistible sleep episodes persist throughout the lifetime but often improve with advancing age due to lifestyle adjustments or natural history of narcolepsy. Sleep episodes are most often relieved by minutes to hours of short naps, which may restore normal wakefulness for several minutes to a couple hours before the next episode occurs.

It is often patients' reports of dreaming and occasionally sleep paralysis during short naps that indicate the intrusion of REM sleep.

POSSIBLE MECHANISMS OF EXCESSIVE DAYTIME SLEEPINESS IN NARCOLEPSY

Degeneration of hypothalamic neurons producing orexin (hypocretin) is the primary cause of human narcolepsy. In patients with type 1 narcolepsy, postmortem studies have consistently demonstrated greater than 85% loss of the hypocretin-producing neurons across the hypothalamus.[6] Although low CSF hypocretin-1 level is not seen in type 2 narcolepsy as defined, limited studies indicated type 2 cases may be caused by less extensive injury to the hypocretin neurons, with an approximately 33% loss of the hypocretin neurons.[29] Orexin is crucial to promote wakefulness and maintaining a long, consolidated waking period. Accordingly, administration of orexin has a robust wake-promoting effect and leads to a remarkable improvement of EDS and decrease in non-REM sleep and REM sleep.[30,31] Lack of wake-promoting substance orexin is the major mechanism of EDS in narcolepsy. Histamine also has wake-promoting effect; reduction in CSF histamine levels in patients with narcolepsy reflect the severity of EDS independently of orexin status.[32–34] Endogenous sleep-promoting substances, such as adenosine, hormones, cytokines, peptides, and endozepines, in the brain also induce sleep in animal studies.[35] Among them, prostaglandin D2 (PGD2) has been recognized as the most potent endogenous somnogen. It is synthesized from prostaglandin H2 by the enzyme of lipocalin-type prostaglandin D synthase (L-PGDS). In humans, alterations in the L-PGDS level seem to be involved in the pathogenesis of EDS in patients with narcolepsy.[36]

Patients with narcolepsy fall asleep readily at night, but their nocturnal sleep is fragmented. PSG studies consistently reveal frequent arousals, higher wake time after sleep onset, frequent shifts to wake or increased non-REM stage 1 sleep and overall decreased sleep efficiency. Sleep fragmentation can worsen other manifestations of narcolepsy, especially EDS. The American Academy of Sleep Medicine (AASM) endorses disrupted nocturnal sleep as part of a narcolepsy symptom pentad and recommends controlling disrupted sleep in patients with narcolepsy to be a treatment of target.[37] Medications may consolidate sleep and improve daytime symptoms of EDS have also been introduced to clinical use. Deficiency of orexin system may induce a destabilized sleep-wake transition mechanism and impair maintenance of sleep during nighttime in narcolepsy.

HLADQ0602 is a near prerequisite for developing narcolepsy cataplexy across multiple ethnic groups. The risk of developing narcolepsy is 7-fold to 25-fold higher in subjects heterozygous for this genotype, and homozygosity for HLA-DQB1*06:02 increases the risk an additional 2-fold to 4-fold.[38] Normal subjects carrying this HLA allele (25% of the general population) were subjectively sleepier and more fatigued; they showed greater sleep fragmentation and decreased sleep homeostatic pressure during baseline sleep and partial sleep deprivation.[39] Thus, HLADQ0602 may represent a genetic biomarker for predicting such individual differences in basal and sleep loss conditions. Because only 40% to 50% of narcolepsy type 2 cases carry DQB1*06:02, its influence on EDS in these patients remains to be established. The HLADQ0602/DQB1*03:01 combination increases narcolepsy risk and the presence of DQB1*03:01 reduces age of EDS onset in Chinese population,[40] so the association is stronger in patients with early-onset narcolepsy. DQB1*03:01 frequency is high in China and variable across Europe, possibly explaining why an unusually large number of cases with childhood onset are reported in Chinese population.

EXCESSIVE DAYTIME SLEEPINESS IN THE DIAGNOSIS OF NARCOLEPSY

The importance of EDS in narcolepsy diagnosing is highlighted by excessive sleepiness present in virtually 100% of patients and sleepiness as usually the first initial symptom of narcolepsy. In ICSD-3, the diagnosis for both type 1 and type 2 narcolepsy has been primarily based on the presence of daytime sleepiness occurring almost daily for at least 3 months.[1] Clarifying the complaint of EDS through history and subjective severity scale evaluation, such as the ESS, is the first step to the diagnosis of narcolepsy; additional tests that confirm the diagnosis include nocturnal PSG followed by a daytime MSLT, which can quantify EDS severity objectively and identify SOREMPs. Refreshing daytime naps are characteristic of narcolepsy, and this is of diagnostic value. Driven by many patients requiring lifelong treatment with potentially addictive medications, the utility of these objective methods to narcolepsy diagnosis is further reinforced in the ICSD-3[1] as indicated by the facts that: first, nocturnal PSG was used not only as a measurement for sleep duration and a differentiated tool for the diagnosis of concomitant sleep disorders of EDS, such as periodic leg movement disorder and sleep deprivation. SOREMP within 15 minutes of onset of nocturnal sleep on the preceding PSG counted as 1 of the required 2 SOREMPs on the MSLT and is added to the diagnostic criteria for narcolepsy, with a very high specificity. Second, in ICSD-3, MSLT is required for diagnosis of type 1 narcolepsy with cataplexy. In contrast, this test is not considered necessary if clear, definite cataplexy is present in ICSD-2. Third, it is strongly recommended that

the MSLT be preceded by at least 1 week of actigraphic recording with a sleep log to establish whether the results could be biased by insufficient sleep, shift work, or another circadian sleep disorder.

It is important to categorize narcolepsy as type 1 or type 2. Type 1 is a distinct phenomenon with consensus on presentation and diagnostic criteria. Type 2, however, remains an evolving diagnosis. As discussed previously, both qualitative and qualitative evaluation of EDS could not differentiate type 1 and type 2 narcolepsy[18,19]; further measurements, such as CSF hypocretin-1 and HLADQ 0602 testing, may be needed.

Type 1 narcolepsy became defined as a narrow disease entity with either documented low CSF hypocretin-1 or clear cataplexy and a positive MSLT. The diagnosis of type 1 narcolepsy with cataplexy is straightforward because cataplexy can often be elicited by a careful history taking; however, determining if cataplexy is truly present is often challenging. Therefore, PSG followed by MSLT in those with cataplexy but no CSF hypocretin measurement is required to make a diagnosis of type 1 narcolepsy in ICSD-3. As defined, hypocretin deficiency can currently be documented by CSF sampling, and CSF hypocretin-1 below 110 pg/mL is highly specific (99%) and sensitive (87%) for cases of narcolepsy cataplexy; the problem is that most patients have not undergone CSF examination in clinical settings. Hypocretin deficiency may be predicted by the appearance of typical cataplexy plus positive HLADQ0602 gene marker, with a probability of 98%. Currently, possible indications for considering measuring CSF Hcrt-1 levels as a diagnostic procedure for type 1 narcolepsy are the presence of disorders, such as obstructive sleep apnea (OSA), or situations when MSLT is difficult to conduct or interpret, for example, in young children who are unable to follow MSLT instructions; individuals with severe or complex psychiatric, neurologic, or medical disorders that could compromise the validity of the MSLT results; and those on drugs substantially alter sleep latency and the occurrence of REM sleep.[41–43]

Type 2 narcolepsy does not have hypocretin deficiency by definition in ICSD-3. A majority are cases of cataplexy but with a positive MSLT as defined in ICSD-2. It is a clinical diagnosis or rather a diagnosis of exclusion. Many symptoms of narcolepsy are nonspecific, and cataplexy is absent. Biomarkers are lacking, and CSF hypocretin-1 levels are almost always normal. Ruling out other sleep disorders is a major aspect of diagnosing type 2 narcolepsy. The diagnosis critically hinges on clinical findings and the MSLT. With the recognition of rapid transitions into REM sleep (REM latency ≤15 minutes) on PSG and the establishment of the MSLT as a diagnostic test, together fueled by the growth of sleep medicine, more and more cases without cataplexy are labeled as narcolepsy.[44,45] Reflecting this, a majority of cases series until 1990 had cataplexy, whereas currently a minority have cataplexy.[46] MSLT remains the most important test for the diagnosis of type 2 narcolepsy, although a positive MSLT result is not specific. If the MSLT shows equivocal results, repeating it after a time interval may be helpful for diagnosis. Unlike true type 1 narcolepsy, patients without cataplexy generally do not have repeatable findings. In patients with suspected type 2 narcolepsy, there has been less interest in measuring hypocretin, because levels are usually normal. Only approximately 40% to 50% of type 2 patients carry DQB1*06:02.4,30; testing for this allele is not helpful for diagnosing. In patients with other evidence for type 2 narcolepsy, however, the presence of DQB1*06:02 may slightly strengthen diagnostic certainty. It cannot be used to predict with high probability a patient's CSF Hcrt-1 levels, but if the patient is HLA negative, CSF Hcrt-1 levels almost certainly are normal and the lumbar puncture is unnecessary,[47] because the probability of low levels of CSF hypocretin-1 in HLA-negative cases without cataplexy is estimated to be far less than 1%.[48] On the other hand, approximately 24% of narcoleptics without cataplexy have a low CSF Hcrt-1 concentration, and almost all of these are positive for the HLA DQB1*0602; in HLA-positive patients with chronic EDS and positive MSLT results but no cataplexy, hypocretin levels can help confirm the diagnosis of narcolepsy and distinguish between type 1 and type 2 narcolepsy.

DIFFERENTIATING EXCESSIVE DAYTIME SLEEPINESS IN NARCOLEPSY FROM OTHER SLEEP DISORDERS

Narcolepsy is commonly confounded with other forms of EDS, such as idiopathic hypersomnia (IH), recurrent hypersomnia, hypersomnia associated with depression, sleep-disordered breathing (SDB), and chronic sleep deprivation.[49] The presence of cataplexy is the key factor to single out type 1 narcolepsy from the other forms of hypersomnia. Rare disorders, such as Neimann-Pick disease type C, Prader-Willi syndrome, and Norrie disease, also exhibits cataplexy.[50–52] Some of the narcolepsy without cataplexy cases, especially in children, may develop true cataplexy later in the course of the illness. The major challenges exist in the diagnosing of type 2 narcolepsy.[47] In addition to the presence of 2 or more sleep-onset REM periods on the MSLT or preceding PSG, the refreshing value of short naps is of considerable diagnostic value, because this may differentiate patients with narcolepsy from patients with IH, who take long and unrefreshing naps. IH also demonstrates higher sleep efficiency than narcolepsy on PSG. EDS associated with a psychiatric disorder should be considered in patients with a psychiatric condition, most typically depression. The complaint of EDS and prolonged sleep may vary from day to day and is often associated with poor sleep at night. The MSLT does not demonstrate a short mean sleep latency. Chronic fatigue syndrome is characterized by persistent or relapsing fatigue that does not resolve with sleep or rest. Patients clearly complain of fatigue rather than EDS, and the mean MSLT sleep latency is normal. Long sleepers feel fully refreshed and do not experience EDS if they are allowed to sleep as long as they need. Detailed neurologic examinations, including brain MRI scan, may be helpful to rule out hypersomnolence due to other medical disorders, in particular, posttraumatic hypersomnolence, residual hypersomnolence after adequate treatment of sleep apnea, and sleep fragmentation due to pain. Shift work commonly leads to circadian phase delay and chronic sleep deprivation that can affect the MSLT regarding both SL and SOREMPs; in addition to a careful history, actigraphy and sleep logs might be the best measures to discriminate shift work from type 2 narcolepsy. Chronic sleep deprivation or insufficient sleep syndrome presents longer sleep duration on weekends and holidays compared with weekdays, as assessed by sleep logs or actigraphy; extending a patient's sleep before testing may reverse the short sleep latency on MSLT. The presence of other sleep disorders, such as SDB, does not preclude a diagnosis of narcolepsy because SDB is prevalent in narcolepsy, and no improvement of EDS after adequate PAP treatment supports the diagnosis of narcolepsy.

MANAGEMENT OF EXCESSIVE DAYTIME SLEEPINESS IN NARCOLEPSY

Because a definitive cause of narcolepsy has yet to be identified, the goal of all therapeutic approaches is relief of symptoms and allowing patients to have a full personal and professional life. When selecting medications, clinicians must consider possible side effects because narcolepsy is a lifelong illness and patients have to receive medication for years. Tolerance or addiction may occur with some compounds. The treatment of narcolepsy must balance the maintenance of an active life with the avoidance of side effects and tolerance to medications.[53]

Nonpharmacologic treatments include optimizing nocturnal sleep duration, good sleep hygiene with a regular sleep schedule, and planning scheduled daytime naps. Diet and exercise to avoid obesity are necessary, especially for type 1 narcoleptics. Support for patients and families through organized patient advocacy and support groups is often reported by patients as helpful in providing information and in combatting the sometimes negative public perception of people who are sleepy. Patients are at increased risk of motor vehicle accidents, and counseling about this risk and the need to avoid driving while sleepy is important.

Improving nocturnal sleep and treatment of concurrent sleep disorders is also important for improving daytime sleepiness. Benzodiazepine receptor agonists like zolpidem may improve sleep quality in some patients, especially those with long awake time during night. Although data are mixed regarding the potential benefit of CPAP on sleepiness in narcolepsy with OSA, adequate treatment of OSA definitely improves long-term outcomes. If restless legs syndrome and periodic limb movements in sleep significantly impair sleep, specific treatment of these problems may be beneficial.

Behavior intervention alone seems insufficient to control sleepiness; almost all patients require medications for EDS (see Shinichi Takenoshita and Seiji Nishino's article, "Pharmacologic Managements of Excessive Daytime Sleepiness," in this issue). These include traditional sympathomimetic stimulants, such as methylphenidate and dextroamphetamine, and nonamphetamine wakefulness-promoting agents, including modafinil and armodafinil. Sodium oxybate is considered a standard therapy for EDS, cataplexy, and disrupted sleep in narcolepsy by the American Academy of Sleep Medicine.[54] One of the major problems in long-term use is that tolerance may develop, requiring escalating doses and leading to ineffectiveness at the highest dose. In some patients, effectiveness can be restored by a drug holiday, that is, no medications for several days, for example during weekends, although this is not encouraged for cataplexy treatment. Although these medications are not Food and Drug Administration approved for children, they are used off-label in this population.[55] Their interaction with oral contraception is important to consider in women of childbearing potential, because contraception efficacy may decrease.

There are emerging medications for EDS treatment. Hypocretin agonists administered via the intranasal route had some limited success to date.[31] Pitolisant, a histamine-3 receptor inverse agonist, stimulates histamine release and promotes wakefulness.[56] Atomoxetine, a selective noradrenergic reuptake inhibitor, has been reported effective in improving daytime sleepiness, particularly in children.[57,58] Hypersomnolent patients demonstrate a positive allosteric modulator of γ-aminobutyric acid (GABA)$_A$ receptors in their CSF, and clarithromycin is a negative allosteric modulator of GABA$_A$ receptors; data from a randomized, placebo-controlled trial of clarithromycin for hypersomnolence confirmed a significant benefit on subjective sleepiness.[59]

ACKNOWLEDGMENTS

This work was supported by research grants from the Ministry of Science and Technology (2015 CB856405), NSFC (81420108002) to Dr F. Han.

REFERENCES

1. American Academy of Sleep Medicine. International classification of sleep disorders. 3rd edition. Darien (IL): American Academy of Sleep Medicine; 2014.
2. Hublin C, Kaprio J, Partinen M, et al. Daytime sleepiness in an adult, Finnish population. J Intern Med 1996;239:417–23.
3. Lin L, Faraco J, Li R, et al. The sleep disorder canine narcolepsy is caused by a mutation in the hypocretin (orexin) receptor 2 gene. Cell 1999;98:365–76.
4. Chemelli RM, Willie JT, Sinton CM, et al. Narcolepsy in orexin knockout mice: molecular genetics of sleep regulation. Cell 1999;98:437–51.
5. Nishino S, Ripley B, Overeem S, et al. Hypocretin (orexin) deficiency in human narcolepsy. Lancet 2000;355:39–40.
6. Thannickal TC, Moore RY, Nienhuis R, et al. Reduced number of hypocretin neurons in human narcolepsy. Neuron 2000;27:469–74.
7. Hublin C, Kaprio J, Partinen M, et al. The prevalence of narcolepsy: an epidemiological study of the Finnish Twin Cohort. Ann Neurol 1994;35:709–16.
8. Ohayon MM, Priest RG, Zulley J, et al. Prevalence of narcolepsy symptomatology and diagnosis in the European general population. Neurology 2002;58:1826–33.
9. Wing YK, Li RH, Lam CW, et al. The prevalence of narcolepsy among Chinese in Hong Kong. Ann Neurol 2002;51:578–84.
10. Silber MH, Krahn LE, Olson EJ, et al. The epidemiology of narcolepsy in Olmsted County, Minnesota: a population-based study. Sleep 2002;25(2):197–202.
11. Longstreth WT Jr, Koepsell TD, Ton TG, et al. The epidemiology of narcolepsy. Sleep 2007;30:13–26.

12. Singh M, Drake CL, Roth T. The prevalence of multiple sleep-onset REM periods in a population-based sample. Sleep 2006;29:890–5.

13. Mignot E, Lin L, Finn L, et al. Correlates of sleep-onset REM periods during the multiple sleep latency test in community adults. Brain 2006;129:1609–23, 25.

14. Mignot E. Genetic and familial aspects of narcolepsy. Neurology 1998;50:S16–22.

15. Morrish E, King MA, Smith IE, et al. Factors associated with a delay in the diagnosis of narcolepsy. Sleep Med 2004;5(1):37–41.

16. Mignot E, Hayduk R, Black J, et al. HLA DQB1*0602 is associated with cataplexy in 509 narcoleptic patients. Sleep 1997;20(11):1012–20.

17. Guilleminault C, Mignot E, Partinen M. Controversies in the diagnosis of narcolepsy. Sleep 1994;17(Suppl 8):S1–6.

18. Takei Y, Komada Y, Namba K, et al. Differences in findings of nocturnal polysomnography and multiple sleep latency test between narcolepsy and idiopathic hypersomnia. Clin Neurophysiol 2012;123:137–41.

19. Leu-Semenescu S, De Cock VC, Le Masson VD, et al. Hallucinations in narcolepsy with and without cataplexy: contrasts with Parkinson's disease. Sleep Med 2011;12:497–504.

20. Dauvilliers Y, Montplaisir J, Molinari N, et al. Age at onset of narcolepsy in two large populations of patients in France and Quebec. Neurology 2001;57:2029–33.

21. Luca G, Haba-Rubio J, Dauvilliers Y, et al. Clinical, polysomnographic and genome-wide association analyses of narcolepsy with cataplexy: a European Narcolepsy Network study. J Sleep Res 2013;22:482–95.

22. Han F, Lin L, Li J, et al. Presentations of primary hypersomnia in Chinese children. Sleep 2011;34:627–32.

23. Han F, Chen E, Wei H, et al. Childhood narcolepsy in North China. Sleep 2001;24:321–4.

24. Wu HJ, Zhuang JH, Stone WS, et al. Symptomatology and occurrences aspects of narcolepsy: a retrospective study of 162 patients during a decade in eastern China. Sleep Med 2014;15(6):607–13.

25. Wing YK, Chen L, Fong SY, et al. Narcolepsy in Southern Chinese patients: clinical characteristics, HLA typing and seasonality of birth. J Neurol Neurosurg Psychiatry 2008;79:1262–7.

26. Chen YH, Huang YS, Chien WH, et al. Association analysis of the major histocompatibility complex, class II, DQ b1 gene, HLA-DQB1, with narcolepsy in Han Chinese patients from Taiwan. Sleep Med 2013;14:1393–7.

27. Han F, Lin L, Warby SC, et al. Narcolepsy onset is seasonal and increased following the 2009 H1N1 pandemic in China. Ann Neurol 2011;70:410–7.

28. Partinen M, Saarenpää-Heikkilä O, Ilveskoski I, et al. Increased incidence and clinical picture of childhood narcolepsy following the 2009 H1N1 pandemic vaccination campaign in Finland. PLoS One 2012;7:e33723.

29. Thannickal TC, Nienhuis R, Siegel JM. Localized loss of hypocretin (orexin) cells in narcolepsy without cataplexy. Sleep 2009;32:993–8.

30. John J, Wu MF, Siegel JM. Systemic administration of hypocretin-1 reduces cataplexy and normalizes sleep and waking durations in narcoleptic dogs. Sleep Res Online 2000;3(1):23–8.

31. Weinhold SL, Seeck-Hirschner M, Nowak A, et al. The effect of intranasal orexin-A (hypocretin-1) on sleep, wakefulness and attention in narcolepsy with cataplexy. Behav Brain Res 2014;262:8–13.

32. Bassetti CL, Baumann CR, Dauvilliers Y, et al. Cerebrospinal fluid histamine levels are decreased in patients with narcolepsy and excessive daytime sleepiness of other origin. J Sleep Res 2010;19(4):620–3.

33. Kanbayashi T, Kodama T, Kondo H, et al. CSF histamine contents in narcolepsy, idiopathic hypersomnia and obstructive sleep apnea syndrome. Sleep 2009;32(2):181–7.

34. Nishino S, Sakurai E, Nevsimalova S, et al. Decreased CSF histamine in narcolepsy with and without low CSF hypocretin-1 in comparison to healthy controls. Sleep 2009;32(2):175–80.

35. Rye DB, Bliwise DL, Parker K, et al. Modulation of vigilance in the primary hypersomnias by endogenous enhancement of GABAA receptors. Sci Transl Med 2012;4(161):161ra151.

36. Jordan W, Tumani H, Cohrs S, et al. Narcolepsy increased L-PGDS (beta-trace) levels correlate with excessive daytime sleepiness but not with cataplexy. J Neurol 2005;252(11):1372–8.

37. Roth T, Dauvilliers Y, Mignot E, et al. Disrupted nighttime sleep in narcolepsy. J Clin Sleep Med 2013;9(9):955–65.

38. Pelin Z, Guilleminault C, Risch N, et al. HLADQB1*06:02 homozygosity increases relative risk for narcolepsy but not disease severity in two ethnic groups. US Modafinil in Narcolepsy Multicenter Study Group. Tissue Antigens 1998;51:96–100.

39. Goel N, Banks S, Mignot E, et al. DQB1*0602 predicts interindividual differences in physiologic sleep, sleepiness, and fatigue. Neurology 2010;75(17):1509–19.

40. Han F, Faraco J, Dong XS, et al. Genome wide analysis of narcolepsy in China implicates novel immune loci and reveals changes in association prior to versus after the 2009 H1N1 influenza pandemic. PLoS Genet 2013;9:e1003880.

41. Bourgin P, Zeitzer JM, Mignot E. CSF hypocretin-1 assessment in sleep and neurological disorders. Lancet Neurol 2008;7:649–62.

42. Dauvilliers Y, Arnulf I, Mignot E. Narcolepsy with cataplexy. Lancet 2007;369:499–511.

43. Han F. Sleepiness that cannot be overcome: narcolepsy and cataplexy. Respirology 2012;17(8): 1157–65.

44. Andlauer O, Moore H, Jouhier L, et al. Nocturnal rapid eye movement sleep latency for identifying patients with narcolepsy/hypocretin deficiency. JAMA Neurol 2013;70:891–902.

45. Aldrich MS, Chervin RD, Malow BA. Value of the multiple sleep latency test (MSLT) for the diagnosis of narcolepsy. Sleep 1997;20:620–9.

46. Sturzenegger C, Bassetti CL. The clinical spectrum of narcolepsy with cataplexy: a reappraisal. J Sleep Res 2004;13:395–406.

47. Baumann CR, Mignot E, Lammers GJ, et al. Challenges in diagnosing narcolepsy without cataplexy: a consensus statement. Sleep 2014;37(6):1035–42.

48. Han F, Lin L, Schormair B, et al. HLA DQB1*06:02 negative narcolepsy with hypocretin/orexin deficiency. Sleep 2014;37:1601–8.

49. Dauvilliers Y. Differential diagnosis in hypersomnia. Curr Neurol Neurosci Rep 2006;6:156–62.

50. Oyama K, Takahashi T, Shoji Y, et al. Niemann-Pick disease type C: cataplexy and hypocretin in cerebrospinal fluid. Tohoku J Exp Med 2006;209:263–7.

51. Weselake SV, Foulds JL, Couch R, et al. Prader-Willi syndrome, excessive daytime sleepiness, and narcoleptic symptoms: a case report. J Med Case Rep 2014;8:127.

52. Koch H, Craig I, Dahlitz M, et al. Analysis of the monoamine oxidase genes and the Norrie disease gene locus in narcolepsy. Lancet 1999;353:645–6.

53. Mignot EJ. A practical guide to the therapy of narcolepsy and hypersomnia syndromes. Neurotherapeutics 2012;9(4):739–52.

54. The Xyrem International Study Group. A double-blind, placebo-controlled study demonstrates sodium oxybate is effective for treatment of excessive daytime sleepiness in narcolepsy. J Clin Sleep Med 2005;1:391–7.

55. Roth T. Narcolepsy: treatment issues. J Clin Psychiatry 2007;68(Suppl 13):16–9.

56. Dauvilliers Y, Bassetti C, Lammers GJ, et al. Pitolisant versus placebo or modafinil in patients with narcolepsy: a double-blind, randomised trial. Lancet Neurol 2013;12(11):1068–75.

57. Zhang S, Ding C, Wu H, et al. Clinical effect of atomoxetine hydrochloride in 66 children with narcolepsy. Zhonghua Er Ke Za Zhi 2015;53(10):760–4 [in Chinese].

58. Bart Sangal R, Sangal JM, Thorp K. Atomoxetine improves sleepiness and global severity of illness but not the respiratory disturbance index in mild to moderate obstructive sleep apnea with sleepiness. Sleep Med 2008;9(5):506–10.

59. Trotti LM, Saini P, Bliwise DL, et al. Clarithromycin in γ-aminobutyric acid-Related hypersomnolence: a randomized, crossover trial. Ann Neurol 2015; 78(3):454–65.

Idiopathic Hypersomnia

Lynn Marie Trotti, MD, MSc

KEYWORDS

- Idiopathic hypersomnia • Narcolepsy • Excessive daytime sleepiness • Multiple sleep latency test
- Sleep drunkenness

KEY POINTS

- Idiopathic hypersomnia (IH) is thought to be a rare disorder, but population-based estimates of prevalence are limited. Symptoms of IH are not uncommon.
- The differential diagnosis includes insufficient sleep time, circadian rhythm disorders, narcolepsy without cataplexy, hypersomnolence associated with psychiatric disease and medical conditions.
- Current diagnostic schema for IH diagnosis are imperfect, such that some patients do not meet criteria but still have problematic sleepiness.
- First-line treatment is generally modafinil, which is supported by 2 randomized, controlled trials showing efficacy. Psychostimulants are often used for IH treatment, although data supporting their use are sparse.
- Medication-refractory symptoms or medication intolerance prevents control of symptoms in one-quarter of IH patients; alternate treatment options are available, including clarithromycin.

INTRODUCTION

Idiopathic hypersomnia (IH) is a chronic neurologic disorder that manifests as pathologic daytime sleepiness with or without prolonged sleep durations. Population-based estimates of the frequency of IH are difficult to obtain, given the requirements for electrophysiologic testing and ruling out of other disorders that may cause similar symptoms. Clinic-based estimates of IH prevalence are limited by differing referral patterns and biases, such that estimates of the relative frequency of IH to narcolepsy with cataplexy vary substantially, anywhere from 1:10 to greater than 1:1.[1–5] As such, the true prevalence of IH is unknown. Using a questionnaire-based algorithm, Ohayon and colleagues[6] have demonstrated that the symptom of excessive sleepiness, associated with irresistible daytime naps, multiple naps in the same day, nonrestorative nocturnal sleep of at least 9 hours, or difficulty waking after sleep, is present in 0.5% of the population. Although presumably not all of these individuals would meet diagnostic criteria for IH, it is clear that the symptoms of IH are not uncommon.

As the name "idiopathic" hypersomnia implies, the pathophysiology of IH is presently unknown. Hypocretin deficiency, known to cause narcolepsy type 1, is not present in patients with IH.[7] Cerebrospinal fluid from patients with IH, and several other central disorders of hypersomnolence, has been shown to enhance activity at gamma-aminobutyric acid (GABA)-A receptors in vitro, in excess of that of cerebrospinal fluid from controls.[8] Although this enhancement of GABAergic transmission has not been shown to be causal to sleepiness or long sleep durations in patients with IH, biological plausibility is demonstrated by the known GABAergic mechanisms of sleep onset

Disclosures: This work was supported by K23NS083748 from the National Institutes of Health. Dr L.M. Trotti reports funds to her institution (but no personal funds) from Jazz Pharma and Balance Therapeutics, outside the submitted work. Dr L.M. Trotti is the Chair of the Medical Advisory Board of the Hypersomnia Foundation, which is discussed in this work.
Department of Neurology, Emory Sleep Center, Emory University School of Medicine, 12 Executive Park Drive Northeast, Atlanta, GA 30329, USA
E-mail address: Lbecke2@emory.edu

and maintenance, as well as the prominent role of GABA-A receptor agonists and modulators in the production of pharmacologic sleep and anesthesia.[9–12] Further, symptoms of IH are reversible in some patients with use of GABA-receptor antagonists or negative allosteric modulators (see Treatment Resistance).[8,13,14]

A family history of excessive sleepiness, IH, or another central disorder of hypersomnolence is seen in 34% to 38% of IH patients,[4,15,16] with parent–child transmission suggested by the finding that 12.5% of IH patients have at least 1 parent who routinely sleeps more than 9.5 hours per night.[17] Taken together, these reports suggest a genetic contribution to IH. However, the strong association between narcolepsy type 1 and HLA DQB1*0602 is not observed in patients with IH, in whom the rate of positivity for this allele ranges from 8% to 27%, depending on the population, and approximates the rate in controls.[4,18–20] An immune system dysregulation, unique from that implicated in narcolepsy type 1, might be present in patients with IH, as suggested by their significantly increased rates of comorbid inflammatory or allergic disorders[17,21] and altered immunoglobulin G profile compared with controls.[22] Disruption of autonomic nervous system functioning, with a shift toward increased vagal tone, has been noted in patients with IH compared with controls, possibly contributing to some of the vegetative symptoms (faintness, orthostatic hypotension, Raynaud syndrome) that are commonly observed in IH patients.[17,23,24]

Classically, sleep efficiency is greater than 90% in patients with IH,[4,16,18,24,25] although some studies have reported mean values in the high 80s.[15,19] The tendency for high sleep efficiency is somewhat at odds with the recently proposed hypothesis that patients with IH have fragmented sleep, as evidenced by more sleep stage changes, more N1 sleep, and more awakenings per hour than either controls or patients with narcolepsy type 1.[26] Abnormalities in slow wave sleep percentage have been proposed but inconsistently observed.[1,4,16,18,19,25,26] A single, small study has suggested an increase in spindle activity in IH patients compared with those with narcolepsy (type unspecified).[27]

PATIENT EVALUATION OVERVIEW
Core Diagnostic Features of Idiopathic Hypersomnia

Daytime sleepiness, defined as an irresistible need to sleep or episode of daytime sleep, is the core diagnostic feature of IH. Current diagnostic criteria in the *International Classification of Sleep Disorders* (ICSD), third edition,[24] require a combination of sleepiness for at least 3 months, not better explained by another disorder or substance, and specific polysomnographic or actigraphic criteria (**Box 1**).

Ancillary Symptoms of Idiopathic Hypersomnia

Several ancillary features are commonly seen in people with IH.

Long sleep duration
Earlier editions of the ICSD explicitly defined a subset of IH defined by long sleep times (ie, >10 hours for the main sleep period). Although current criteria do not distinguish those with long sleep from those without, long sleep times can be used to confirm an IH diagnosis.[24]

Prolonged and unrefreshing naps
Similar to long sleep at night, naps during the day tend to be of long duration in patients with IH.[4,15,24] Patients with IH often find naps to be unrefreshing.[4,15–18,24] The clinical consequence of this is that, unlike in patients with narcolepsy

---

Box 1
Idiopathic hypersomnia diagnostic criteria

All of the following criteria must be met

1. Daily daytime sleepiness, defined as an "irrepressible need to sleep" or daytime sleep, that has been present at least 3 months

2. No cataplexy

3. No MSLT evidence for narcolepsy (ie, <2 sleep-onset REM periods on the overnight PSG and daytime MSLT considered together)

4. Electrophysiologic evidence of hypersomnolence, defined as either (or both) of:

   a. Mean sleep latency on MSLT of at least 8 minutes

   b. At least 11 hours of sleep per 24 hours, documented on a single 24-hour PSG or averaged across at least 7 days of actigraphic monitoring during ad lib sleep

5. Insufficient sleep is ruled out (including immediately before 24-hour PSG, if performed)

6. No other disorder or substance use better explains the symptoms

Abbreviations: MSLT, multiple sleep latency test; PSG, polysomnogram; REM, rapid eye movement.
   Data from International classification of sleep disorders. 3rd edition. Darien (IL): American Academy of Sleep Medicine; 2014.

type 1, patients with IH often do not benefit from prescribed or scheduled naps as part of their management.

Sleep inertia or sleep drunkenness

Patients with IH often demonstrate prolonged and pronounced difficulty with awakening from nocturnal sleep and daytime naps. This symptom is sometimes referred to as "sleep drunkenness," to distinguish it from the milder and physiologic state of sleep inertia seen even in healthy controls.[28] Sleep drunkenness occurs in nearly one-half of IH patients[28,29] and presents a clinical challenge because patients may have difficulty awakening enough to take their wake-promoting medications. Dosing of stimulant medications 1 hour before planned awakening (which often requires assistance from a family member), or even dosing of stimulants at bedtime, may be necessary to overcome this symptom.[28,30] Although not yet tested in a controlled fashion, melatonin at bedtime has been advocated for use in IH patients with sleep drunkenness[18,31]; this has had mixed results in our clinical experience but is a relatively low-risk intervention.

"Brain fog" and cognitive dysfunction

Subjective reports from patients with IH suggest that cognitive dysfunction is frequently present. Memory problems are reported by 79% of IH patients and attention problems by 55%. A feeling of one's mind going blank (58%) or making a mistake in a habitual activity (61%) are also reported commonly by IH patients, more so than by controls for all of these symptoms.[17] A small study suggests that cognitive symptoms in patients with IH may be sufficiently pronounced that 1 in 5 patients also meets criteria for attention deficit disorder.[32]

DIAGNOSTIC TESTING FOR IDIOPATHIC HYPERSOMNIA

The diagnosis of IH rests heavily on objective monitoring of sleep time and "sleepability" (ie, the speed with which people fall asleep when attempting to do so, on multiple sleep latency testing [MSLT]) (see **Box 1**). Previous versions of the ICSD have required an MSLT mean sleep latency of less than 8 minutes for the diagnosis of IH.[33] However, data have shown that it is common for patients with clinical diagnoses of IH to demonstrate mean sleep latencies longer than this 8 minute threshold,[4,18] including 71% of those with long sleep times.[18] Therefore, current ICSD criteria for IH also include an objectively measured sleep time of at least 660 minutes (by 24-hour polysomnography [PSG] or averaged across at least 1 week of actigraphy),

which can be used to confirm an IH diagnosis in patients with a mean sleep latency of greater than 8 minutes.[24] Whether or not the current criteria fully capture the spectrum of IH remains to be determined. Indeed, the ICSD-3 notes that there may be patients who meet all criteria for IH except the objective documentation criterion (ie, not meeting MSLT, 24-hour PSG, or actigraphy criteria), and that these patients may still be clinically considered to have IH, especially if other causes of symptoms have been excluded comprehensively.[24] Although this situation is reported to be rare by the ICSD-3, a prospective series of consecutive patients with a clinical diagnosis of IH found 29% (30/105) to have neither a mean sleep latency of less than 8 minutes nor at least 660 minutes of sleep during 24-hour monitoring.[18] In 100 consecutive patients evaluated for excessive daytime sleepiness, in whom psychiatric diagnoses, medication effects, insufficient sleep duration, and other sleep disorders had been excluded carefully, 33% had mean sleep latency of greater than 8 minutes; in 24-hour ad lib PSG of these 33 patients, mean sleep time was less than 500 minutes,[19] suggesting that many of these patients would remain excluded from a diagnosis under current criteria. Yet, those who did not meet IH diagnostic criteria were indistinguishable from those who did meet criteria on all measured sleep variables.[19]

Differential Diagnosis of Idiopathic Hypersomnia

Because sleepiness is a core feature of multiple disorders, because there is currently no validated biomarker that is diagnostic of IH, and because ancillary symptoms of IH can be seen in other disorders, the differential diagnosis of IH can be challenging. In some cases, for example, the differentiation between IH and insufficient sleep syndrome, careful attention to history and diagnostic testing can distinguish these disorders convincingly. In other cases, a diagnosis is rendered based on phenomenology and best clinical judgment, but important unanswered questions remain about pathophysiologic overlap. Differential diagnostic considerations include insufficient sleep syndrome, the narcolepsies, delayed sleep phase syndrome (DSPS), hypersomnia associated with a psychiatric disorder, and hypersomnia owing to a medical disorder.

Insufficient sleep syndrome versus idiopathic hypersomnia

Insufficient sleep duration can result in daytime sleepiness that mimics the sleepiness reported by patients with IH and that results in MSLT findings consistent with IH. However, the combination of clinical history, sleep logs, and actigraphic monitoring generally allows this diagnosis to be ruled in or out with a reasonable degree of certainty. Patients reporting sleepiness who are found to have insufficient sleep durations should be advised to extend sleep times to at least 8 hours, and then reassessed for resolution of sleepiness after several weeks on the new schedule.

The narcolepsies (types 1 and 2) versus idiopathic hypersomnia

Clinical features of IH and narcolepsy type 1 are fairly distinct: patients with IH do not have cataplexy, whereas patients with narcolepsy type 1 do; patients with IH have high sleep efficiency with few nocturnal awakenings, whereas patients with narcolepsy type 1 have fragmented nocturnal sleep; patients with IH have long and unrefreshing naps, whereas patients with narcolepsy type 1 generally find short naps to be restorative.

In contrast, the distinction between IH and narcolepsy type 2 can be considerably more difficult. Cataplexy is absent in both disorders. Other components of the "narcolepsy tetrad," namely, sleep paralysis and sleep-related hallucinations, are commonly seen in patients with narcolepsy type 2, but their presence in approximately one-quarter of IH patients prevents them from being useful features to rule out a diagnosis of IH (**Table 1**). Long sleep times may be present in narcolepsy type 2.[34] Sleep drunkenness, although relatively understudied in narcolepsy type 2 versus IH, seems to be about as common in both disorders.[28] Fragmented nocturnal sleep, although common in narcolepsy type 1, is no more common in narcolepsy type 2 patients than in IH patients (limited to those narcolepsy type 2 who were HLA DQB1*0602 negative in 1 study).[1,25,35] In cluster analysis (ie, independent of preexisting assumptions about diagnosis), symptoms and MSLT findings combined result in 3 clear clusters: a cluster of those with narcolepsy type 1, a cluster of those with IH and long sleep times, and a cluster containing both those with narcolepsy type 2 and IH without long sleep times.[36]

As a result of this symptom overlap, the differentiation between IH and narcolepsy type 2 rests entirely on the presence or absence of at least 2 sleep-onset rapid eye movement periods (SOREMs) on PSG/MSLT (with 0–1 SOREMs in patients with IH). In light of this, the limitations of the MSLT on this measure are particularly important. The test–retest reliability of multiple SOREMs in patients reporting problematic daytime sleepiness in the absence of cataplexy is relatively poor, with 31% of patients changing across the threshold of 2 or more SOREMs between 2 MSLTs.[37] This

Table 1
Features of the "narcolepsy tetrad" in patients with IH

Feature	Frequency in IH Patients
Daytime sleepiness	100% (by definition)
Cataplexy	0% (by definition)
Sleep paralysis[a]	
Bassetti & Aldrich,[16] 1997	17/42 (40%)
Anderson et al,[4] 2007	3/77 (4%)
Ali et al,[15] 2009	7/69 (10%)
Sasai et al,[5] 2009	13/59 (22%)
Vernet et al,[18] 2009	21/75 (28%)
Sasai-Sakuma et al,[25] 2015	114/395 (29%)
Sleep paralysis total	175/717 (24%)
Sleep-related hallucinations[a]	
Bassetti & Aldrich,[16] 1997	18/42 (43%)
Anderson et al,[4] 2007	4/77 (5%)
Ali et al,[15] 2009	3/66 (4%)
Sasai et al,[5] 2009	15/59 (25%)
Vernet & Arnulf,[18] 2009	18/75 (24%)
Sasai-Sakuma et al,[25] 2015	129/395 (33%)
Hallucinations total	187/714 (26%)

Abbreviation: IH, idiopathic hypersomnia.
[a] In series where only a percentage affected was reported (rather than the number affected), the number of affected patients was calculated assuming the total number of IH patients was used to generate the percentage (ie, could not account for the possibility of missing data).

finding is mirrored in the general population, in which the finding of multiple SOREMs has a kappa of only 0.1, that is, repeatability is only minimally higher than expected by chance alone.[38] At present, it is unknown if IH and narcolepsy type 2 are truly separate disorders, if they are the same disorder but seem to be distinct because of limitations of MSLT measurement, or if they may reflect a common pathophysiology occurring in people with different underlying rapid eye movement sleep propensity.

Delayed sleep phase syndrome versus idiopathic hypersomnia

In patients with delayed sleep phase syndrome, preferred circadian timing for sleep is later than what is optimal for functioning in society, for example, a person who will tend to sleep from 3 AM until 11 AM if able to do so absent external forces but must awaken for work at 8 AM. As a result of the misalignment between preferred circadian timing and external obligations, patients with DSPS are frequently sleep deprived and have substantial daytime sleepiness.

The difficulty in distinguishing IH from DSPS springs from several key issues. First, patients with DSPS frequently present with the combination of daytime sleepiness and sleep drunkenness, that is, a combination of symptoms classically seen in people with IH. In patients with DSPS, the etiology of sleep drunkenness is presumed to be the combination of chronic sleep deprivation (making it difficult to awaken because of increased homeostatic sleep pressure) and the circadian misalignment (making it difficult to awaken because the circadian drive is to sleep at the time of attempted awakening). Second, patients with IH are known to have a tendency toward a delayed sleep phase[18] and the presence of an evening chronotype in patients with IH increases their likelihood of displaying sleep drunkenness.[17] Recent work has shown that the amplitude of circadian clock gene expression over the circadian period is decreased in skin fibroblasts from IH patients compared with controls[39] and that patients with central disorders of hypersomnolence (including IH) are more likely than controls to have a polymorphism in circadian gene CRY1,[40] adding support to the hypothesis of altered circadian function as a key component of IH pathophysiology or symptomatology. Thus, the presence of sleep drunkenness cannot rule out DSPS and the presence of a delayed sleep schedule cannot rule out IH.

Sleepiness in patients with DSPS is thought to result from chronic sleep deprivation caused by attempting to function in a world that is out of alignment with the preferred phase. This implies that patients with DSPS who are allowed to sleep a sufficient duration of hours should have improvement in daytime sleepiness. As such, history, sleep logs, and actigraphy with ad lib sleep are very important in distinguishing these 2 disorders. A patient who cannot fall asleep until 3 AM and who is sleepy when sleeping from 3 to 8 AM but whose sleepiness resolves when allowed to sleep from 3 to 11 AM likely has DSPS alone, whereas a patient who routinely sleeps from 3 AM until 11 AM and is sleepy despite this may have both IH and a tendency toward a delayed sleep phase.

Hypersomnia associated with a psychiatric disorder versus idiopathic hypersomnia

One of the most challenging differential diagnostic considerations in IH is the entity of hypersomnia associated with a psychiatric disorder. Although the ICSD-3 explicitly refrains from assigning causality in the diagnosis, noting that hypersomnia "associated with" a psychiatric disorder may be more correct than hypersomnia "due to" a psychiatric disorder, criteria still require a judgment about whether the main diagnosis is IH (in which psychiatric disease may be comorbid) or whether it is primarily psychiatric. Both sets of criteria require the exclusion of the other disorder.[41] Current criteria suggest that this distinction may revolve around sleep quality and mean sleep latency test results,[24] although the specificity of these findings based on existing data has been questioned.[42]

Hypersomnia due to a medical disorder versus idiopathic hypersomnia

Certain medical and neurologic disorders are known to result in daytime sleepiness. Two well-characterized examples are Parkinson's disease and myotonic dystrophy.[43,44] In many cases, the comorbid medical disorder has already been diagnosed when a patient presents with excessive sleepiness, and the diagnosis of hypersomnia due to a medical disorder is made relatively easily. However, in some cases, sleepiness may present before the apparent onset of the other disorder, such that an index of suspicion for incident medical disorders should be maintained in patients with IH. This lag between onset of sleepiness and onset of other symptoms of a medical disorder is perhaps best described in patients with Parkinson's disease, in whom sleepiness is known to predict the subsequent onset of the movement disorder 4 to 12 years later.[45–47]

Other medical conditions are also implicated in causing sleepiness, with varying levels of evidence. Our routine laboratory screen (in addition to a comprehensive history) for such disorders in patients being evaluated for IH includes a complete blood count, full iron panel (iron, total iron binding capacity, percent saturation, and ferritin), vitamin B_{12}, thyroid-stimulating hormone (with additional thyroid testing if this results in the high-normal or high range), and free and total carnitine.

Although the treatment of some of medical conditions associated with hypersomnolence results in improvement in sleepiness, it is important to keep in mind that this is not always the case. For example, the treatment of Parkinson's disease patients with dopamine agonists may worsen, rather than lessen, daytime sleepiness.[48,49] In these cases, management of sleepiness may be an important, but separate, clinical goal. **Table 2** summarizes the clinical features in IH and these disorders with similar symptoms.

Table 2
Clinical features and differential diagnosis of IH

	IH	NT2	ISS	DSPS	Psychiatric	Medical
Sleepiness	Present	Present	Present	Present	Present	Present
Long sleep times	Frequently	May be present	Absent by definition	Absent if allowed to habitually sleep at preferred schedule[24]	May be present, although distinction between time asleep and time in bed may be important[61]	May be present
Sleep inertia	Frequently present	Frequently present (based on small series)	Limited data	Commonly present	Commonly present[62–64]	Limited data
Depressive or other mood symptoms	May be present	May be present	May be present as a consequence of chronic short sleep[24]	May be present[24]	Present by definition	May be present (eg, Parkinson's disease)
Mean sleep latency on MSLT	<8 min by definition (if MSLT criteria are used for diagnosis)	<8 min by definition	May be decreased[24]; short sleep increases likelihood of MSL <8 min with 2+ SOREMs[38]	Limited data; sleep latencies may increase over the course of the day[65]	<8 min in 25% of patient with psychiatric hypersomnolence[42]	PD: wide-ranging estimates for MSL across studies; 20%–24% of PD patients unselected for sleepiness have MSL <8 min[66] MD: wide-ranging estimates across studies; 13%–92% have MSL <8 min (generally higher in those reporting EDS)[67]
Sleep onset REM periods on PSG/MSLT	0–1 by definition	≥2 by definition	≥2 may occur[24]; short sleep increases likelihood of mean sleep latency <8 min with 2+ SOREMs[38]	Limited data	Seem to be rare; 2+ SOREMs reported in 2/25 patients with bipolar and hypersomnolence; other studies have reported no SOREMs in patients with psychiatric hypersomnia[42]	PD: Up to one-third of sleepy PD patients have ≥2 SOREMs[66] MD: ≥2 SOREMs in 33%–60% of sleepy MD patients and 25%–35% of MD patients unselected for EDS[67]

Abbreviations: DSPS, delayed sleep phase syndrome; EDS, excessive daytime sleepiness; IH, idiopathic hypersomnia; ISS, insufficient sleep syndrome; MD, myotonic dystrophy; Medical, hypersomnolence owing to a medical disorder; MSL, mean sleep latency; MSLT, multiple sleep latency test; NT2, narcolepsy type 2; PD, Parkinson's disease; PSG, polysomnography; Psychiatric, hypersomnolence associated with a psychiatric disorder; REM, rapid eye movement; SOREM, sleep-onset REM period.

NONPHARMACOLOGIC TREATMENT OPTIONS

Quality of life and daytime functioning can be profoundly affected in patients with IH, even after treatment.[50–52] Although the distinction between IH with mood dysfunction and hypersomnia associated with a psychiatric disorder can be challenging,[41] symptoms of depression are encountered commonly in people with IH and may add to the burden of disease.[52] In light of these factors, increasing attention has recently been paid to the possible role of nonpharmacologic therapy as adjunct treatment in patients with IH.[52] The vast majority of IH patients (96.1%) endorse using at least 1 nonpharmacologic strategy for management of their illness.[52] The most commonly used nonpharmacologic strategies include caffeine (endorsed by 82.2% of IH patients), daytime naps (81.4%), and scheduling of nocturnal sleep (75.2%). Yet, the effectiveness of nonpharmacologic strategies for IH, on a 1 to 10 scale where 10 is most effective, is universally rated as poor. Most effective were caffeine (only 3.3 ± 2.6 out of 10), nicotine (3.2 ± 2.9 out of 10), and scheduled nocturnal sleep (3.0 ± 2.3 out of 10); daytime naps, exercise, diet, temperature manipulations, chewing gum, mindfulness, and yoga all received numerically lower scores.[52] Patients with IH reported nearly all interventions as less effective than did patients with narcolepsy in the same study.

Safety counseling is an important nonpharmacologic aspect of the clinical care of patients with IH, just as it is in patients with narcolepsy.[53] Such counseling revolves around 2 key issues: (1) medication side effects or interactions and (2) driving and other safety-critical activities. Routine treatment of IH patients raises several potential medication concerns. First, amphetamines carry "black box" warnings regarding their potential for abuse, dependence, drug diversion, and cardiovascular side effects. Second, modafinil and armodafinil may interfere with the effectiveness of hormonal birth control. Patients with central disorders of hypersomnolence, including IH, also have an increased risk of motor vehicle accidents[54] and treatment may not fully abolish this risk.[55] Other safety-critical tasks (eg, use of heavy machinery, power tools) may be compromised in some patients. Performance on maintenance of wakefulness testing (MWT) predicts on-road driving performance in patients with IH and narcolepsy,[55,56] and may be useful to guide decision making, when available.

As with other chronic diseases, support groups and patient advocacy groups may be beneficial. Education regarding the availability of local, national, and online resources (eg, the Hypersomnia Foundation, www.hypersomniafoundation.org) should be part of patient counseling when appropriate.

Spontaneous remission of IH has been reported to occur in approximately 20% of cases in which this measure is reported (**Table 3**), but factors that predict such remission remain incompletely defined.

PHARMACOLOGIC TREATMENT OPTIONS

There are currently no medications approved by the US Food and Drug Administration specifically for the treatment of IH and, until relatively recently, there were no published, randomized, controlled trials (RCTs) of any treatment for IH. The most recent practice parameter from the American Academy of Sleep Medicine, which was published in 2007 before the publication of the first 3 RCTs of IH, recommended modafinil as an option for the treatment of IH,[57] based on an open-label clinical series showing reduction in drowsiness and sleep attacks in 15 IH patients.[58] Other medications recommended in this practice parameter, based on their beneficial effects on sleepiness in patients with narcolepsy but absence of data in patients with IH, were amphetamine, methamphetamine, dextroamphetamine, and methylphenidate.[57] Clinical series of IH patients treated with these medications are found in **Table 4**.

The first RCT to include patients with IH was published in 2014.[55] This crossover trial compared modafinil (400 mg, divided into 2 doses) and

Table 3
Spontaneous remission rates in idiopathic hypersomnia

Study	Sample Size	Remission Rate (%)	Time Period
Kim et al,[68] 2016	24	32.5	5.5 y after diagnosis
Anderson et al,[4] 2007	77	14	Followed ≥1 y
Bassetti & Aldrich,[16] 1997	35	25.7	Followed ≥1 y
Total	136	20.3	—

Table 4
Modafinil and traditional psychostimulants for IH treatment: case series

	Sample Size with IH	Response Rate	Duration of Follow-up
Modafinil			
Lavault et al,[60] 2011	n = 104 prescribed modafinil (monotherapy in 96.1%); mean max dose 318 ± 192 mg	Major to moderate improvement in 67/75 patients with CGI data available	4.0 ± 5.0 y
Ali et al,[15] 2009	n = 50 prescribed modafinil; mean daily dose 367.4 ± 140.9 mg	25/50 remained on modafinil at EOM 18/25 complete symptom relief	Median 2.4 y (4.7 IQR)
Anderson et al,[4] 2007	n = 54 initially prescribed modafinil; mean daily dose 400 mg (range, 100–1000 mg)	39/54 remained on modafinil monotherapy 24/39 responders	3.8 ± 2.1 y
Bastuji & Jouvet,[58] 1988	n = 18 prescribed modafinil monotherapy; dose range 200–500 mg/d	83% improved; 11% lost to follow-up; 6% discontinued for side effects	2 mo
Modafinil total	n = 226	124/197 (63%) remained on modafinil with good response	—
Methylphenidate			
Ali et al,[15] 2009	n = 61 prescribed methylphenidate; mean daily dose 50.9 ± 27.3 mg	40/61 remained on methylphenidate at EOM 25/40 complete symptom relief 41% remained on methylphenidate with complete response	Median 2.4 y (4.7 IQR)
Amphetamine-dextroamphetamine			
Ali et al,[15] 2009	n = 8 prescribed amphetamine-dextroamphetamine; mean daily dose 79.3 ± 30.6 mg[a]	4/8 remained on amphetamine-dextroamphetamine at EOM 2/4 complete response 25% remained on amphetamine-dextroamphetamine with complete response	Median 2.4 y (4.7 IQR)
Dextroamphetamine			
Ali et al,[15] 2009	n = 7 prescribed dextroamphetamine; mean daily dose 35.7 ± 44.4 mg	2/7 remained on dextroamphetamine monotherapy, both poor responders	Median 2.4 y (4.7 IQR)
Anderson et al,[4] 2007	n = 8 prescribed dextroamphetamine monotherapy; mean daily dose 30 mg	5/8 responders	3.8 ± 2.1 y
Dextroamphetamine Total	n = 15	5/15 (33%) responded to dextroamphetamine	—

None of these medications are approved for use in idiopathic hypersomnia by the US Food and Drug Administration.
Abbreviations: CGI, clinical global impression; EOM, end of monitoring; IH, idiopathic hypersomnia; IQR, interquartile range.
[a] Maximum Food and Drug Administration recommended dose for amphetamine-dextroamphetamine for use in narcolepsy is 60 mg/d.

Table 5
Treatment options for treatment-refractory IH

Class and Medications	Dosage	Level of Evidence for Use in IH	Availability	Side Effects/Other Considerations
GABA-A receptor antagonists/negative modulators				
Clarithromycin[13,69]	500 mg with breakfast and lunch; up to 1000 mg bid in some cases	One cross-over RCT showing improvement in subjective sleepiness vs placebo; included 10 IH patients (of 20 total subjects); clinical series of treatment-refractory patients (25 IH patients of 53 total) showed benefit in 64%, with 38% of patients continuing therapy	Widespread	Antibiotic resistance, superinfection, taste perversion, GI symptoms
Flumazenil[14]	Transdermal cream or sublingual lozenges	Clinical series of treatment-refractory patients (36 IH patients of 153 total) demonstrated benefit in 63%, with 39% continuing therapy	Must be compounded; limited	Long-term effects not fully known; seizures and arrhythmias known to occur with intravenous use
GABA-B/gamma-hydroxybutyrate agonists				
Sodium oxybate[70]	Titrated up to 4.5 g twice nightly (separated by 2.5–4.0 h); mean dose in IH patients 4.3 g/night; lower than in patients with NT1	Clinical series of treatment-refractory patients (comparing 46 IH patients to 47 patients with NT1) demonstrated mean ESS decrease of 3.5 ± 4.5 points, but with 53% dropout rate	Within United States, must be dispensed by centralized pharmacy under FDA REMS program	Black box warnings for central nervous system depression, respiratory depression, and abuse; drug diversion possibility (sodium salt of gamma-hydroxybutyrate)
Histaminergic				
Pitolisant[71]	5–50 mg/d, taken once in the morning	Clinical series of treatment-refractory patients (including 65 IH patients of 78 total) demonstrating 36% responder rate and 37% continuing therapy	Not available in United States for any indication; EMA authorization for use in narcolepsy	GI symptoms, weight gain, insomnia, headache seen in >10% of hypersomnia patients

(continued on next page)

Table 5
(continued)

Class and Medications	Dosage	Level of Evidence for Use in IH	Availability	Side Effects/Other Considerations
Miscellaneous				
Mazindol, a nonamphetamine stimulant[72]	1–6 mg/d, average 3.6 ± 1.2 mg	Clinical series of treatment-refractory patients (including 37 IH patients of 139 total) demonstrated 4.8 point reduction in ESS; 84% of IH group continued therapy	Not available in the United States for any indication; EMA orphan designation	Echocardiogram recently required but no valvulopathy or pulmonary hypertension in the 45 patients studied; QT prolongation, dry mouth, palpitations, ventricular hyperexcitability, anorexia, nervousness, headaches
Levothyroxine[73]	25 µg/d	Clinical series of 9 previously untreated IH patients (with normal thyroid function) demonstrated reduction in sleep time from 12.9 to 8.5 h and reduction of 5.5 points on ESS at 8 wk	Widespread	None seen in Ref.[73]; known serious effects include arrhythmias, heart failure, hypertension, angina, and seizures
Transcranial direct current stimulation[74]	3 stimulations per week × 4 wk, performed between 8 and 11 AM to avoid disturbing nocturnal sleep	Pilot study of 8 previously untreated IH patients showed 5.75 point decrease in ESS, 7/8 reporting improvement in sleepiness, and improvements in reaction times on attention test	Limited	Not reported in Ref.[74]; headache, sensory discomfort, and skin burns may occur[75]

None of these treatments are approved by the US FDA for the treatment of IH. Some of these medications (ie, pitolisant, mazindol) are not approved by the US FDA for any indication.

Abbreviations: EMA, European Medications Agency; ESS, Epworth Sleepiness Scale; FDA, Food and Drug Administration; REMS, Risk Evaluation and Mitigation Strategy; GABA, gamma-aminobutyric acid; GI, gastrointestinal; IH, idiopathic hypersomnia; NT1, narcolepsy type 1; RCT, randomized, controlled trial.

placebo on the ability to maintain wakefulness on MWT and driving performance on an on-road driving test. Fourteen patients with IH were included in the total sample of 27 patients. Use of modafinil significantly decreased inappropriate line crossings on the driving test, that is, it improved driving safety, compared with placebo, but did not normalize performance to that of controls. Similarly, modafinil improved ability to maintain wakefulness on MWT, but treated patients remained significantly sleepier than controls.[55]

In an parallel group RCT including 33 IH patients (without long sleep time per ICSD-2 criteria), modafinil (200 mg, divided into 2 doses) decreased subjective sleepiness measured with Epworth Sleepiness Scale scores compared with placebo. Differences in MWT between modafinil and placebo were not significant, although the modafinil group had significant improvements in maintenance of wakefulness compared with their own baseline.[59]

TREATMENT RESISTANCE

Clinical series of IH patients reveal that many patients do well with monotherapy, but approximately one-quarter of patients have treatment-resistant symptoms despite use of standard therapies. In a series of 85 IH patients (by ICSD-2 criteria), 58% required only 1 treatment for their symptoms, and 65% of patients were ultimately able to achieve complete control of symptoms.[15] An additional 26% had partial relief of symptoms, with 9% demonstrating a poor response. In another series, using somewhat less stringent diagnostic criteria, 18 of 25 patients (72%) demonstrated satisfactory symptom control with unspecified stimulant use.[16] Among 54 patients meeting ICSD-2 criteria other than MSLT mean sleep latency, 32 (61%) were considered responders to monotherapy or combined therapy.[4] Considering only modafinil, response rates of 83% (n = 18)[58] and 89.3% (for at least moderate improvement, n = 75)[60] have been reported. In an Internet survey of 129 patients self-reporting a diagnosis of IH, medication effectiveness was rated only 5.4 out of 10 (±1.9, where 10 is most effective), significantly lower than effectiveness rated by patients with narcolepsy in the same survey.[52] Across the entire hypersomnolent group (ie, people with either type of narcolepsy or IH), medication side effects prevented consistent use of pharmacotherapy for excessive daytime sleepiness in 23% of patients.[52]

In cases with treatment-refractory sleepiness or intolerance to standard treatments, alternate pharmacologic strategies are needed. A number of different classes of medications have been proposed for the treatment of IH, including GABA-A receptor antagonists/negative modulators (clarithromycin and flumazenil), GABA-B/gamma hydroxybutyrate receptor agonists, histamine H3 inverse agonists, levothyroxine, nonamphetamine stimulants, and transcranial direct stimulation (**Table 5**). Of these interventions, only clarithromycin has been evaluated in an RCT including patients with IH.[13] In this study, clarithromycin 500 mg taken with breakfast and lunch resulted in a significant improvement in Epworth Sleepiness Scale scores and other subjective measures of IH symptoms, but did not improve psychomotor vigilance.[13]

SUMMARY

IH causes severe daytime sleepiness and impairs quality of life. Currently available medications insufficiently control symptoms in a substantial proportion of patients. Although recent work has provided clinicians with some direction in terms of pharmacologic and nonpharmacologic strategies, much work remains to be done. In particular, a clear knowledge of IH pathophysiology has the potential to open new avenues for the targeted, and more effective, treatments that are urgently needed.

REFERENCES

1. Takei Y, Komada Y, Namba K, et al. Differences in findings of nocturnal polysomnography and multiple sleep latency test between narcolepsy and idiopathic hypersomnia. Clin Neurophysiol 2012; 123(1):137–41.
2. Bassetti C, Gugger M, Bischof M, et al. The narcoleptic borderland: a multimodal diagnostic approach including cerebrospinal fluid levels of hypocretin-1 (orexin A). Sleep Med 2003;4(1):7–12.
3. Pizza F, Vandi S, Detto S, et al. Different sleep onset criteria at the multiple sleep latency test (MSLT): an additional marker to differentiate central nervous system (CNS) hypersomnias. J Sleep Res 2011; 20(1 Pt 2):250–6.
4. Anderson KN, Pilsworth S, Sharples LD, et al. Idiopathic hypersomnia: a study of 77 cases. Sleep 2007;30(10):1274–81.
5. Sasai T, Inoue Y, Komada Y, et al. Comparison of clinical characteristics among narcolepsy with and without cataplexy and idiopathic hypersomnia without long sleep time, focusing on HLA-DRB1(*) 1501/DQB1(*)0602 finding. Sleep Med 2009;10(9): 961–6.
6. Ohayon MM, Reynolds CF 3rd, Dauvilliers Y. Excessive sleep duration and quality of life. Ann Neurol 2013;73(6):785–94.

7. Mignot E, Lammers GJ, Ripley B, et al. The role of cerebrospinal fluid hypocretin measurement in the diagnosis of narcolepsy and other hypersomnias. Arch Neurol 2002;59(10):1553–62.

8. Rye DB, Bliwise DL, Parker K, et al. Modulation of vigilance in the primary hypersomnias by endogenous enhancement of GABAA receptors. Sci Transl Med 2012;4(161):161ra51.

9. Franks NP. General anaesthesia: from molecular targets to neuronal pathways of sleep and arousal. Nat Rev Neurosci 2008;9(5):370–86.

10. Franks NP, Zecharia AY. Sleep and general anesthesia. Can J Anaesth 2011;58(2):139–48.

11. Rudolph U, Knoflach F. Beyond classical benzodiazepines: novel therapeutic potential of GABAA receptor subtypes. Nat Rev Drug Discov 2011;10(9):685–97.

12. Lu J, Greco MA. Sleep circuitry and the hypnotic mechanism of GABAA drugs. J Clin Sleep Med 2006;2(2):S19–26.

13. Trotti LM, Saini P, Bliwise DL, et al. Clarithromycin in gamma-aminobutyric acid-Related hypersomnolence: a randomized, crossover trial. Ann Neurol 2015;78(3):454–65.

14. Trotti LM, Saini P, Koola C, et al. Flumazenil for the treatment of refractory hypersomnolence: clinical experience with 153 patients. J Clin Sleep Med 2016;12(10):1389–94.

15. Ali M, Auger RR, Slocumb NL, et al. Idiopathic hypersomnia: clinical features and response to treatment. J Clin Sleep Med 2009;5(6):562–8.

16. Bassetti C, Aldrich MS. Idiopathic hypersomnia. A series of 42 patients. Brain 1997;120(8):1423–35.

17. Vernet C, Leu-Semenescu S, Buzare MA, et al. Subjective symptoms in idiopathic hypersomnia: beyond excessive sleepiness. J Sleep Res 2010;19(4):525–34.

18. Vernet C, Arnulf I. Idiopathic hypersomnia with and without long sleep time: a controlled series of 75 patients. Sleep 2009;32(6):753–9.

19. Pizza F, Moghadam KK, Vandi S, et al. Daytime continuous polysomnography predicts MSLT results in hypersomnias of central origin. J Sleep Res 2013;22(1):32–40.

20. Miyagawa T, Toyoda H, Kanbayashi T, et al. An association analysis of HLA-DQB1 with narcolepsy without cataplexy and idiopathic hypersomnia with/without long sleep time in a Japanese population. Hum Genome Var 2015;2:15031.

21. Barateau L, Lopez R, Arnulf I, et al. Comorbidity between central disorders of hypersomnolence and immune-based disorders. Neurology 2017;88(1):93–100.

22. Tanaka S, Honda M. IgG abnormality in narcolepsy and idiopathic hypersomnia. PLoS One 2010;5(3):e9555.

23. Sforza E, Roche F, Barthelemy JC, et al. Diurnal and nocturnal cardiovascular variability and heart rate arousal response in idiopathic hypersomnia. Sleep Med 2016;24:131–6.

24. International classification of sleep disorders. 3rd edition. Darien (IL): American Academy of Sleep Medicine; 2014.

25. Sasai-Sakuma T, Kinoshita A, Inoue Y. Polysomnographic assessment of sleep comorbidities in drug-naive narcolepsy-spectrum disorders–a Japanese cross-sectional study. PLoS One 2015;10(8):e0136988.

26. Pizza F, Ferri R, Poli F, et al. Polysomnographic study of nocturnal sleep in idiopathic hypersomnia without long sleep time. J Sleep Res 2013;22(2):185–96.

27. Delrosso LM, Chesson AL, Hoque R. Manual characterization of sleep spindle index in patients with narcolepsy and idiopathic hypersomnia. Sleep Disord 2014;2014:271802.

28. Trotti LM. Waking up is the hardest thing I do all day: sleep inertia and sleep drunkenness. Sleep Med Rev 2016. [Epub ahead of print]. http://dx.doi.org/10.1016/j.smrv.2016.08.005.

29. Kretzschmar U, Werth E, Sturzenegger C, et al. Which diagnostic findings in disorders with excessive daytime sleepiness are really helpful? A retrospective study. J Sleep Res 2016;25(3):307–13.

30. Roth B, Nevsimalova S, Rechtschaffen A. Hypersomnia with "sleep drunkenness". Arch Gen Psychiatry 1972;26(5):456–62.

31. Montplaisir J, Fantini L. Idiopathic hypersomnia: a diagnostic dilemma. A commentary of "idiopathic hypersomnia" (M. Billiard and Y. Dauvilliers). Sleep Med Rev 2001;5(5):361–2.

32. Oosterloo M, Lammers GJ, Overeem S, et al. Possible confusion between primary hypersomnia and adult attention-deficit/hyperactivity disorder. Psychiatry Res 2006;143(2–3):293–7.

33. International classification of sleep disorders: diagnostic and coding manual. 2nd edition. Darien (IL): American Academy of Sleep Medicine; 2005.

34. Vernet C, Arnulf I. Narcolepsy with long sleep time: a specific entity? Sleep 2009;32(9):1229–35.

35. Sasai-Sakuma T, Inoue Y. Differences in electroencephalographic findings among categories of narcolepsy-spectrum disorders. Sleep Med 2015;16(8):999–1005.

36. Sonka K, Susta M, Billiard M. Narcolepsy with and without cataplexy, idiopathic hypersomnia with and without long sleep time: a cluster analysis. Sleep Med 2015;16(2):225–31.

37. Trotti LM, Staab BA, Rye DB. Test-retest reliability of the multiple sleep latency test in narcolepsy without cataplexy and idiopathic hypersomnia. J Clin Sleep Med 2013;9(8):789–95.

38. Goldbart A, Peppard P, Finn L, et al. Narcolepsy and predictors of positive MSLTs in the Wisconsin sleep cohort. Sleep 2014;37(6):1043–51.

39. Lippert J, Halfter H, Heidbreder A, et al. Altered dynamics in the circadian oscillation of clock

genes in dermal fibroblasts of patients suffering from idiopathic hypersomnia. PLoS One 2014; 9(1):e85255.

40. Schirmacher A, Hor H, Heidbreder A, et al. Sequence variants in circadian rhythmic genes in a cohort of patients suffering from hypersomnia of central origin. Biol Rhythm Res 2011;42(5):407–16.

41. Trotti LM. Another strike against sleepability. J Clin Sleep Med 2016;12(4):467–8.

42. Plante DT. Sleep propensity in psychiatric hypersomnolence: a systematic review and meta-analysis of multiple sleep latency test findings. Sleep Med Rev 2017;31:48–57.

43. Chahine LM, Amara AW, Videnovic A. A systematic review of the literature on disorders of sleep and wakefulness in Parkinson's disease from 2005 to 2015. Sleep Med Rev 2016. [Epub ahead of print]. http://dx.doi.org/10.1016/j.smrv.2016.08.001.

44. Laberge L, Gagnon C, Dauvilliers Y. Daytime sleepiness and myotonic dystrophy. Curr Neurol Neurosci Rep 2013;13(4):340.

45. Gao J, Huang X, Park Y, et al. Daytime napping, nighttime sleeping, and Parkinson disease. Am J Epidemiol 2011;173(9):1032–8.

46. Chen H, Schernhammer E, Schwarzschild MA, et al. A prospective study of night shift work, sleep duration, and risk of Parkinson's disease. Am J Epidemiol 2006;163(8):726–30.

47. Abbott RD, Ross GW, White LR, et al. Excessive daytime sleepiness and subsequent development of Parkinson disease. Neurology 2005;65(9):1442–6.

48. Bliwise DL, Trotti LM, Wilson AG, et al. Daytime alertness in Parkinson's disease: potentially dose-dependent, divergent effects by drug class. Mov Disord 2012;27(9):1118–24.

49. Trotti LM, Bliwise DL. Treatment of the sleep disorders associated with Parkinson's disease. Neurotherapeutics 2014;11(1):68–77.

50. Avis KT, Shen J, Weaver P, et al. Psychosocial characteristics of children with central disorders of hypersomnolence versus matched healthy children. J Clin Sleep Med 2015;11(11):1281–8.

51. Ozaki A, Inoue Y, Hayashida K, et al. Quality of life in patients with narcolepsy with cataplexy, narcolepsy without cataplexy, and idiopathic hypersomnia without long sleep time: comparison between patients on psychostimulants, drug-naive patients and the general Japanese population. Sleep Med 2012;13(2):200–6.

52. Neikrug AB, Crawford MR, Ong JC. Behavioral sleep medicine services for hypersomnia disorders: a survey study. Behav Sleep Med 2017; 15(2):158–71.

53. Krahn LE, Hershner S, Loeding LD, et al. Quality measures for the care of patients with narcolepsy. J Clin Sleep Med 2015;11(3):335.

54. Pizza F, Jaussent I, Lopez R, et al. Car crashes and central disorders of hypersomnolence: a French study. PLoS One 2015;10(6):e0129386.

55. Philip P, Chaufton C, Taillard J, et al. Modafinil improves real driving performance in patients with hypersomnia: a randomized double-blind placebo-controlled crossover clinical trial. Sleep 2014;37(3): 483–7.

56. Philip P, Chaufton C, Taillard J, et al. Maintenance of wakefulness test scores and driving performance in sleep disorder patients and controls. Int J Psychophysiol 2013;89(2):195–202.

57. Morgenthaler TI, Kapur VK, Brown T, et al. Practice parameters for the treatment of narcolepsy and other hypersomnias of central origin. Sleep 2007; 30(12):1705–11.

58. Bastuji H, Jouvet M. Successful treatment of idiopathic hypersomnia and narcolepsy with modafinil. Prog Neuropsychopharmacol Biol Psychiatry 1988; 12(5):695–700.

59. Mayer G, Benes H, Young P, et al. Modafinil in the treatment of idiopathic hypersomnia without long sleep time-a randomized, double-blind, placebo-controlled study. J Sleep Res 2015;24(1): 74–81.

60. Lavault S, Dauvilliers Y, Drouot X, et al. Benefit and risk of modafinil in idiopathic hypersomnia vs. narcolepsy with cataplexy. Sleep Med 2011; 12(6):550–6.

61. Plante DT, Finn LA, Hagen EW, et al. Subjective and objective measures of hypersomnolence demonstrate divergent associations with depression among participants in the Wisconsin sleep cohort study. J Clin Sleep Med 2016;12(4):571–8.

62. Ritter PS, Marx C, Lewtschenko N, et al. The characteristics of sleep in patients with manifest bipolar disorder, subjects at high risk of developing the disease and healthy controls. J Neural Transm (Vienna) 2012;119(10):1173–84.

63. Kanady JC, Harvey AG. Development and validation of the Sleep Inertia Questionnaire (SIQ) and assessment of sleep inertia in analogue and clinical depression. Cognit Ther Res 2015;39(5):601–12.

64. Cassano GB, Benvenuti A, Miniati M, et al. The factor structure of lifetime depressive spectrum in patients with unipolar depression. J Affect Disord 2009;115(1–2):87–99.

65. Thorpy MJ, Korman E, Spielman AJ, et al. Delayed sleep phase syndrome in adolescents. J Adolesc Health Care 1988;9(1):22–7.

66. Ataide M, Franco CM, Lins OG. Daytime sleepiness and Parkinson's disease: the contribution of the multiple sleep latency test. Sleep Disord 2014;2014: 767181.

67. Dauvilliers YA, Laberge L. Myotonic dystrophy type 1, daytime sleepiness and REM sleep dysregulation. Sleep Med Rev 2012;16(6):539–45.

68. Kim T, Lee JH, Lee CS, et al. Different fates of excessive daytime sleepiness: survival analysis for remission. Acta Neurol Scand 2016;134(1):35–41.

69. Trotti LM, Saini P, Freeman AA, et al. Improvement in daytime sleepiness with clarithromycin in patients with GABA-related hypersomnia: clinical experience. J Psychopharmacol 2013;28(7):697–702.

70. Leu-Semenescu S, Louis P, Arnulf I. Benefits and risk of sodium oxybate in idiopathic hypersomnia versus narcolepsy type 1: a chart review. Sleep Med 2016;17:38–44.

71. Leu-Semenescu S, Nittur N, Golmard JL, et al. Effects of pitolisant, a histamine H3 inverse agonist, in drug-resistant idiopathic and symptomatic hypersomnia: a chart review. Sleep Med 2014; 15(6):681–7.

72. Nittur N, Konofal E, Dauvilliers Y, et al. Mazindol in narcolepsy and idiopathic and symptomatic hypersomnia refractory to stimulants: a long-term chart review. Sleep Med 2013;14(1):30–6.

73. Shinno H, Ishikawa I, Yamanaka M, et al. Effect of levothyroxine on prolonged nocturnal sleep time and excessive daytime somnolence in patients with idiopathic hypersomnia. Sleep Med 2011; 12(6):578–83.

74. Galbiati A, Abutalebi J, Iannaccone S, et al. The effects of transcranial direct current stimulation (tDCS) on idiopathic hypersomnia: a pilot study. Arch Ital Biol 2016;154(1):1–5.

75. Lefaucheur JP, Antal A, Ayache SS, et al. Evidence-based guidelines on the therapeutic use of transcranial direct current stimulation (tDCS). Clin Neurophysiol 2017;128(1):56–92.

The "Known Unknowns" of Kleine-Levin Syndrome
A Review and Future Prospects

Saad M. Al Suwayri, MD, MHPE, SBIM[a],
Ahmed S. BaHammam, MD, FRCP[b],*

KEYWORDS

- Kleine-Levin syndrome • Autoimmunity • Biomarker • Hypersomnia • Sleep disorder

KEY POINTS

- Kleine-Levin syndrome (KLS) is a debilitating sleep disorder of unknown etiology and limited treatment options are available.
- The published literature mainly comprises case reports and small clinical series with no clinical trials that have been conducted to date.
- Our review identifies KLS immunopathogenesis, next-generation genetics, multimodal functional imaging, and clinical drug trials as important knowledge gaps.
- A centralized registry of afflicted individuals must be established with a biorepository to facilitate clinical research.

INTRODUCTION

Kleine-Levin syndrome (KLS) is a rare, relapsing–remitting, debilitating sleep disorder that primarily affects adolescents.[1] Patients with KLS experience an alternating pattern of major hypersomnia lasting 1 to a few weeks accompanied by cognitive, behavioral, and psychiatric disturbances and periods of normalcy.[1] Kleine first described 2 adolescent boys with recurrent hypersomnia, hyperphagia, and cognitive disturbance in 1925,[2] with Lewis (1926)[3] and Levin (1929)[4] describing similar cases not long after. In their description of 2 naval personnel with periodic somnolence and "morbid hunger" in 1942, Critchley and Hoffmann coined the eponymous Kleine-Levin syndrome.[5]

Since then, and despite its rarity at only approximately 2 cases per million in Western populations,[6] numerous KLS cases and case series have been described in the literature, and readers are referred to the many excellent recent reviews on KLS[1,7–13] that include very useful clinical practice reviews.[14] For this reason, the clinical details and symptoms of KLS are not discussed here (**Box 1**) presents the clinical characteristics of KLS. Instead, to clarify recommendations on avenues for future clinical research on KLS, herein we systematically review the following 3 areas of importance in KLS that are not as well-documented in the literature: genetics studies, functional imaging studies, and biochemical studies. In doing so, we identify 5 "known unknowns" and make suggestions and recommendations for future research in these areas, not least is the establishment of a multinational registry to coordinate

Disclosure statement: The authors have nothing to disclose.
[a] Department of Internal Medicine, College of Medicine, Al Imam Mohammad Ibn Saud Islamic University (IMSIU), PO Box 7544, Othman bin Afan Road, Riyadh, Saudi Arabia; [b] University Sleep Disorders Center, Department of Medicine, College of Medicine, King Saud University, Box 225503, Riyadh 11324, Saudi Arabia
* Corresponding author.
E-mail addresses: ashammam2@gmail.com; ashammam@ksu.edu.sa

Box 1
Clinical characteristics of Kleine-Levin syndrome

- Periodic hypersomnia
- Depersonalization, derealization, and aggression
- Sensory disturbances
- Compulsive hyperphagia
- Disinhibition and hypersexuality, which are more common among men
- Apathy during the attack
- Most patients do not recall the episodes
- Attacks are usually triggered by infection, fever, sleep deprivation, menses, alcohol intake, vaccination, and head trauma
- Usually, attacks last between 1 and 3 weeks, with recurrence every few months (usually, occur every 2–3 months)
- Usually, the frequency and severity of attacks decrease as the patient gets older

clinical trials and a biorepository to facilitate translational research.

SEARCH STRATEGY

The PubMed database was searched to September 2016 for all articles on KLS using the following search terms: "Kleine-Levin syndrome"[-MeSH Terms] OR ("kleine-levin"[All Fields] AND "syndrome"[All Fields]) OR "kleine-levin syndrome"[All Fields] OR ("Kleine"[All Fields] AND "Levin"[All Fields] AND "syndrome"[All Fields]) OR "Kleine Levin syndrome"[All Fields]. We identified 373 in total, 286 of which were in English. These articles were reviewed for relevance to the topics of KLS genetics, functional imaging, and biochemistry (cerebrospinal fluid [CSF] and serum) and, in total, 79 studies were included in this review.

SYMPTOMS AND DEFINITION

In a recent update,[15] the latest *International Classification of Sleep Disorders* (3rd Edition; ICSD-3[16]) places KLS as a subcategory of central disorders of hypersomnolence. The diagnostic criteria for KLS changed little from ICSD-2 to ICSD-3, but the historic term Kleine-Levin syndrome was preferred to recurrent hypersomnia, because the condition is extremely homogeneous in presentation and features and, as such, the eponymous title remains. The ICDS-2 menstrual-related hypersomnia now appears as a subtype of KLS. With this in mind, KLS is defined as follows:

A. The patient experiences at least 2 recurrent episodes of excessive sleepiness and sleep duration, each persisting for 2 days to 5 weeks;
B. Episodes recur usually more than once a year and at least once every 18 months;
C. The patient has normal alertness, cognitive function, behavior, and mood between episodes;
D. The patient must demonstrate at least one of the following during episodes:
   1. Cognitive dysfunction,
   2. Altered perception,
   3. Eating disorder, or
   4. Disinhibited behavior.
E. The hypersomnolence and related symptoms are not better explained by another sleep disorder; other medical, neurologic, or psychiatric disorders (especially bipolar disorder); or the use of drugs or medications. All the criteria must be met to diagnose an individual with KLS.

THE ETIOLOGY AND GENETICS OF KLEINE-LEVIN SYNDROME

The etiology of KLS remains uncertain, but is likely to be multifactorial, although no causative genes have been identified. Nevertheless, there is evidence that the disease has a genetic component, with the first degree relatives of affected individuals having an 800-fold to 4000-fold increased risk of developing KLS.[17] Multiplex families with KLS have been described,[18–21] including monozygotic twins,[22,23] and there is a slightly higher prevalence in Ashkenazi Jews, which suggests a founder effect.[24] In a recent more comprehensive comparison of 21 patients from 10 multiplex families and 239 patients with sporadic KLS, there were no autoimmune, neurologic, psychiatric, HLA, or karyotypic differences between the groups.[25] Clinically, the disease characteristics were similar between familial and sporadic cases, except for a few minor markers of severity that suggested that the familial form might be slightly less severe (eg, slightly fewer episodes per year and less inhibited speech in familial cases).[25] In our recent review of the literature,[26] we identified 17 definitive familial cases of KLS in 9 papers,[18–23,27–29] including a consanguineous Saudi family with 6 affected individuals.[18] Similar to Nguyen and colleagues,[25] we did not identify significant differences between familial or sporadic cases.

Unbiased genome-wide association studies of patients with KLS have yet to be conducted, but several papers describe the presence of HLA locus polymorphisms in association with KLS, and polymorphisms in tryptophan hydroxylase and catechol-*O*-methyltransferase have also been examined owing to the hypothesis that KLS may arise from abnormalities in central serotonin and dopamine metabolism.[30] These studies are summarized in **Table 1**. HLA was chosen as a candidate locus because of its known tight association with the related narcolepsy with cataplexy (HLA-DQB1*0602, DR2 haplotype),[31] but in this initial study, only 1 of the 11 patients carried HLA-DR2. Nevertheless, several (but not all) subsequent studies have shown evidence of HLA-DR1 and DR2 haplotypes, including in some sibling pairs, although the largest study to compare HLA haplotype distributions between familial and sporadic cases failed to find a significant difference between groups.[25] Other genes are likely responsible for KLS susceptibility and a thorough genetic examination of familial cases and unaffected family members is likely to be helpful in identifying them.

IMAGING AND BIOCHEMISTRY IN PATIENTS WITH KLEINE-LEVIN SYNDROME
Imaging Studies

Despite the stereotyped nature of KLS, a specific structural pathology has yet to be identified in the brains of patients with KLS via computed tomography scans or MRI. Brains largely appear normal with classical imaging modalities,[32–34] although in 1 case, MRI revealed a large and asymmetrical mammillary body in an 18-year-old man with typical KLS,[35] and, in another, a cystic lesion was noted in the pineal gland.[36] An early case report detected a hypodense lipid-rich area in the interpeduncular cistern via computed tomography scanning.[37] Autopsy studies of the brains of 3 KLS patients revealed no hypothalamic abnormalities, although in 2 patients, inflammatory infiltrates were noted in the thalamus[38] and the

Table 1
Genetic studies of patients with Kleine-Levin syndrome

Study	Number of Patients	Locus/Technique Used	Results
Visscher et al,[68] 1990	2	HLA typing	No DR2 haplotype
Manni et al,[69] 1993	2	HLA typing	HLA-DR1, DQ1 haplotype
Hasegawa et al,[70] 1998	1	Cytogenetic analysis	Metaphase chromosomes mosaic for 45X/46XX and showed premature centromere division and chromatid pulling
Dauvilliers et al,[30] 2002	30	Tryptophan hydroxylase	No association
Dauvilliers et al,[30] 2002	30	Catechol-O-methyltransferase	No association
Dauvilliers et al,[30] 2002	30	HLA-DQB1	HLA-DQB1*0201 allele frequency significantly increased in KLS patients, 3 homozygous
BaHammam et al,[18] 2008	6 related family members	HLA-A, B, C, DRB1, DQB1	HLA-DQB1*02 homozygosity present in 4/6 affected and 2/6 unaffected family members
Rocamora et al,[21] 2010	2 siblings with menstrual-related hypersomnia	HLA typing	HLA-DQB1*0501
Huang et al,[71] 2012	12	HLA typing	HLA-DQB1, DQB1/0602 in 3/12
Katz et al,[19] 2002	2 (twins)	HLA typing	Shared HLA-DR2, DQ1, and DR5 haplotypes
Nguyen et al,[25] 2016	260 (21 familial, 239 sporadic)	HLA typing	No significant difference in distribution between familial and sporadic
Ueno et al,[23] 2012	2 (twins)	HLA typing	No DQB1*02 loci

Abbreviation: HLA, human leukocyte antigen.

diencephalon and midbrain,[39] and in another patient, a small locus coeruleus and decreased substantia nigra pigmentation was identified.[40] The other case did exhibit structural abnormalities of the hypothalamus, amygdala, and temporal lobe gray matter.[41]

However, functional brain imaging studies that have used a variety of imaging modalities have revealed a spectrum of perfusion, pathway, and metabolic changes in the brains of KLS patients. These are summarized in **Table 2**. Single-photon positron emission CT (SPECT) scanning has been used most commonly for this purpose. Although many studies reported abnormal perfusion patterns in the hypothalamus that might corroborate the hypothesis that KLS represents a disorder of diencephalic or hypothalamic function,[38,41–45] it is clear that the perfusion and metabolic deficits are present in both cortical and subcortical regions in many cases. This pattern may explain not only the hypersomnolent phenotype, but also the behavioral changes. Decreased orbitofrontal and anterior parasagittal brain metabolism, for instance, might be responsible for apathy, disinhibition, and inappropriate sexual behavior, whereas decreased posterior abnormalities might alter perception. Functional MRI (fMRI)[46] has been useful for mapping neuronal connectivity in affected individuals, with some but not all studies showing decreased thalamic connectivity and others implicating other pathways such as the frontal eye fields (see **Table 2**). Only 1 study to date has leveraged the full benefits of fMRI with perfusion and spectroscopy. Billings and colleagues[47] examined the brain of a 20-year-old-woman with KLS with fMRI and detected a 25% reduction in medial thalamic perfusion, increased glutamine metabolites in the left thalamus, and a paradoxic right-sided cortical response. These studies are, however, hampered by small numbers of subjects, an absence of quantitative analysis, and a lack of control groups.

Chemical Biomarkers

Together, functional imaging studies and CSF biomarker studies support the hypothesis that the hypersomnolence in at least some KLS cases is caused by transient hypothalamic dysfunction.[48] One hypothesis of KLS pathophysiology postulates that an environmental trigger results in blood–brain barrier dysfunction, immune-mediated hypothalamic dysfunction, and hypocretin neuron inhibition.[30,48,49] Another hypothesis that is based on biochemical findings is that symptomatic KLS patients have reduced hypothalamic dopaminergic tone.[50] Therefore, several biochemical parameters have been measured in both the serum and CSF of affected individuals, with CSF hypocretin-1, a hypothalamic neuropeptide, the most commonly studied molecule because of its known role in sleep regulation and almost undetectable concentrations in the CSF of patients with the related sleep disorder narcolepsy.[51] These studies are summarized in **Table 3**. Similar to the imaging studies, results are variable, with some but not all patients showing decreased (but not absent) hypocretin-1 in their CSF and some other isolated disturbances in hypothalamic–pituitary axis hormones that are consistent with a hypothalamic disturbance. Of particular note, however, and despite a putative autoimmune etiology (discussed elsewhere in this article), a comprehensive study of serum inflammatory cytokines did not reveal evidence of systemic inflammation.[52]

TREATMENT

The Cochrane systematic review of the pharmacologic treatment of KLS is now in its third edition, and the latest version was published in 2016.[53] No studies met the inclusion criteria of being randomized controlled trials or quasi-randomized controlled trials, which highlights the critical need for therapeutic trials of pharmacologic agents in patients with KLS in the double-blind, placebo-controlled setting. Given the comprehensive nature of the Cochrane review, a systemic review of the therapeutics that have been tested in KLS patients will not be revisited here, and the interested readers are referred to this up-to-date review.[53] Briefly, however, several treatments have been tested that are reported to alleviate specific symptoms (**Box 2**). In the absence of a definitive pharmacologic treatment, current best practice focuses on the creation of a supportive environment for the patient, preferably at home, to ensure safety during symptomatic periods, to ensure self-care, and to prevent suicide or the sequelae of mood disorders. Arnulf[1] recommends a trial of amantadine at the start of an episode, sublingual bromazepam during an episode to alleviate intense anxiety, and/or a short trial of risperidone if behavior indicates neuroleptic treatment, and perhaps prolonged release lithium in cases that are characterized by long episodes with a target serum level of 0.8 to 1.2 mmol/L.[1]

THE "KNOWN UNKNOWNS" AS A BASIS FOR FUTURE ADVANCES IN KLEINE-LEVIN SYNDROME

Although the preceding discussion and review of the literature highlight that the etiology and

Table 2
Functional imaging studies of patients with Kleine-Levin syndrome

Study	Imaging Modality	Number of Patients	Perfusion/Activation Pattern During Relapse	Perfusion Pattern During Remission
Lu et al,[36] 2000	SPECT	1	Hypoperfusion in basal ganglia, hypothalamus, right frontotemporal lobe	N/A
Landtblom et al,[35] 2002	SPECT	1	Hypoperfusion of left frontal and temporal lobes during relapse	Slight frontotemporal hypoperfusion at 2 mo with temporal changes persisting at 7 years
Portilla et al,[72] 2002	SPECT	1	Mesiotemporal hypoperfusion	Mesiotemporal hypoperfusion
Landtblom et al,[73] 2003	SPECT	4	Hypoperfusion of temporal and frontotemporal regions in 2/4 cases, normal in 2/4	
Huang et al,[32] 2005	SPECT	7	Thalamic hypoperfusion in all cases and temporal, frontal, and basal ganglia hypoperfusion in some cases	Normal thalami perfusion but some persistent hypoperfusion in other areas
Hong et al,[74] 2006	SPECT	1	Hypoperfusion frontal and temporal lobes, thalami, hypothalami	Right mesial temporal region
Poryazova et al,[75] 2007	MRS	1	Lower NAA/Cr ratios and higher Glu-Gln/Cr in both thalami during episode and higher NAA/Cr ratio in hypothalamus during episode	N/A
Hoexter et al,[76] 2010 (extension of[77])	SPECT with Tc99m-TRODAT-1	1 (7 controls)	Dopamine transporter availability was reduced in the left striatum, right striatum, lower than when asymptomatic	Dopamine transporter availability was reduced in the left striatum, right striatum
Billings et al,[47] 2011	fMRI with perfusion, MRS	1	25% reduction in medial thalamic perfusion, increased glutamine in left thalamus and basal ganglia, paradoxic right-sided cortical response	Normal
Huang et al,[33] 2012	SPECT	30	66.7% asymmetric hypoperfusion left thalamus, 11.1% right thalamus, 11.1% left basal ganglia, 22.2% right basal ganglia	N/A

(continued on next page)

Table 2
(continued)

Study	Imaging Modality	Number of Patients	Perfusion/Activation Pattern During Relapse	Perfusion Pattern During Remission
Lo et al,[78] 2012	FDG-PET	1	Lower metabolism in the right thalamus, right hypothalamus, left hypothalamus, right caudate nucleus, right striatum, left striatum	Higher metabolism in the right thalamus, right hypothalamus, left hypothalamus, right caudate nucleus, right striatum, left striatum
Haba-Rubio et al,[79] 2012	FDG-PET	2	Decreased hypothalamic, orbitofrontal, and frontal parasagittal metabolism, increased anterior caudate nuclei, cingulate gyrus, and premotor cortex	N/A
Vigren et al,[80] 2013	fMRI and MRS	14 (15 controls)	Negative correlation between thalamic fMRI activation and thalamic NAA levels in affected subjects	N/A
Vigren et al,[81] 2014	SPECT	24	Temporal/ frontotemporal hypoperfusion in 48% of patients	Temporal/ frontotemporal hypoperfusion in 56% of patients
Engström et al,[63] 2014 (extension study of[82])	fMRI	18 (26 controls)	Reduced activation in medial frontal and anterior cingulate cortices; increased activation in the left thalamus, the left dorsolateral prefrontal cortex and left inferior frontal cortex, left precuneus, left cuneus, right superior parietal cortex, right putamen	N/A
Dauvilliers et al,[83] 2014	FDG-PET	4 (15 controls)	Increased metabolism paracentral, precentral, and postcentral areas, supplementary motor area, medial frontal gyrus, thalamus and putamen during symptomatic episodes, and decreased metabolism in occipital and temporal gyri	Hypermetabolism in frontal and temporal cortices, posterior cingulate, and precuneus, with no detected hypometabolism

(continued on next page)

Table 2
(continued)

Study	Imaging Modality	Number of Patients	Perfusion/Activation Pattern During Relapse	Perfusion Pattern During Remission
Kas et al,[84] 2014	Brain perfusion scintigraphy	41 (15 controls)	Persistent hypoperfusion in the hypothalamus, thalamus, caudate nucleus, and cortical associated areas and right dorsomedial prefrontal cortex and right parietotemporal junction	Persistent hypoperfusion in the hypothalamus, thalamus, caudate nucleus, and cortical associated areas
Engström et al,[85] 2014	fMRI	1 (14 controls)	Decreased thalamic connectivity, especially the thalamus–brainstem	Normal thalamic connectivity
Engström et al,[86] 2016	fMRI	12 (14 controls)	Lower connectivity between pons and frontal eye field, but not the thalamus	N/A
Xie et al,[34] 2016	FDG-PET	1	Symmetric hypometabolism in the thalamus and hypothalamus	N/A

Abbreviations: FDG-PET, fluorodeoxyglucose positron emission tomography; fMRI, functional magnetic resonance imaging; MRS, magnetic resonance spectroscopy; N/A, not applicable; NAA, *N*-acetylaspartate; SPECT, single-positron emission computer tomography.

pathophysiology of KLS are far from being well-understood, a few patterns and themes can clearly be identified that help distinguish knowledge gaps that can be used to focus future clinical and experimental studies. The following are the "known unknowns": Kleine-Levin syndrome may be an autoimmune disease; the genetics of Kleine-Levin syndrome are poorly defined; Kleine-Levin Syndrome is characterized by abnormal brain function, but this does not seem to be limited to the hypothalamus; hypocretin-1 levels are decreased in a proportion of patients with Kleine-Levin Syndrome, but the identification of an ideal blood or cerebrospinal fluid biomarker has proven elusive; and there are currently no rational or evidence-based pharmaceuticals available for Kleine-Levin syndrome patients.

Kleine-Levin Syndrome May Be an Autoimmune Disease

Evidence summary
KLS is commonly preceded by a flulike illness, upper respiratory tract infection, or gastroenteritis (in 38.2% of cases in 1 large systematic review of 186 cases[54]), although preceding head trauma (9%), alcohol use (5.4%), and comorbid autoimmune

disease or sarcoidosis are also reported triggers. Although systemic inflammation (measured by cytokines[52] or C-reactive protein[24]) seems to be absent in affected individuals, the limited autopsy data that are available suggest that patients may have local brain inflammation. This is further supported by the association with the HLA-DQB1*201 homozygous genotype (see **Table 1**). Given the variable but reproducible decreases in CSF hypocretin-1 levels that are observed in KLS patients, the autoimmune target may be the hypocretin-producing cells of the brain and in particular the hypothalamus,[55] and a recent case was reported in which the concentration of circulating GAD65 antibodies was 9-fold higher in a patient with KLS than in controls.[56]

Future prospects
In many ways, the infection-triggered autoimmune hypothesis closely mirrors the theory of the development of multiple sclerosis, in which several viruses are thought to trigger the disease by initiating immune responses to host antigens via multiple mechanisms, such as molecular mimicry, bystander activation, or epitope spreading.[57] In addition to the hypocretin-producing cells in the

Table 3
Biochemical biomarkers of KLS

Study	Number of Patients	Assay	Levels During Relapse	Levels During Remission
Livrea et al,[87] 1977	1	CSF homovanillic acid, 5-HIAA, 3-methoxy-4-hydroxyphenylethylene glycol	Increased dopamine turnover	N/A
Koerber et al,[40] 1984	1	CSF 5-HT and 5-HIAA	Elevated CSF 5-HT and 5-HIAA	N/A
Hart,[88] 1985	1	Glucose, creatinine, BUN, cholesterol, uric acid, T3, T4, TSH, serum ACTH, FSH, LH, GH	Normal	N/A
Thompson et al,[89] 1985	1	Melatonin, cortisol, and prolactin over 24 h	Normal rhythms	Abnormal cortisol rhythm (absent morning peak)
Gadoth et al,[90] 1987	1	GH, 11-OHCS, prolactin, FSH, LH, TSH	Paradoxic GH response to TRH, high prolactin and abnormal LH, 11-OHCS, and prolactin during sleep	N/A
Fukinishi et al,[91] 1989	1	Growth hormone, prolactin, cortisol	Abnormal growth hormone pattern (absent peak) during sleep	N/A
Fernandez et al,[92] 1990	1	ACTH and cortisol	Abolished ACTH and cortisol responses to insulin-induced hypoglycemia, absent TSH and diminished prolactin responses to TRH	Normalized responses to challenge
Chesson et al,[50] 1991	1	Serum TSH, cortisol, prolactin, growth hormone	TSH and prolactin increased and growth hormone and cortisol decreased compared with asymptomatic period	N/A
Hasegawa et al,[70] 1998	1	7-Ketosteroid, 17-hydroxycorticosteroid, GH, TSH, FSH, prolactin, aldosterone, and ACTH; CSF sugar, homovanillic acid, vanillylmandelic acid, 5-HIAA, serotonin, aminobutyric acid	Normal	N/A

Study	n	Measurements	Results (patients)	Controls
Mayer et al,[93] 1998	5	GH, melatonin, TSH, cortisol, FSH	2/4 decreased GH Increased melatonin	N/A
Janicki et al,[28] 2001	1	Serum carnitine, TSH, melatonin, cortisol, glucose, insulin, FSH, LH	Low serum carnitine	N/A
Dauvilliers et al,[51] 2003	4	CSF hypocretin-1	1/4 2-fold decrease	Normal
Podesta et al,[94] 2006	1 (47 controls)	CSF hypocretin-1	282 pg/mL	581 pg/mL
Arnulf et al,[24] 2008	108 (108 controls)	Serum CRP and leptin	No difference between patients and controls after controlling for BMI	N/A
Li et al,[95] 2013	42 (53 controls)	CSF hypocretin-1	Lower hypocretin in KLS patients than controls (185 vs 320 pg/mL)	No difference between KLS patients and controls
Rout et al,[56] 2014	1	GAD65 autoantibodies	9-fold higher than controls	N/A
Kornum et al,[52] 2015	52 (8 controls)	51 serum cytokines	Higher sVCAM1 (soluble vascular cell adhesion molecule-1) than controls	No difference to when symptomatic
Lopez et al,[49] 2015	2	CSF hypocretin-1, histamine, tele-methylhistamine	Low hypocretin in both patients, 1 patient 2-fold histamine decrease	Normal
Wang et al,[96] 2016	57	CSF hypocretin-1	31% lower than during remission in 34/57 patients	Persistent low levels during remission in 3/57 patients
Cho et al,[97] 2016	1	CSF hypocretin-1	174 pg/mL	284 pg/mL

Abbreviations: 11-OHCS, 11-hydroxycorticosteroid; 5-HIAA, 5-hydroxyindoleacetic acid; 5-HT, 5-hydroxytryptamine; ACTH, adrenocorticotrophic hormone; BMI, body mass index; BUN, blood urea nitrogen; CRP, C-reactive protein; CSF, cerebrospinal fluid; FSH, follicle-stimulating hormone; GH, growth hormone; KLS, Kleine-Levin syndrome; LH, luteinizing hormone; N/A, not applicable; sVCAM1, soluble Vascular cell adhesion protein 1; T3, triiodothyronine; T4, thyroxine; TRH, thyroid-releasing hormone; TSH, thyroid-stimulating hormone.

Box 2
The main drugs that have been tested in Kleine-Levin syndrome patients

Drug	Outcome
Stimulants/ amphetamines	Improved sleepiness but no other symptoms[98]
Antidepressants	No effect in preventing relapse, except in a case that was treated with the monoamine oxidase inhibitor moclobemide[99]
Antiepileptics	Improvements with carbamazepine[100,101]
Lithium	Improved abnormal behavior and symptom recovery[20,102]

Adapted from de Oliveira MM, Conti C, Prado GF. Pharmacological treatment for Kleine-Levin syndrome. Cochrane Database Syst Rev 2016(5):CD006685.

brain, a recent report of a patient with anti-*N*-methyl-D-aspartate encephalitis with features of KLS raises the possibility that the *N*-methyl-D-aspartate receptor may be another candidate target of the immune response.[58] Great progress has been made in multiple sclerosis research owing to the availability of mouse models (such as experimental autoimmune encephalitis) that recapitulate human KLS, and the development of other environmental or genetic models of KLS would be of great use for preclinical research. In that regard, it is interesting to note that hypocretin-1 knockout mice exhibit disordered cataplexy-type bouts of REM sleep.[59]

The Genetics of Kleine-Levin Syndrome Are Poorly Defined

Evidence summary
Genetic studies of KLS patients have hitherto mainly been limited to HLA typing (see **Table 1**). The disease requires a full genetic characterization.

Future prospects
The recent advances in next-generation sequencing technologies and their application to tissue-based research provide an excellent opportunity to characterize fully individual genomes and to perform genome-wide association studies in cohorts of patients with KLS and other sleep disorders.[60,61] In addition to linkage or association studies, sequencing or microarray-based transcriptomic studies could be performed on blood samples or tissues from patients and, where available, brain autopsy material. For these types of studies to be performed, coordinated, multicenter,

and multinational tissue banking initiatives are required, such as those that have been implemented successfully in other rare diseases, including pediatric liver tumors.[62]

Kleine-Levin Syndrome Is Characterized by Abnormal Brain Function, but This Does Not Seem to Be Limited to the Hypothalamus

Evidence summary
The data that are summarized in **Table 2** strongly suggest that, regardless of etiology, most if not all KLS patients exhibit functional brain abnormalities. Although the early studies suggested the existence of more localized hypothalamic changes, it is now clear that KLS patients experience quite a widespread brain dysfunction in both cortical and subcortical regions.

Future prospects
The presence of reproducible functional changes in KLS patients raises the possibility that these changes could be used as imaging biomarkers. Given the data that are shown in **Table 2**, which show a rather heterogeneous pattern of perfusion changes by SPECT, the sensitivity and specificity of an SPECT-based assay are likely to be poor. Therefore, fMRI might be better suited to the development of a diagnostic or prognostic test, especially if they are combined with a simultaneous working memory assessment.[63] Furthermore, there have been recent advances in ultra-high–resolution MRI that might improve the sensitivity of fMRI.[46] Alternatively, the assay characteristics might be improved via a multimodal approach, for instance, fMRI combined with SPECT, PET, or MR spectroscopy, to leverage the benefits of each approach. Regardless of the approach that is selected, there will need to be vigorous testing of the assay under different clinical scenarios to (i) establish the optimal modality, combination of modalities, or testing scenario (eg, during wakefulness or sleep) and (ii) determine the accuracy and validity of the assay. Given the small numbers of patients with KLS, this will require a coordinated, multicenter approach.

Hypocretin-1 Levels Are Decreased in a Proportion of Patients with Kleine-Levin Syndrome, but the Identification of an Ideal Blood or Cerebrospinal Fluid Biomarker Has Proven Elusive

Evidence summary
Hypocretin-1 is the most studied biomarker in the CSF of KLS patients, with most studies showing decreases in hypocretin-1 expression in at least a proportion of the patients who were studied.

Future prospects

Given that KLS may be characterized by more subtle decreases in hypocretin-1 than other hypersomnolence disorders such as narcolepsy, highly sensitive and specific methods with which to measure CSF hypocretin-1 are essential for future biomarker studies to detect any changes. The majority of previous studies have used a hypocretin-1 I^{125} radioimmunoassay,[64] which is considered to be the clinical gold standard, although other methods, including enzyme immunoassay[65] and fluorescence immunoassay,[66] are also available. However, radioimmunoassay uses radioactive materials and may cross-react with other matrix constituents and suffers from low reliability and accuracy. A recent advance in this regard has been the development of a new quantitative mass spectrometry assay (multiple reaction monitoring),[67] which was highly correlated with radioimmunoassay tests in samples from the same patients but with a wider range of detection. Together with its lack of cross-reactivity and robustness and the inclusion of internal controls, multiple reaction monitoring may become more useful for the sensitive and specific detection of hypocretin-1 in patients with KLS in future clinical diagnostic studies.

There Are Currently No Rational or Evidence-Based Pharmaceuticals Available for Kleine-Levin Syndrome Patients

Evidence summary

The recent Cochrane review[53] highlights the lack of evidence for the use of particular therapeutics in patients with KLS, with only low-quality evidence available from case reports or small series.

Future prospects

The debilitating episodes, severe behavioral abnormalities, and effects on patients' function and quality of life mandate an urgent call for the performance of double-blind, placebo-controlled, randomized, controlled trials of drugs to prevent or improve the symptoms of KLS. The immunopathology of KLS suggests that drugs that modulate or target the immune system are worthy of further testing in clinical trials. Because KLS is a rare disease, clinical trial efforts will require a consortium-based, multinational approach. Properly designed and coordinated trials will also allow for the standardized collection and analysis of tissue samples for ancillary genetic and biochemical studies.

SUMMARY

KLS is a rare, debilitating, homogeneous disease. These features provide both opportunities and barriers to the diagnosis and management of KLS. Here, via an extensive review of the literature, we have identified the following 5 key areas that require clinical academic attention to make progress on behalf of those afflicted by KLS: immunopathogenesis, genetics, imaging, biomarker discovery, and clinical trials. If clinicians have a high enough index of suspicion for KLS and are aware of the diagnostic criteria, its homogeneity should allow for the centralized registration of a relatively uniform population of afflicted individuals to facilitate clinical research. Furthermore, the disease uniformity should make the identification of associated genetic or imaging biomarkers easier. These clinical efforts also require concurrent laboratory efforts to model the disease and generate preclinical data for clinical translation.

ACKNOWLEDGMENTS

The work was supported by the Strategic Technologies Program of the National Plan for Sciences and Technology and Innovation in the Kingdom of Saudi Arabia (08-MED511-02).

REFERENCES

1. Arnulf I. Kleine-Levin syndrome. Sleep Med Clin 2015;10(2):151–61.
2. Kleine W. Periodische Schlafsucht. Monatsschr Psychiatr Neurol 1925;57:285–320.
3. Lewis ND. The psychoanalytic approach to the problem of children under twelve years of age. Psychoanal Rev 1926;13:424–43.
4. Levin M. Narcolepsy (Gelineau's syndrome) and other varieties of morbid somnolence. Arch Neurol Psychiatr 1929;6(22):1172–200.
5. Critchley M, Hoffman HL. The syndrome of periodic somnolence and morbid hunger (Kleine-Levin syndrome). Br Med J 1942;1(4230):137–9.
6. Lavault S, Golmard JL, Groos E, et al. Kleine-Levin syndrome in 120 patients: differential diagnosis and long episodes. Ann Neurol 2015;77(3):529–40.
7. Arnone JM, Conti RP. Kleine-Levin syndrome: an overview and relevance to nursing practice. J Psychosoc Nurs Ment Health Serv 2016;54(3):41–7.
8. Lisk DR. Kleine-Levin syndrome. Pract Neurol 2009;9(1):42–5.
9. Billiard M. Recurrent hypersomnias. Handb Clin Neurol 2011;99:815–23.
10. Billiard M, Jaussent I, Dauvilliers Y, et al. Recurrent hypersomnia: a review of 339 cases. Sleep Med Rev 2011;15(4):247–57.
11. Billiard M. Kleine–Levin syndrome. Sleep medicine. New York: Springer; 2015. p. 229–36.
12. Miglis MG, Guilleminault C. Kleine-Levin syndrome: a review. Nat Sci Sleep 2014;6:19–26.

13. Miglis MG, Guilleminault C. Kleine-Levin syndrome. Curr Neurol Neurosci Rep 2016;16(6):60.

14. Sum-Ping O, Guilleminault C. Kleine-Levin syndrome. Curr Treat Options Neurol 2016;18(6):24.

15. Sateia MJ. International classification of sleep disorders-third edition: highlights and modifications. Chest 2014;146(5):1387–94.

16. American Academy of Sleep Medicine. International classification of sleep disorders—third edition (ICSD-3). Darien (IL):: American Academy of Sleep Medicine; 2014.

17. Arnulf I, Rico TJ, Mignot E. Diagnosis, disease course, and management of patients with Kleine-Levin syndrome. Lancet Neurol 2012;11(10): 918–28.

18. BaHammam AS, GadElRab MO, Owais SM, et al. Clinical characteristics and HLA typing of a family with Kleine-Levin syndrome. Sleep Med 2008; 9(5):575–8.

19. Katz JD, Ropper AH. Familial Kleine-Levin syndrome: two siblings with unusually long hypersomnic spells. Arch Neurol 2002;59(12):1959–61.

20. Poppe M, Friebel D, Reuner U, et al. The Kleine-Levin syndrome - effects of treatment with lithium. Neuropediatrics 2003;34(3):113–9.

21. Rocamora R, Gil-Nagel A, Franch O, et al. Familial recurrent hypersomnia: two siblings with Kleine-Levin syndrome and menstrual-related hypersomnia. J Child Neurol 2010;25(11):1408–10.

22. Peraita-Adrados R, Vicario JL, Tafti M, et al. Monozygotic twins affected with Kleine-Levin syndrome. Sleep 2012;35(5):595–6.

23. Ueno T, Fukuhara A, Ikegami A, et al. Monozygotic twins concordant for Kleine-Levin syndrome. BMC Neurol 2012;12:31.

24. Arnulf I, Lin L, Gadoth N, et al. Kleine-Levin syndrome: a systematic study of 108 patients. Ann Neurol 2008;63(4):482–93.

25. Nguyen QT, Groos E, Leclair-Visonneau L, et al. Familial Kleine-Levin syndrome: a specific entity? Sleep 2016;39(8):1535–42.

26. Al Suwayri SM. Kleine-Levin syndrome. Familial cases and comparison with sporadic cases. Saudi Med J 2016;37(1):21–8.

27. Bonkalo A. Hypersomnia. A discussion of psychiatric implications based on three cases. Br J Psychiatry 1968;114(506):69–75.

28. Janicki S, Franco K, Zarko R. A case report of Kleine-Levin syndrome in an adolescent girl. Psychosomatics 2001;42(4):350–2.

29. Suwa K, Toru M. A case of periodic somnolence whose sleep was induced by glucose. Folia Psychiatr Neurol Jpn 1969;23(4):253–62.

30. Dauvilliers Y, Mayer G, Lecendreux M, et al. Kleine-Levin syndrome: an autoimmune hypothesis based on clinical and genetic analyses. Neurology 2002; 59(11):1739–45.

31. Mignot E. Genetic and familial aspects of narcolepsy. Neurology 1998;50(2 Suppl 1):S16–22.

32. Huang YS, Guilleminault C, Kao PF, et al. SPECT findings in the Kleine-Levin syndrome. Sleep 2005;28(8):955–60.

33. Huang YS, Guilleminault C, Lin KL, et al. Relationship between Kleine-Levin syndrome and upper respiratory infection in Taiwan. Sleep 2012;35(1):123–9.

34. Xie H, Guo J, Liu H, et al. Do the symptoms of Kleine-Levin syndrome correlate with the hypometabolism of the thalamus on FDG PET? Clin Nucl Med 2016;41(3):255–6.

35. Landtblom AM, Dige N, Schwerdt K, et al. A case of Kleine–Levin syndrome examined with SPECT and neuropsychological testing. Acta Neurol Scand 2002;105(4):318–21.

36. Lu ML, Liu HC, Chen CH, et al. Kleine-Levin syndrome and psychosis: observation from an unusual case. Neuropsychiatry Neuropsychol Behav Neurol 2000;13(2):140–2.

37. Argenta G, Bozzao L, Petruzzellis MC. First CT findings in the Kleine-Levin-Critchley syndrome. Ital J Neurol Sci 1981;2(1):77–9.

38. Carpenter S, Yassa R, Ochs R. A pathologic basis for Kleine-Levin syndrome. Arch Neurol 1982;39(1): 25–8.

39. Fenzi F, Simonati A, Crosato F, et al. Clinical features of Kleine-Levin syndrome with localized encephalitis. Neuropediatrics 1993;24(5):292–5.

40. Koerber RK, Torkelson R, Haven G, et al. Increased cerebrospinal fluid 5-hydroxytryptamine and 5-hydroxyindoleacetic acid in Kleine-Levin syndrome. Neurology 1984;34(12):1597–600.

41. Takrani LB, Cronin D. Kleine-Levin syndrome in a female patient. Can Psychiatr Assoc J 1976;21(5): 315–8.

42. Critchley M. Periodic hypersomnia and megaphagia in adolescent males. Brain 1962;85:627–56.

43. Gadoth N, Kesler A, Vainstein G, et al. Clinical and polysomnographic characteristics of 34 patients with Kleine-Levin syndrome. J Sleep Res 2001; 10(4):337–41.

44. Malhotra S, Das MK, Gupta N, et al. A clinical study of Kleine-Levin syndrome with evidence for hypothalamic-pituitary axis dysfunction. Biol Psychiatry 1997;42(4):299–301.

45. Billiard M. The Kleine-Levin syndrome: a paramedian thalamic dysfunction? Sleep 2005;28(8):915–6.

46. Engstrom M, Hallbook T, Szakacs A, et al. Functional magnetic resonance imaging in narcolepsy and the kleine-levin syndrome. Front Neurol 2014; 5:105.

47. Billings ME, Watson NF, Keogh BP. Dynamic fMRI changes in Kleine-Levin syndrome. Sleep Med 2011;12(5):532.

48. Dauvilliers Y, Lopez R. Time to find a biomarker in Kleine-Levin syndrome. Sleep Med 2016;21:177.

49. Lopez R, Barateau L, Chenini S, et al. Preliminary results on CSF biomarkers for hypothalamic dysfunction in Kleine-Levin syndrome. Sleep Med 2015;16(1):194–6.

50. Chesson AL Jr, Levine SN, Kong LS, et al. Neuroendocrine evaluation in Kleine-Levin syndrome: evidence of reduced dopaminergic tone during periods of hypersomnolence. Sleep 1991;14(3):226–32.

51. Dauvilliers Y, Baumann CR, Carlander B, et al. CSF hypocretin-1 levels in narcolepsy, Kleine-Levin syndrome, and other hypersomnias and neurological conditions. J Neurol Neurosurg Psychiatry 2003;74(12):1667–73.

52. Kornum BR, Rico T, Lin L, et al. Serum cytokine levels in Kleine-Levin syndrome. Sleep Med 2015;16(8):961–5.

53. de Oliveira MM, Conti C, Prado GF. Pharmacological treatment for Kleine-Levin syndrome. Cochrane Database Syst Rev 2016;(5):CD006685.

54. Arnulf I, Zeitzer JM, File J, et al. Kleine-Levin syndrome: a systematic review of 186 cases in the literature. Brain 2005;128(Pt 12):2763–76.

55. Ebrahim IO, Howard RS, Kopelman MD, et al. The hypocretin/orexin system. J R Soc Med 2002;95(5):227–30.

56. Rout UK, Michener MS, Dhossche DM. GAD65 autoantibodies in Kleine-Levin syndrome. J Neuropsychiatry Clin Neurosci 2014;26(2):E49–51.

57. Libbey JE, Cusick MF, Fujinami RS. Role of pathogens in multiple sclerosis. Int Rev Immunol 2014;33(4):266–83.

58. Feigal J, Lin C, Barrio G, et al. Anti-N-Methyl-d-Aspartate receptor encephalitis presenting with features of Kleine-Levin syndrome and demyelination. Psychosomatics 2016;57(3):310–4.

59. Willie JT, Chemelli RM, Sinton CM, et al. Distinct narcolepsy syndromes in Orexin receptor-2 and Orexin null mice: molecular genetic dissection of non-REM and REM sleep regulatory processes. Neuron 2003;38(5):715–30.

60. Dauvilliers Y, Tafti M. The genetic basis of sleep disorders. Curr Pharm Des 2008;14(32):3386–95.

61. Raizen DM, Wu MN. Genome-wide association studies of sleep disorders. Chest 2011;139(2):446–52.

62. Czauderna P, Haeberle B, Hiyama E, et al. The Children's Hepatic tumors International Collaboration (CHIC): novel global rare tumor database yields new prognostic factors in hepatoblastoma and becomes a research model. Eur J Cancer 2016;52:92–101.

63. Engstrom M, Karlsson T, Landtblom AM. Thalamic activation in the Kleine-Levin syndrome. Sleep 2014;37(2):379–86.

64. Dauvilliers Y, Arnulf I, Mignot E. Narcolepsy with cataplexy. Lancet 2007;369(9560):499–511.

65. Liguori C, Placidi F, Albanese M, et al. CSF beta-amyloid levels are altered in narcolepsy: a link with the inflammatory hypothesis? J Sleep Res 2014;23(4):420–4.

66. Schmidt FM, Kratzsch J, Gertz HJ, et al. Cerebrospinal fluid melanin-concentrating hormone (MCH) and hypocretin-1 (HCRT-1, orexin-A) in Alzheimer's disease. PLoS One 2013;8(5):e63136.

67. Hirtz C, Vialaret J, Gabelle A, et al. From radioimmunoassay to mass spectrometry: a new method to quantify orexin-A (hypocretin-1) in cerebrospinal fluid. Sci Rep 2016;6:25162.

68. Visscher F, van der Horst AR, Smit LM. HLA-DR antigens in Kleine-Levin syndrome. Ann Neurol 1990;28(2):195.

69. Manni R, Martinetti M, Ratti MT, et al. Electrophysiological and immunogenetic findings in recurrent monosymptomatic-type hypersomnia: a study of two unrelated Italian cases. Acta Neurol Scand 1993;88(4):293–5.

70. Hasegawa Y, Morishita M, Suzumura A. Novel chromosomal aberration in a patient with a unique sleep disorder. J Neurol Neurosurg Psychiatry 1998;64(1):113–6.

71. Huang CJ, Liao HT, Yeh GC, et al. Distribution of HLA-DQB1 alleles in patients with Kleine-Levin syndrome. J Clin Neurosci 2012;19(4):628–30.

72. Portilla P, Durand E, Chalvon A, et al. SPECT-identified hypoperfusion of the left temporomedial structures in a Kleine-Levin syndrome. Rev Neurol 2002;158(5 Pt 1):593.

73. Landtblom AM, Dige N, Schwerdt K, et al. Short-term memory dysfunction in Kleine-Levin syndrome. Acta Neurol Scand 2003;108(5):363–7.

74. Hong SB, Joo EY, Tae WS, et al. Episodic diencephalic hypoperfusion in Kleine-Levin syndrome. Sleep 2006;29(8):1091–3.

75. Poryazova R, Schnepf B, Boesiger P, et al. Magnetic resonance spectroscopy in a patient with Kleine-Levin syndrome. J Neurol 2007;254(10):1445–6.

76. Hoexter MQ, Shih MC, Felicio AC, et al. Greater reduction of striatal dopamine transporter availability during the symptomatic than asymptomatic phase of Kleine-Levin syndrome. Sleep Med 2010;11(9):959.

77. Hoexter MQ, Shih MC, Mendes DD, et al. Lower dopamine transporter density in an asymptomatic patient with Kleine-Levin syndrome. Acta Neurol Scand 2008;117(5):370–3.

78. Lo YC, Chou YH, Yu HY. PET finding in Kleine-Levin syndrome. Sleep Med 2012;13(6):771–2.

79. Haba-Rubio J, Prior JO, Guedj E, et al. Kleine-Levin syndrome: functional imaging correlates of hypersomnia and behavioral symptoms. Neurology 2012;79(18):1927–9.

80. Vigren P, Tisell A, Engstrom M, et al. Low thalamic NAA-concentration corresponds to strong neural

activation in working memory in Kleine-Levin syndrome. PLoS One 2013;8(2):e56279.

81. Vigren P, Engstrom M, Landtblom AM. SPECT in the Kleine-Levin syndrome, a possible diagnostic and prognostic aid? Front Neurol 2014;5:178.

82. Engstrom M, Vigren P, Karlsson T, et al. Working memory in 8 Kleine-Levin syndrome patients: an fMRI study. Sleep 2009;32(5):681–8.

83. Dauvilliers Y, Bayard S, Lopez R, et al. Widespread hypermetabolism in symptomatic and asymptomatic episodes in Kleine-Levin syndrome. PLoS One 2014;9(4):e93813.

84. Kas A, Lavault S, Habert MO, et al. Feeling unreal: a functional imaging study in patients with Kleine-Levin syndrome. Brain 2014;137(Pt 7):2077–87.

85. Engstrom M, Karlsson T, Landtblom AM. Reduced thalamic and pontine connectivity in kleine-levin syndrome. Front Neurol 2014;5:42.

86. Engstrom M, Landtblom AM, Karlsson T. New hypothesis on pontine-frontal eye field connectivity in Kleine-Levin syndrome. J Sleep Res 2016; 25(6):716–9.

87. Livrea P, Puca FM, Barnaba A, et al. Abnormal central monoamine metabolism in humans with "true hypersomnia" and "sub-wakefulness". Eur Neurol 1977;15(2):71–6.

88. Hart EJ. Kleine-Levin syndrome: normal CSF monoamines and response to lithium therapy. Neurology 1985;35(9):1395–6.

89. Thompson C, Obrecht R, Franey C, et al. Neuroendocrine rhythms in a patient with the Kleine-Levin syndrome. Br J Psychiatry 1985;147:440–3.

90. Gadoth N, Dickerman Z, Bechar M, et al. Episodic hormone secretion during sleep in Kleine-Levin syndrome: evidence for hypothalamic dysfunction. Brain Dev 1987;9(3):309–15.

91. Fukunishi I, Hosokawa K. A female case with the Kleine-Levin syndrome and its physiopathologic aspects. Jpn J Psychiatry Neurol 1989;43(1):45–9.

92. Fernandez JM, Lara I, Gila L, et al. Disturbed hypothalamic-pituitary axis in idiopathic recurring hypersomnia syndrome. Acta Neurol Scand 1990; 82(6):361–3.

93. Mayer G, Leonhard E, Krieg J, et al. Endocrinological and polysomnographic findings in Kleine-Levin syndrome: no evidence for hypothalamic and circadian dysfunction. Sleep 1998;21(3): 278–84.

94. Podesta C, Ferreras M, Mozzi M, et al. Kleine-Levin syndrome in a 14-year-old girl: CSF hypocretin-1 measurements. Sleep Med 2006;7(8):649–51.

95. Li Q, Wang J, Dong X, et al. CSF hypocretin level in patients with Kleine-Levin syndrome. Sleep Med 2013;14:e47.

96. Wang JY, Han F, Dong SX, et al. Cerebrospinal fluid orexin a levels and autonomic function in Kleine-Levin syndrome. Sleep 2016;39(4):855–60.

97. Cho JW, Kim JH. Recurrent hypersomnia in an 18-year old boy: CSF hypocretin level and MSLT findings. Sleep Med 2016;21:176.

98. Gallinek A. The Kleine-Levin syndrome: hypersomnia, bulimia, and abnormal mental states. World Neurol 1962;3:235–43.

99. Chaudhry HR. Clinical use of moclobemide in Kleine-Levin syndrome. Br J Psychiatry 1992;161: 720.

100. Mukaddes NM, Kora ME, Bilge S. Carbamazepine for Kleine-Levin syndrome. J Am Acad Child Adolesc Psychiatry 1999;38(7):791–2.

101. El Hajj T, Nasreddine W, Korri H, et al. A case of Kleine-Levin syndrome with a complete and sustained response to carbamazepine. Epilepsy Behav 2009;15(3):391–2.

102. Smolik P, Roth B. Kleine-Levin syndrome etiopathogenesis and treatment. Acta Univ Carol Med Monogr 1988;128:5–94.

Neuroimaging of Narcolepsy and Kleine-Levin Syndrome

Seung Bong Hong, MD, PhD

KEYWORDS

- Narcolepsy • Kleine-Levin syndrome • MRI • SPECT • PET

KEY POINTS

- Numerous neuroimaging studies have been performed to characterize the pathophysiology and various clinical features of narcolepsy.
- Brain MRI and various functional imaging tools revealed structural and functional abnormalities located in the hypothalamus, in agreement with a loss of hypocretinergic neurons in narcolepsy.
- In Kleine-Levin syndrome (KLS), subtracted single-photon emission CT (SPECT) showed significant hypoperfusion in the left hypothalamus, bilateral thalami, basal ganglia, bilateral medial and dorsolateral frontal regions, and left temporal lobe during the symptomatic period.
- Brain imaging is a useful tool to investigate and understand the neuroanatomic correlates and brain abnormalities of narcolepsy and other hypersomnias.

Narcolepsy is characterized by excessive daytime sleepiness (EDS), a disruption of sleep-wake behavior, cataplexy (sudden loss of muscle tone provoked by emotional stimuli), and other rapid eye movement (REM) sleep phenomena, such as sleep paralysis and hypnagogic hallucination. Hypocretin-containing neuron numbers are reduced in the hypothalamus of the narcolepsy brain.[1] The neuropeptide hypocretin seems to play a critical role in the neurobiology of narcolepsy.[2–4] Narcolepsy patients suffer from cognitive or emotional problem besides sleep-wake disturbances. To investigate the responsible neuroanatomic substrates for those problems, neuroimaging studies have been actively performed.

STRUCTURAL IMAGING IN NARCOLEPSY
Voxel-Based Morphometry

Differences in brain morphology that are not identifiable by routine visual inspection of individual brain MRI[5–8] can be investigated using voxel-based morphometry (VBM). VBM allows between-group statistical comparisons of tissue composition (gray matter and white matter [WM]) across all brain regions, based on high-resolution scans. Previous VBM studies reported equivocal results in narcolepsy patients.

One study insisted that there were no structural changes in brains of patients with hypocretin-deficient narcolepsy,[9] whereas all other studies reported significant regional decreases in gray matter volumes (GMVs) or gray matter concentration (GMC).[10–14] Two of these studies reported decreases of GMC[10] or GMV[11] in the hypothalamus of narcolepsy patients. These findings suggest that neuronal losses may affect hypocretinergic structures (ie, hypothalamus) as well as some major sites of hypocretin projections (ie, nucleus accumbens). Two other studies found decreases of GMV in 12 narcolepsy patients in inferior temporal/frontal[12] and right prefrontal/frontomesial regions,[13] possibly contributing to cognitive impairments, such as attentional deficits experienced by narcolepsy patients.[15] A recent VBM study revealed that 29 narcolepsy patients showed reduced

Department of Neurology, Samsung Medical Center, Samsung Advanced Institute for Health Sciences & Technology (SAIHST), Sungkyunkwan University School of Medicine, Samsung Biomedical Research Institute (SBRI), 81 Irwon-ro, Gangnam-gu, Seoul 06351, Republic of Korea
E-mail address: sbhong@skku.edu

Sleep Med Clin 12 (2017) 359–368
http://dx.doi.org/10.1016/j.jsmc.2017.03.021
1556-407X/17/© 2017 Elsevier Inc. All rights reserved.

sleep.theclinics.com

GMC in bilateral thalami, left gyrus rectus, bilateral frontopolar gyri, bilateral short insular gyri, bilateral superior frontal gyri, and right superior temporal and left inferior temporal gyri compared with 29 normal controls and, furthermore, small volume correction revealed GMC reduction in bilateral nuclei accumbens, hypothalami, and thalami (**Fig. 1**).[14] In particular, reduced GMC in the hypothalamus and nucleus accumbens in the author and colleagues' study, may support the prior hypothesis that these reductions are associated with EDS and cataplexy in narcolepsy patients. The

author and colleagues' result suggests that those areas with decreased GMC may serve possible roles in wake-sleep controls, attention, or memory. Discrepancies of results among several VBM studies might be due to differences in the analysis processes used (eg, the SPM version, modulated or unmodulated, grand mean scaling, absolute or relative thresholding, and sample size) and clinical characteristics of study patients (hypocretin deficiency, disease duration, medical treatment, and so forth). The patients' characteristics are variable from one study to another. More than half of

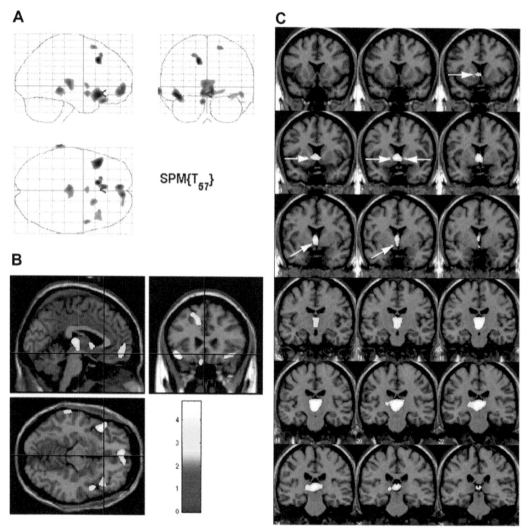

Fig. 1. GMC abnormality in brains of narcolepsy patients. Overall areas showing reduced GMCs are shown in glass brain view (*A*). Decreased gray matter concentrations in narcolepsies with cataplexy in left gyrus rectus, bilateral thalami, bilateral frontopolar gyri, bilateral short insula gyri, bilateral superior frontal gyri, right superior temporal gyrus, and left inferior temporal gyrus are shown as T1 template overlaid MRI at the level of uncorrected *P*<.001 (extent threshold *k*E <100 voxels) (*B*). Bilateral nuclei accumbens (*dotted arrows*), bilateral hypothalamus (*solid arrows*), and bilateral thalami (*arrowhead*) showed reduced GMCs at the level of false discovery rate corrected *P*<.05 with small volume correction (*C*). Superior to inferior panels are arranged in anterior to posterior direction in coronal images. (*Adapted from* Joo EY, Tae WS, Kim ST, et al. Gray matter concentration abnormality in brains of narcolepsy patients. Korean J Radiol 2009;10:555; with permission.)

patients were medicated for EDS in 3 studies,[9,12,13] and in another 2 studies, medication history was not mentioned.[10,11] Only the Joo and colleagues' study included unmedicated, drug-naïve narcolepsy patients.[14] More studies are needed to know whether brain structures is changed by pharmacologic treatment. Among 6 VBM studies, 4 showed GMV changes[11-13] and the other 2[10,14] reported GMC reductions in narcolepsy patients. Optimized VBM can quantify either gray matter differences between subjects: relative distribution of gray matter differences (GMC; no correction for nonlinear normalization) or absolute GMV differences (correction for nonlinear normalization).[16] It is not clear if either GMV or GMC is more sensitive to detect structural abnormalities of brain. On the other hand, the thickness of the cerebral cortex (ranging between 1.5 mm and 4.5 mm) reflects the density and arrangement of cells (neurons, neuroglia, and nerve fibers).[17]

Analysis of Cortical Thickness

The VBM method has some limitations in representing gray matter morphology and localization in the sulcal regions, where the fine details of the anatomy are often obscured by a partial volume effect. Measuring cortical thickness using the cortical surface has been suggested in studies of gray matter morphometry as a strategy for overcoming the limitation of volumetric analyses.[18,19] A cortical-thickness analysis performed at the nodes of a 3-D polygonal mesh has the advantage of providing a direct quantitative index of cortical morphology.[20] In contrast with GMC or GMV analyses, cortical thickness measured from the cortical surfaces differentiates between cortexes of opposing sulcal walls within the same sulcal bed, enabling more precise measurement in deep sulci and analysis of the morphology as a cortical sheet.[20] Localized cortical thinning was found in orbitofrontal gyri, dorsolateral and medial prefrontal cortexes, insula, cingulate gyri, middle and inferior temporal gyri, and inferior parietal lobule of the right and left hemispheres in 28 narcolepsy patients compared with 33 normal controls (**Fig. 2**).[21] Moreover, significant negative correlation was observed between cortical thickness in the left supramarginal gyrus and the score on the Epworth Sleepiness Scale and between the cortical thickness in the left parahippocampal gyrus and the scores of general depressive symptoms on the Beck Depression Inventory. Cortical thinning of the prefrontal and limbic cortices and parietal cortex in narcolepsy may provide a neuroanatomic explanation of the disturbances in attention, memory, emotion, and sleepiness of narcolepsy patients.[21] The results of a cortical thickness analysis may be less subject to variation between laboratories compared with VBM analyses because thickness-measurement procedures are consistent.[22] The spatial distributions of cortical thinning[21] and of the reduced GMCs in VBM study[14] in the authors and colleagues' laboratory were similar even though the population of narcolepsy patients and the study periods were different. Cortical thinning of the dorsolateral prefrontal, orbitofrontal, and temporal cortexes is consistent with the areas in which significant reduced GMCs in narcolepsy patients were observed.[14] The VBM study showed GMC

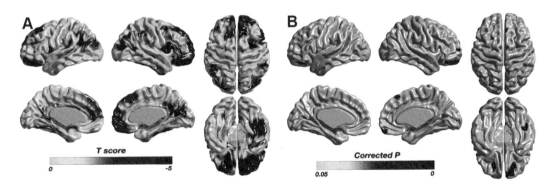

Fig. 2. Measurement of cortical thickness using an automated 3-D algorithm. Statistical t map with t value range of −4.607 to 2.239 and positive values truncated. Most of the cortical area was thinner than in healthy control subjects (A). A significant localized thinning of cortical thickness in patients was found in the orbitorectal gyri, the dorsolateral frontal gyri, the medial frontal gyrus, the cingulate gyrus, the middle and inferior temporal gyri, and the precuneus in the right hemisphere and the dorsolateral frontal gyri, the insular cortex, the posterior parietal lobule, and the middle occipital gyrus in the left hemisphere at the level of false discovery rate corrected $P<.05$ (B). (Adapted from Joo EY, Jeon S, Lee M, et al. Analysis of cortical thickness in narcolepsy patients with cataplexy. Sleep 2011;34:1361; with permission.)

reduction in the bilateral nuclei accumbens, hypothalami, and thalami, which were not included in the measurement of cortical thickness because they are subcortical structures. The similarities between the results of VBM and cortical thickness studies suggest that those findings are more reliable for revealing the neural substrates of clinical symptoms and the pathophysiology of narcolepsy.

Volume Measurement of Amygdala/Hippocampus

Difficulty in cognitive function has been reported as another aspect of brain functional characteristics in narcolepsy.[23] Sophisticated MRI allows in vivo visualization of human brain anatomy with exquisite detail and quantification of morphologic changes. Studies that have investigated the structural integrity of the mesiotemporal lobe structures have been scarce, however, partly due to excessive manual work required for boundary delineation,[24] and identified amygdalar volume reduction in a small cohort of 11 narcolepsy patients compared with controls. Joo and colleagues[25] performed manual labeling of the hippocampus and reported bilateral volume reduction in narcolepsy patients when comparing 36 narcolepsy patients with controls (left hippocampus, 2907.2 mm³ in patients vs 3092.3 mm³ in controls; $P = .005$; right hippocampus, 2990.8 mm³ in patients vs 3184.3 mm³ in

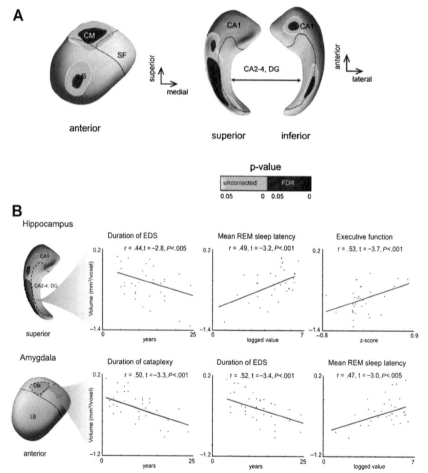

Fig. 3. Morphologic alterations in amygdalo-hippocampal substructures in narcolepsy patients with cataplexy. (A) Vertex (= surface point)-wise group comparison between patients with narcolepsy and healthy controls. Regions of volume decrease in patients relative to controls are shown: the identified atrophy was mapped mainly in hippocampal CA1[a] and in amygdalar CM and LB subfields. [a] Significances are thresholded at the level of false discovery rate less than 0.05. (B) Association between mesiotemporal local volume and clinical parameters and neuropsychological scores in patients with narcolepsy. For each cluster representing significant volume loss in patients relative to controls, the mean volume is correlated with a given clinical parameter. CA, cornu ammonis; CM, centromedial; DG, dentate gyrus; LB, laterobasal; SF, superficial. (Adapted from Kim H, Suh S, Joo EY, et al. Morphological alterations in amygdalo-hippocampal substructures in narcolepsy patients with cataplexy. Brain Imaging Behav 2016;10(4):989–90; with permission.)

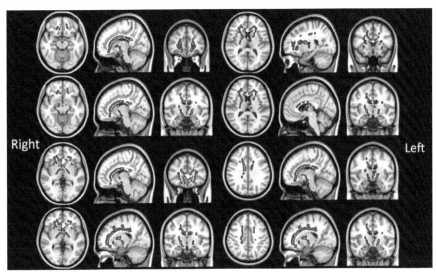

Fig. 4. WM alterations in narcolepsy patients with cataplexy: tract-based special statistics (*red* displays the WM changes of patients relative to controls). Significant fractional anisotrophy (FA) decreases in patients with narcolepsy compared with controls (*P*<.05, threshold free cluster enhancement). The underlay image is the standard Montreal Neurological Institute template. (*Adapted from* Park YK, Kwon OH, Joo EY, et al. White matter alterations in narcolepsy patients with cataplexy: tract-based spatial statistics. J Sleep Res 2016;25(2):186; with permission.)

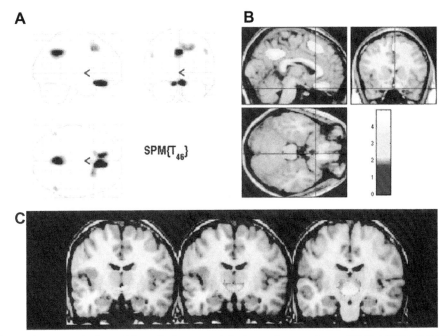

Fig. 5. Glucose hypometabolism of hypothalamus and thalamus in narcolepsy. (*A*) The brain regions showing glucose hypometabolism in narcoleptic patients. The overall hypometabolic areas are shown in glass brain view. (*B*) Hypometabolism in bilateral rectal, subcallosal gyri, right superior frontal gyrus, the medial convexity of right superior frontal gyrus, and in right inferior parietal lobule are shown as a T1 template overlaid MRI at the uncorrected *P*<.001 level. (*C*) Bilateral posterior hypothalami and mediodorsolateral thalamic nuclei show hypometabolism in the level of false discovery rate corrected *P*<.05 with small volume correction. The left-hand side of the images represents the left side of the brain. The order of left to right panels (*C*) is arranged in the anterior to posterior direction in coronal images of the brain. (*Adapted from* Joo EY, Tae WS, Kim JH, et al. Glucose hypometabolism of hypothalamus and thalamus in narcolepsy. Ann Neurol 2004;56:439; with permission.)

controls; $P = .004$). These studies have shown significant association of mesiotemporal lobar volume with clinical symptoms of narcolepsy patients. Amygdalo-hippocampal structures consist of subfields or subnuclear divisions, which are cytoarchitectonically and functionally distinctive. Kim and colleagues[26] demonstrated that subfields atrophy in patients with relative to controls suggests that centromedial area of the amygdala and CA1 of the hippocampus are closely related to the severity of narcolepsy and play a crucial role in the circuitry of cataplexy (**Fig. 3**). Amygdalo-hippocampal subfield analysis may provide new perspectives how neural substrates are associated with key features in narcolepsy.

Diffusion Tensor Imaging: White Matter Exploration

Functional imaging studies showed metabolic[27] and perfusion abnormalities[28] in the hypothalamus-thalamus-orbitofrontal pathway and other brain areas in patients with narcolepsy, demonstrating alterations in the hypocretin pathway. The finding of hypoperfusion WM noted in the frontal and parietal lobes of narcolepsy patients suggested the necessity of appropriate imaging methods to evaluate WM changes. Tract-based spatial statistics (TBSS) were used to localize WM abnormalities with fractional anisotropy (FA) and mean diffusivity (MD) from whole-brain diffusion tensor imaging (DTI). Compared with 26 controls, 22 patients showed significant decreases in FA of WM of the bilateral anterior cingulate, fronto-orbital area, frontal lobe, anterior limb of the internal capsule, and corpus callosum as well as the left anterior and medial thalamus (**Fig. 4**).[29] Although MD values were not different between patients and controls, MD values of WM in the bilateral superior frontal gyri, bilateral fronto-orbital gyri, and right superior parietal gyrus were positively correlated with depressive mood in patients. To avoid the inaccurate alignment between subjects and the ambiguity in choosing the extent of smoothing from DTI-VBM technique, Park and

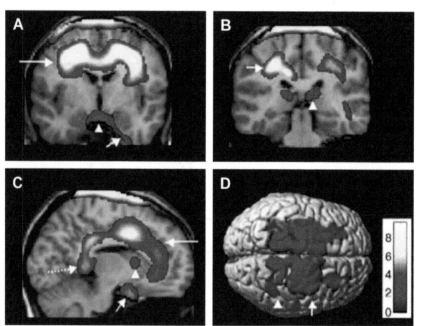

Fig. 6. Cerebral perfusion abnormality in narcolepsy with cataplexy. Brain regions with decreased cerebral perfusion in narcoleptic patients. (*A–C*) In SPM results overlaid on T1 MRI, significant hypoperfusion was observed in bilateral anterior hypothalami (*arrowhead*) and in the right parahippocampal gyrus (*short arrow*). Bilateral cingulate gyri and WMs in bilateral middle frontal gyri (*long arrow*) showed decreased cerebral perfusion (*A*). Hypoperfusion was evident in bilateral posterior thalami (*arrowhead*) and in the WMs of the bilateral postcentral and supramarginal gyri (*arrow*) (*B*). In the sagittal view of right hemisphere, focal hypoperfusion in the caudate nucleus (*arrowhead*) was noted. In the anterior to posterior direction significant hypoperfusion was observed in the subcallosal gyrus (*short arrow*), the cingulate gyrus extending along corpus callosum (*long arrow*), and in the parahippocampal gyrus (*dotted arrow*) (*C*). (*D*) 3-D rendering view showing decreased cerebral perfusion in bilateral paracentral areas (*arrowhead*) and superior/middle frontal gyri (*arrow*). The frontal lobe is on the right and the occipital lobe on the left. These results are significant at false discovery rate corrected $P<.05$. (*Adapted from* Joo EY, Hong SB, Tae WS, et al. Cerebral perfusion abnormality in narcolepsy with cataplexy. Neuroimage 2005;28:410–6; with permission.)

colleagues[29] adopted the DTI-TBSS technique and successfully demonstrated the widespread disruption of WM integrity and prevalent brain degeneration of frontal lobes related to a depressive symptom in narcolepsy.

FUNCTIONAL IMAGING IN NARCOLEPSY AND KLEINE-LEVIN SYNDROME
Cerebral Glucose Metabolism: PET

In 2004, Joo and colleagues[27] reported the alteration of glucose metabolism in narcolepsy patients. The relative difference between cerebral glucose metabolism of 24 narcolepsy patients and 24 normal controls was studied using fluorine-18 (F-18) fluorodeoxyglucose (FDG) PET. Patients with narcolepsy showed significantly reduced cerebral glucose metabolism in bilateral rectal and subcallosal gyri, the medial convexity of right superior frontal gyrus, bilateral precuneus, right inferior parietal lobule, and left supramarginal gyrus (uncorrected $P<.001$). Bilateral posterior hypothalami and mediodorsal thalamic nuclei

showed hypometabolism with significance at the level of corrected $P<.05$, with small volume correction (**Fig. 5**). This PET study may be important to reveal the metabolic impairment of hypothalamus-thalamus-orbitofrontal pathways in the narcolepsy brain for the first time.

Cerebral Perfusion: Single-Photon Emission CT

Several striatal SPECT studies had been performed because evidence indicates that dopaminergic systems are disturbed in narcolepsy and interact with the hypocretin system.[30] Striatal neuroimaging studies of human narcolepsy, however, have produced variable results. Technetium-99m–labeled ethyl cysteinate dimer (ECD) single-photon emission computed tomography (SPECT) has an advantage of investigating the whole brain perfusion pattern.[28] Statistical parametric mapping (SPM) analysis of brain SPECT showed hypoperfusion of the bilateral anterior hypothalami, caudate nuclei, and pulvinar nuclei of thalami, parts of the dorsolateral/ventromedial prefrontal cortices,

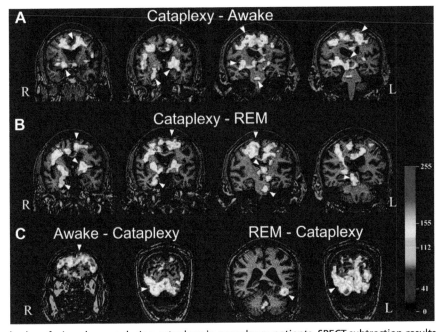

Fig. 7. Cerebral perfusion changes during cataplexy in narcolepsy patients. SPECT subtraction results. (*A*) Hyperperfusion in bilateral premotor cortices, cingulate gyri, sensorimotor cortices, basal ganglia, right amygdala/hippocampus, right insula, both thalami, and brainstem during cataplectic episode compared with baseline awake period (brain SPECT during cataplexy brain SPECT during baseline awake period). (*B*) Hyperperfusion in sensorimotor cortices, cingulate gyri, basal ganglia, thalami, right amygdala/hippocampus, midbrain, and pons during cataplexy compared with REM sleep (brain SPECT during cataplexy brain SPECT during REM sleep). ([*C*] *left 2 images*) Hyperperfusion in prefrontal cortices and occipital lobes during awake period compared with cataplexy (brain SPECT during awake period brain SPECT during cataplexy). ([*C*] *right 2 images*) Hyperperfusion in left posterior basal temporal cortex and bilateral occipital lobes during REM sleep compared with cataplexy attack (brain SPECT during REM sleep brain SPECT during cataplexy). Small arrowheads indicate brain structures described. (*Adapted from* Hong SB, Tae WS, Joo EY. Cerebral perfusion changes during cataplexy in narcolepsy patients. Neurology 2006;66(11):1749; with permission.)

parahippocampal gyri, and cingulate gyri in narcolepsy ($P<.05$ by t test with false discovery rate correction) during wakefulness (**Fig. 6**). Also, reduced cerebral perfusion in subcortical structures and cortical areas in narcolepsy induced the necessity of exploring WM alteration in this disease.

The radiotracer for SPECT, 99mTc-ECD, has a high first-pass brain extraction rate, with maximum uptake achieved within 30 seconds to 60 seconds of an intravenous injection.[31] Radiotracers become trapped in the brain, thereby producing a snapshot of the cerebral perfusion pattern during the event. Hong and colleagues[32] localized cerebral perfusion differences during cataplexy, REM sleep, and a baseline awake period in 2 patients with narcolepsy. To localize brain regions with perfusion changes during cataplexy, SPECT images of REM sleep or images of awake state were compared to images of cataplexy state. During cataplexy, hyperperfusion were shown in right amygdala, bilateral cingulate gyri, basal ganglia, thalami, premotor cortices, sensorimotor cortices,

right insula, and brainstem, and hypoperfusion in prefrontal cortex and occipital lobe (**Fig. 7**). This result suggests that cataplexy is produced by the activation of amygdalo-cortico-basal ganglia–brainstem circuit.

Another SPECT study in narcolepsy was to investigate the effects of modafinil on regional cerebral blood flow (rCBF) in narcolepsy. Modafinil (a diphenylmethyl-sulfinyl-2-acetamide derivative) is a wake-promoting substance used for the treatment of hypersomnolence, in particular that associated with narcolepsy.[33] Brain SPECT was performed twice, during the awake state before and after modafinil or placebo administration, for 4 weeks in 43 drug-naïve narcolepsy patients with cataplexy.[34] Chronic administration of modafinil (mean 207.8 ± 62.3 mg/d) in narcolepsy patients increased rCBF in the bilateral prefrontal cortices, whereas it decreased in the left mesio/basal, temporal, bilateral occipital areas, and cerebellum (**Fig. 8**). This was the first study to investigate the pharmacologic effect on brain and suggested that

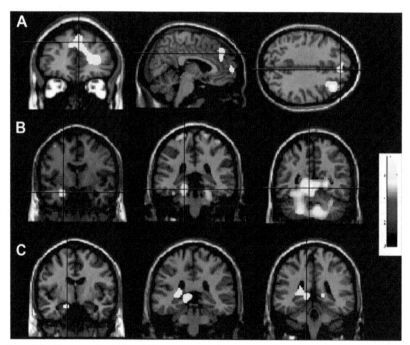

Fig. 8. Effect of modafinil on cerebral blood flow in narcolepsy patients. SPM results demonstrating brain regions with rCBF increase or decrease after modafinil administration in narcolepsy patients. (*A*) According to SPM overlaid on T1 MR images, modafinil administration increased rCBF in bilateral medial prefrontal cortices, right dorsolateral prefrontal cortex at an uncorrected $P<.001$. (*B*) Modafinil administration decreased rCBF in left hippocampus (*left*), bilateral precentral gyri, left fusiform gyrus (*middle*), and bilateral lingual gyri and cerebellum (*right*) in the anterior to posterior direction in coronal MR images at an uncorrected $P<.001$. The result at false discovery rate corrected $P<.05$ is similar to this figure. (*C*) Compared with the on-placebo condition in placebo group, the on-modafinil condition in modafinil group showed rCBF decrease in left hippocampus (*left*) and bilateral parahippocampal gyri (*middle and right*) (uncorrected $P<.05$). The left-hand side of the images represent the left side of the brain. (*Adapted from* Joo EY, Seo DW, Tae WS, et al. Effect of modafinil on cerebral blood flow in narcolepsy patients. Sleep 2008;31(6):871; with permission.)

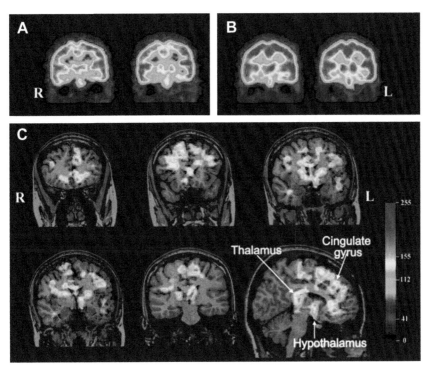

Fig. 9. Episodic diencephalic hypoperfusion in KLS. (*A*) Brain SPECT during a symptomatic period shows hypoperfusion in bilateral frontal (especially medial frontal region), temporal lobes, and thalami/hypothalami. (*B*) Brain SPECT during an asymptomatic period shows recovered cerebral perfusion, except right mesial temporal region. (*C*) SISCOM (subtraction of brain SPECT images between symptomatic and asymptomatic periods and then coregistered to MRI scans) showed significant hypoperfusion in bilateral thalami and basal ganglia, left hypothalamus, both medial frontal regions, bilateral dorsolateral frontal regions, and left temporal lobe during the symptomatic period. (*Adapted from* Hong SB, Joo EY, Tae WS, et al. Episodic diencephalic hypoperfusion in Kleine-Levin syndrome. Sleep 2006;29(8):1091–3; with permission.)

the dose of modafinil that induces a satisfactory wakefulness-promoting response in human narcolepsy also causes regional increase in cerebral blood flow in the bilateral prefrontal cortices.

KLS is a poorly understood neuropsychological disorder typified by intermittent periods of hypersomnia, bulimia, and behavioral disturbances, such as hypersexuality, apathy, and personality changes.[35] A disturbance of diencephalic or hypothalamic function has been proposed because of the character of the symptoms. 99mTc-ECD SPECT was performed in a 22-year-old woman who suffered from recurrent episodes of hypersomnia, apathy, and hyperphagia. During symptomatic and asymptomatic periods, 2 SPECTs were performed, respectively.[36] To localize brain regions with perfusion changes during symptomatic period, asymptomatic SPECT was subtracted from symptomatic SPECT. The subtracted SPECT showed significant hypoperfusion in the left hypothalamus, bilateral thalami, basal ganglia, bilateral medial and dorsolateral frontal regions, and left temporal lobe during the symptomatic period (**Fig. 9**). These cerebral hypoperfusion areas

support the diencephalic hypothesis and clinical symptoms of KLS.

SUMMARY

Neuroimaging studies have provided new information about brain abnormalities in narcolepsy patients. The computer-aided analysis of brain MRI and various functional imaging tools revealed structural and functional abnormalities located in the hypothalamus, in agreement with a loss of hypocretinergic neurons in narcolepsy, as well as in multiple brain structures, possibly in relation with cataplexy and the cognitive and mood disturbances observed in narcolepsy or KLS.

REFERENCES

1. Thannickal TC, Moore RY, Nienhuis R, et al. Reduced number of hypocretin neurons in human narcolepsy. Neuron 2000;27:469–74.
2. Taheri S, Zeitzer JM, Mignot E. The role of hypocretins (orexins) in sleep regulation and narcolepsy. Annu Rev Neurosci 2002;25:283–313.

3. Sakurai T, Amemiya A, Ishii M, et al. Orexins and orexin receptors: a family of hypothalamic neuropeptides and G protein-coupled receptors that regulate feeding behavior. Cell 1998;92:573–85.

4. Nishino S, Ripley B, Overeem S, et al. Hypocretin (orexin) deficiency in human narcolepsy. Lancet 2000;355:39–40.

5. Plazzi G, Montagna P, Provini F, et al. Pontine lesions in idiopathic narcolepsy. Neurology 1996; 46:1250–4.

6. Bassetti C, Aldrich MS, Quint DJ. MRI findings in narcolepsy. Sleep 1997;20:630–1.

7. Frey JL, Heiserman JE. Absence of pontine lesions in narcolepsy. Neurology 1997;48:1097–9.

8. Desseilles M, Dang-Vu TD, Schabus M, et al. Neuroimaging insights into the pathophysiology of sleep disorders. Sleep 2008;31:777–94.

9. Overeem S, Steens SC, Good CD, et al. Voxel-based morphometry in hypocretin-deficient narcolepsy. Sleep 2003;26:44–6.

10. Draganski B, Geisler P, Hajak G, et al. Hypothalamic gray matter changes in narcolepsy patients. Nat Med 2002;8:1186–8.

11. Buskova J, Vaneckova M, Sonka K, et al. Reduced hypothalamic gray matter in narcolepsy with cataplexy. Neuro Endocrinol Lett 2006;27:769–72.

12. Kaufmann C, Schuld A, Pollmacher T, et al. Reduced cortical gray matter in narcolepsy: preliminary findings with voxel-based morphometry. Neurology 2002;58:1852–5.

13. Brenneis C, Brandauer E, Frauscher B, et al. Voxel based morphometry in narcolepsy. Sleep Med 2005;6:531–6.

14. Joo EY, Tae WS, Kim ST, et al. Gray matter concentration abnormality in brains of narcolepsy patients. Korean J Radiol 2009;10:552–8.

15. Rieger M, Mayer G, Gauggel S. Attention deficits in patients with narcolepsy. Sleep 2003;26:36–43.

16. Good CD, Johnsrude IS, Ashburner J, et al. A voxel-based morphometric study of ageing in 465 normal adult human brains. Neuroimage 2001;14:21–36.

17. Parent A, Carpenter MB. Human neuroanatomy. Baltimore (MD): Williams & Wilkins; 1995.

18. Fischl B, Dale AM. Measuring the thickness of the human cerebral cortex from magnetic resonance images. Proc Natl Acad Sci U S A 2000;97:11050–5.

19. Kabani N, Le Goualher G, MacDonald D, et al. Measurement of cortical thickness using an automated 3-D algorithm: a validation study. Neuroimage 2001;13:375–80.

20. Im K, Lee JM, Lee J, et al. Gender difference analysis of cortical thickness in healthy young adults with surface-based methods. Neuroimage 2006;31: 31–8.

21. Joo EY, Jeon S, Lee M, et al. Analysis of cortical thickness in narcolepsy patients with cataplexy. Sleep 2011;34:1357–64.

22. Lin JJ, Salamon N, Lee AD, et al. Reduced neocortical thickness and complexity mapped in mesial temporal lobe epilepsy with hippocampal sclerosis. Cereb Cortex 2007;17:2007–18.

23. Hood B, Bruck D. Metamemory in narcolepsy. J Sleep Res 1997;6(3):205–10.

24. Brabec J, Rulseh A, Horinek D, et al. Volume of the amygdala is reduced in patients with narcolepsy - a structural MRI study. Neuro Endocrinol Lett 2011; 32(5):652–6.

25. Joo EY, Kim SH, Kim ST, et al. Hippocampal volume and memory in narcoleptics with cataplexy. Sleep Med 2012;13(4):396–401.

26. Kim H, Suh S, Joo EY, et al. Morphological alterations in amygdalo-hippocampal substructures in narcolepsy patients with cataplexy. Brain Imaging Behav 2016;10(4):984–94.

27. Joo EY, Tae WS, Kim JH, et al. Glucose hypometabolism of hypothalamus and thalamus in narcolepsy. Ann Neurol 2004;56:437–40.

28. Joo EY, Hong SB, Tae WS, et al. Cerebral perfusion abnormality in narcolepsy with cataplexy. Neuroimage 2005;28:410–6.

29. Park YK, Kwon OH, Joo EY, et al. White matter alterations in narcolepsy patients with cataplexy: tract-based spatial statistics. J Sleep Res 2016;25(2): 181–9.

30. Eisensehr I, Linke R, Tatsch K, et al. Alteration of the striatal dopaminergic system in human narcolepsy. Neurology 2003;60:1817–9.

31. O'Brien TJ, O'Connor MK, Mullan BP, et al. Subtraction ictal SPET co-registered to MRI in partial epilepsy: description and technical validation of the method with phantom and patient studies. Nucl Med Commun 1998;19:31–45.

32. Hong SB, Tae WS, Joo EY. Cerebral perfusion changes during cataplexy in narcolepsy patients. Neurology 2006;66(11):1747–9.

33. Bastuji H, Jouvet M. Successful treatment of idiopathic hypersomnia and narcolepsy with modafinil. Prog Neuropsychopharmacol Biol Psychiatry 1988; 12:695–700.

34. Joo EY, Seo DW, Tae WS, et al. Effect of modafinil on cerebral blood flow in narcolepsy patients. Sleep 2008;31(6):868–73.

35. Gadoth N, Dickerman Z, Bechar M, et al. Episodic hormone secretion during sleep in Kleine-Levin syndrome: evidence for hypothalamic dysfunction. Brain Dev 1987;9(3):309–15.

36. Hong SB, Joo EY, Tae WS, et al. Episodic diencephalic hypoperfusion in Kleine-Levin syndrome. Sleep 2006;29(8):1091–3.

Sleep-Disordered Breathing and Excessive Daytime Sleepiness

Ken He, MD[a,b], Vishesh K. Kapur, MD, MPH[c,*]

KEYWORDS

- Sleep disorders • Sleep apnea • Excessive daytime sleepiness • Persistent sleepiness
- Hypersomnolence • Hypersomnia • Therapy • Treatment resistance

KEY POINTS

- Excessive daytime sleepiness is common in obstructive sleep apnea, although a significant number of patients lack this complaint.
- Excessive daytime sleepiness may coexist with other forms of sleep-related breathing disorders, but the evidence regarding this is less robust than for obstructive sleep apnea.
- Multiple methods are available to evaluate sleepiness, all of which have limitations including inconsistent correlation to presence and severity of obstructive sleep apnea.
- Data on amelioration of sleepiness with treatment of obstructive sleep apnea are most robust for positive airway pressure therapy, but improvement is seen with other treatment modalities.
- Before initiating pharmacotherapy for persistent sleepiness despite adequate control of obstructive sleep apnea, alternative causes of sleepiness should be evaluated and treated.

INTRODUCTION

The term sleep-disordered breathing encompasses the full spectrum of sleep-related respiratory disturbances. Sleep-related breathing disorders (SRBD) represent the subset that meets International Classification of Sleep Disorders Third Edition (ICSD-3) criteria as a disorder; abnormalities such as snoring or catathrenia are examples of entities not included under the term SRBD.[1] The ICSD-3 describes 4 different, but interrelated types of SRBD: (1) obstructive sleep apnea (OSA) syndrome, central sleep apnea (CSA) syndromes, sleep-related hypoventilation (SRH) disorders, and sleep-related hypoxemia disorder.[1] SRBD in the various forms may manifest as abnormal airflow, oxygen desaturation, or hypercarbia that can be associated with excessive daytime sleepiness (EDS). For OSA, EDS is a frequently reported symptom that is included as a possible clinical feature in the ICSD-3 diagnostic criteria, but a significant number of OSA patients do not report this symptom. Here we discuss the relationship between EDS and SRBD focusing primarily on OSA. We review patient factors related to EDS, treatment options, evaluation and treatment of persistent sleepiness despite treated OSA, and future developments.

Disclosure Statement: The authors have nothing to disclose.
[a] Division of General Internal Medicine, University of Washington, Seattle, WA 98195, USA; [b] Hospital and Sleep Medicine Sections, VA Puget Sound Health Care System, S-111-Pulm, 1660 South Columbian Way, Seattle, WA 98108, USA; [c] Division of Pulmonary, Critical Care and Sleep Medicine, University of Washington, Seattle, WA 98104, USA
* Corresponding author. UW Medicine Sleep Center, Harborview Medical Center, 325 Ninth Avenue, Box 359803, Seattle, WA 98104.

EXCESSIVE DAYTIME SLEEPINESS

A standard definition for EDS is lacking. It is often described as the inability to stay awake and alert during the day when the circadian sleep drive promotes alertness.[2] EDS can manifest as falling asleep unintentionally during routine daily activities or the subjective perception of sleepiness. Patients who do not report subjective sleepiness may nevertheless have objective sleepiness and vice versa. To further complicate matters, patients use a diverse vocabulary to describe the feeling of sleepiness including fatigue, tiredness, unrested, and lack of energy. Patients with EDS have lower quality of life, decreased workplace productivity, and increased risk of work-related injury.[3,4] In the United States, a general population survey noted a prevalence of 18% based on Epworth Sleepiness Scale (ESS) score of $\geq$10.[5] Population-based surveys from the National Sleep Foundation found that about 30% of respondents suffer from enough EDS to interfere with their quality of life.[6] Methods have been developed over the last 4 decades to subjectively and objectively measure EDS. The ESS is the most commonly used subjective instrument to assess EDS in clinical practice and research applications.[7] The Multiple Sleep Latency Test (MSLT) and Maintenance of Wakefulness Test (MWT) are well-established objective measures for EDS but are used infrequently in clinical practice because of their resource intensity and limited utility in the evaluation of patients with SRBD.[8]

EXCESSIVE DAYTIME SLEEPINESS IN SLEEP-RELATED BREATHING DISORDERS

OSA is the most common type of SRBD and also the disorder for which the most is known about with regard to EDS.

Obstructive Sleep Apnea Disorders

OSA is characterized by upper airway narrowing or closure during sleep with continued respiratory effort.[1] It is commonly thought that repetitive obstructions with and without intermittent nocturnal hypoxemia lead to sleep fragmentation, cortical arousals, awakenings, and inability to achieve and sustain more restful sleep stages resulting in EDS. The Wisconsin Sleep Cohort reported the prevalence of OSA syndrome (Apnea-hypopnea index [AHI] $\geq$5 with sleepiness) to be 4% in men and 2% in women.[9] Several other population studies on OSA associated with EDS found prevalences of 3% to 7% in men and 2% to 5% in women.[10] A more recent large population-based study found a prevalence of OSA syndrome

(AHI $\geq$5 and ESS score $\geq$11) of 13% in men and 6% in women.[11] The higher prevalence is attributed to the increased prevalence of obesity and changes in the diagnostic and scoring criteria for OSA. OSA prevalence when defined by AHI alone is several-fold higher, indicating that a large percentage of OSA subjects do not complain of EDS.[9,11,12] The relationship between OSA and EDS is seem to be influenced by a host of factors and subject to considerable interindividual variability in susceptibility to sleepiness.

Central Sleep Apnea Syndromes

CSA syndromes are characterized by recurrent cessation or attenuation of respiratory effort during sleep.[1] CSA can be the result of distinct disease processes, most commonly heart failure (HF), atrial fibrillation, stroke, chronic kidney disease, and medications.[1] Recent analyses show a CSA prevalence of 0.9% to 3.5%.[13,14] Other systematic reviews report the prevalence of CSA to be 24% in the setting of opioid use—averaging 200 mg of morphine equivalent daily dose and 8% for treatment emergent CSA (TECSA).[15,16] There are little data on the relationship between CSA and EDS, which suggests that CSA may not be independently associated with EDS. A community-based study reported that those with CSA had a level of sleepiness comparable to those without SRBD and lower than those with OSA despite having higher AHI.[14] Furthermore, a study in stable HF patients found that the prevalence of EDS in those with CSA was not statistically different (16% vs 11%) than in those without CSA; EDS was associated with HF severity rather than sleep parameters.[17] Finally, a study in patients with atrial fibrillation found those with CSA had a lower prevalence of EDS than those with OSA.[18]

Sleep-Related Hypoventilation Disorders

The hallmark of SRH is abnormally elevated arterial pressure of carbon dioxide during sleep, although hypoventilation may also be present during waking hours.[1] Most of data regarding EDS and SRH come from patients with obesity hypoventilation syndrome (OHS). Because 90% of those with OHS also have OSA, it is unclear whether hypoventilation is playing an independent role.[19] OHS subjects were reported to have more EDS and higher ESS score compared with isolated OSA. However, this finding may be attributed to higher body mass index (BMI) and worse sleep parameters,[20] as one study found resolution of symptom differences after adjusting for obesity.[21] Yet another study found significantly higher ESS score in OHS patients compared with OSA patients matched for body mass index, AHI, and oxygen desaturation index, but the former had greater exposure to hypoxemia.[22] Small studies in OHS patients found correlation of EDS with hypercarbia and subsequent improvement of both parameters on therapy.[23,24]

Sleep-Related Hypoxemia Disorder

This last category is a diagnosis of exclusion, reached after other SRBDs that cause hypoxemia during sleep are ruled out. There are sparse data regarding EDS in this disorder, and association remains unclear.

PATHOPHYSIOLOGY OF EXCESSIVE DAYTIME SLEEPINESS IN OBSTRUCTIVE SLEEP APNEA

Although superficially it seems reasonable to presume that sleep disruption from respiratory events are central to the etiology of EDS in OSA, the underlying mechanisms remain to be fully elucidated. A diverse collection of mechanisms has been implicated. Rodent models show that chronic intermittent hypoxemia increases levels of harmful enzymes that cause oxidative damage to brain regions involved in regulation of wakefulness.[25,26] In humans with OSA, markedly reduced hippocampal volumes are associated with increased ESS score.[27] One study that found this association did not find an association of OSA severity or hypoxemia to hippocampal volumes.[28] Reduced regional cerebral blood flow during wakefulness to brain areas is associated with subjective sleepiness in older subjects with severe OSA.[29] Epigenetically, changes in DNA methylation patterns of specific genes are associated with EDS in subjects with OSA.[30] Yet another proposed mechanism implicates cardiac autonomic dysregulation caused by arousals as a pathway to EDS.[31]

PATIENT EVALUATION

This section focusses on the evaluation of the OSA patient, as this is the most common type of SRBD and the type most closely associated with EDS.

History

EDS can manifest as either falling asleep unintentionally or simply a perception of feeling sleepy. Inquiry should be made regarding the likelihood of falling asleep during sedentary activities and situations in which diminished alertness may be dangerous. Verification by a third party such as family members is especially helpful in patients that have poor awareness of lapses into sleep. In the medical lexicon, fatigue is distinct from sleepiness; sleepiness typically manifests during sedentary activities, whereas fatigue limits physical activities without affecting mental alertness. Nevertheless, patients frequently use these terms interchangeably to describe the state of feeling sleepy.[32,33] Chervin[34] reported that fatigue, tiredness, and lack of energy were all more commonly reported than sleepiness in OSA patients. In subjects with moderate-to-severe OSA, several individuals reported feeling unrested, tired, or worn out despite not having an elevated ESS score or feeling sleepy.[35]

The signs and symptoms of OSA are well described; important ones include habitual snoring, witnessed apneas, gasping/choking episodes, and nocturia. Insufficient sleep opportunity is a common cause of sleepiness; therefore, it is important to inquire about sleep-wake schedules. Differences of greater than 1 hour between weekdays and weekends can indicate sleep restriction owing to work responsibilities. Several medical conditions can contribute to or mimic sleepiness; some of the more common types to consider include depression, hypothyroidism, iron deficiency, and vitamin D deficiency. Identification of prescription and nonprescription use of sedatives or alerting substances is also important.

Physical

Patients, while waiting to be roomed and during the medical interview, may manifest sleepiness. They may be engaged in activities to avoid falling asleep such as standing during the encounter or consuming caffeine-laden beverages. Obesity is associated with sleepiness independent of OSA.[36,37]

Epworth Sleepiness Scale

The ESS is the most widely used tool to assess sleepiness in research and clinical practice.[7] However, the ESS measures sleep propensity based on recall of situational dozing episodes rather than subjective sleepiness.[38] Thus, patients with poor sleep perception may underestimate their degree of sleepiness. An extensive number of studies evaluated the validity of ESS in the assessment of EDS in OSA and the correlation to OSA severity, although these relationships remain unclear. Although some studies show an association between the ESS score and objective sleepiness or OSA severity,[39–41] other studies found no relationship.[42–44] A community-based sample showed an association between elevated ESS score and OSA severity, although only some subjects with moderate-to-severe OSA had an ESS score greater than the normal threshold.[35,41]

Multiple Sleep Latency and Maintenance of Wakefulness Tests

The MSLT is the most commonly used objective measure of sleepiness in clinical practice. The MWT was subsequently developed to objectively measure the ability to stay awake. In OSA patients, the MSLT is poorly correlated to subjective sleep measures,[34,45] although studies found an association between OSA severity and shorter mean sleep latency (MSL).[40,44] Even fewer data exist on use of MWT in OSA. Lack of normative data on both tests and the wide range of MSL thresholds used to signify abnormal degree of sleepiness limits their utility.[2] In addition, subjects can volitionally alter their MSLT/MWT sleep latency.[46] Because of their resource-intensive nature and limited utility, these tests should not be routinely used to assess EDS in OSA nor to measure response to therapy. In some cases, MWT may be requested by licensing authorities in individuals with OSA in whom ability to remain alert constitutes an occupational safety issue; however, there is little evidence that MWT results are associated with real-world performance.[8,47,48]

Laboratory Evaluation

Laboratory testing in the initial evaluation of EDS in OSA is not indicated unless symptoms support an alternative or coexistent cause of EDS that requires evaluation. Comprehensive laboratory testing should be considered for patients with persistent sleepiness despite adequate control of OSA to look for alternative causes of EDS or fatigue. These tests include metabolic panel, blood counts, thyroid function, testosterone level in men, iron studies, urine drug screen, and vitamin levels such as B12 and D.[49–51] Case reports show resolution of EDS and fatigue in subjects without sleep disorders after correction of vitamin deficiencies.[52–54]

Polysomnography Correlates

Studies have evaluated whether specific polysomnography (PSG) indices are associated with EDS in OSA. Objective sleepiness as measured by MSLT was most strongly associated with supine AHI, non–rapid eye movement sleep AHI, apnea burden, and obstructive respiratory events in a sleep center cohort.[55,56] Other studies highlight the role of hypoxemia as reflected by lower nadir or mean oxygen saturation and higher oxygen desaturation index.[57–62] Other PSG determinants of EDS reported include longer total sleep time, shorter sleep latency, greater sleep efficiency, and greater snoring severity.[58,59,62–64] The association of sleep stage distribution and arousal index with sleepiness are not consistently seen.[58,59,64] There are conflicting findings regarding the associations between specific PSG parameters and sleepiness.

RESPONSE TO THERAPY
Therapies for Obstructive Sleep Apnea

Positive airway pressure
There is robust evidence based on randomized controlled trials (RCT) that continuous positive airway pressure (CPAP) therapy for OSA improves subjective EDS. The findings regarding objective sleepiness are more variable, but also support improvement. A meta-analysis of 10 studies with 712 participants found nearly a 4-point improvement of ESS score in the CPAP group compared with control.[65] Several studies from this meta-analysis found CPAP prolonged MSL by 2.4 minutes on MWT but not on MSLT.[65] Weaver and colleagues[66] found in those with moderate or severe OSA, a dose-response relationship is present; increasing duration of CPAP use was associated with a higher percentage of subjects with normalized ESS score and MSL on MSLT. ESS score improvement was also found in nonsevere OSA in an RCT comparing active CPAP with sham CPAP.[67] More advanced PAP delivery modes to treat OSA include auto-titrating PAP (APAP), bi-level PAP (BPAP), and expiratory pressure relief. Three separate meta-analyses comparing change in ESS score with APAP against CPAP indicate no significant or clinically marginal ($\leq$0.5) superiority of APAP.[68–70] Similarly, BPAP and expiratory pressure relief were not found to have superior outcomes to CPAP.[71–73]

Oral repositioning devices
The most widely used type of oral repositioning device is the mandibular advancement device (MAD). MADs have become accepted as a second-line therapy for OSA. Studies find, on average, that reduction in ESS score after initiation of MAD is comparable to that of CPAP, although improvement in OSA is not uniform across patients.[74,75] Therefore, confirming MAD efficacy via a sleep study is recommended when EDS persists. Custom and titratable MADs have been found to improve EDS, but prefabricated MADs have not.[75,76] The tongue-retaining device (TRD) is an alternative type of oral repositioning device that anteriorly displaces the tongue using suction. A small retrospective case series found therapy with TRDs improved ESS score.[77] However, tongue-retaining devices are less well tolerated than MADs because of greater side effects such as soft tissue irritation, dry mouth, and excessive

salivation. Consequently, TRDs are uncommonly used in clinical practice.[78]

Sleep surgery

Surgical therapies for OSA can be divided into airway (nasal, upper pharyngeal, lower pharyngeal/laryngeal, global upper airway) and nonairway (bariatric) procedures. Therapies can be done in isolation or combined either simultaneously or in a stepwise fashion. Although benefits do not depend on long-term adherence, efficacy may diminish over time. The evidence supporting surgery is limited by a paucity of RCTs and studies evaluating the effect of a single procedure, as patients often have multilevel or prior surgeries. A meta-analysis of various upper airway surgeries, consisting primarily of case series, reported improved EDS after maxillomandibular advancement, uvulopharyngopalatoplasty, and radiofrequency ablation with more invasive surgeries yielding greater benefit.[79] As for bariatric surgery, a RCT by Dixon and colleagues[80] of 60 obese patients with OSA found improved ESS score from baseline but no significant difference in ESS score between surgery and medical weight loss groups despite greater weight loss with surgery.

Pharmacologic therapy

There are no approved drug treatments for OSA. A meta-analysis of 30 trials concerning 25 drugs found small studies of low-quality evidence with only 4 studies specifically addressing EDS.[81] None found a significant change in ESS score with drug therapy except for a single RCT of 21 subjects without Alzheimer's treated with donepezil at 1 month versus placebo that showed ESS score reduction of 2.9.[82] Separately, a study of subjects with OSA and allergic rhinitis treated with nasal mometasone alone or combined with desloratadine found a significant ESS score reduction.[83]

Positional therapy

Positional therapies run the gamut from tennis balls and foam bumps to electronic wearables that discourage supine sleep. A meta-analysis of positional therapy for positional OSA found no difference in ESS score in those treated with positional therapy compared to CPAP or nonstandard therapy.[84]

Lifestyle modification

Exercise and weight loss are beneficial in ameliorating OSA. Meta-analyses show exercise improves OSA severity and ESS score despite nonsignificant impact on body weight.[85,86] In another meta-analysis of diet and exercise for OSA, pooled RCT data did not show a significant change in ESS score, whereas pooled non-RCT pre-post study data did.[87]

Expiratory positive airway pressure

Application of one-way valves at the nasal airway to generate expiratory positive airway pressure (EPAP) improves OSA. An RCT found that ESS score improved by 2.7 in patients treated with nasal EPAP relative to sham EPAP.[88] A meta-analysis of 18 studies on nasal EPAP found improvement of ESS score by 2.5 after treatment compared with baseline.[89]

Hypoglossal Nerve Stimulator

Hypoglossal nerve stimulation synchronized with the respiratory cycle results in tongue protrusion, which can improve OSA. Several systems have been developed with at least one showing consistent data in durable reduction of OSA severity and improved ESS score.[90,91] Meta-analysis of 6 studies found reduction in ESS score of 4.4 at 12 months compared with baseline.[92]

Myofunctional therapy

Myofunctional therapy (MT) includes airway training exercises such as specific vocalizations, singing, and playing instruments (eg, didgeridoo) that target the oral cavity and oropharyngeal structures as a method to treat OSA. A meta-analysis of 9 studies found reduction in ESS score by nearly 7 compared with baseline after MT.[93] A more recent study of 20 patients with mild-to-moderate OSA treated with MT for 3 months had significant reduction of ESS score by 2, and 14 of 16 patients with EDS noticed improvement at 3 months.[94] A study of 100 men with OSA randomly assigned to placebo, MT, CPAP, or CPAP with MT found significant reduction in ESS at 3 months in all active groups compared with baseline and placebo (MT with 5.6-point improvement relative to placebo). Only the MT group had sustained improvement in ESS score after a 3-week washout period.[95] In contrast, an RCT of 39 patients treated with MT (intervention) versus nasal dilator strips plus respiratory exercises (control) found no change in ESS score in either group at 3 months despite significant reduction of snoring in the MT group.[96]

Combination therapies

Given the number of available therapies for OSA, there are several permutations of combined therapies that are possible. As a starting point (TRD), lifestyle modification is recommended regardless of additional therapies. One goal of combining therapies is to enhance effectiveness and tolerability of the more efficacious treatment, usually PAP. Studies report use of positional therapy,[97] topical nasal steroids,[98] nasal surgery,[99] and myofunctional therapy to enhance CPAP adherence.[95] In one study, 10 patients intolerant of CPAP, who had residual events with MAD, tolerated combined therapy, allowing a 2-cm lowering of CPAP. Residual AHI and ESS score were reduced more than with MAD alone.[100]

Therapies for Central Sleep Apnea

The outcomes of PAP treatment of CSA have been studied predominantly in patients with HF and Cheyne-Stokes breathing. Improvement in EDS has not been consistently seen in this population. Fewer studies evaluate PAP therapy in TECSA and CSA related to opioid use. A meta-analysis including 301 patients found that adaptive servo ventilation (ASV) was superior to subtherapeutic ASV, CPAP, or BPAP in reducing AHI in HF patients, although improvement in ESS was not significantly different.[101] Most recently, the Treatment of Predominant Central Sleep Apnea by Adaptive Servo Ventilation in Patients With Heart Failure (SERVE-HF) trial evaluated the impact of ASV in those with HF, and predominant CSA showed statistically significant but clinically marginal reduction in ESS score by 0.5 with ASV compared with control at 3 months (both groups had mean baseline ESS score close to 7). Improved ESS score was not sustained, and no difference was seen at end of the study at 48 months.[102] Similarly, a systematic review on the effect of ASV on ESS score in HF with CSA/Cheyne-Stokes breathing patients showed mean ESS score was normal at baseline and did not change significantly with ASV.[103] ASV is no longer recommended for CSA/Cheyne-Stokes breathing–predominant sleep apnea in systolic HF because of concerns related to increased cardiovascular mortality.

In TECSA, residual events improve over time with CPAP alone in about 90% of cases.[104] ASV can reduce residual AHI and ESS score in these patients but is not necessarily superior to CPAP.[105] A retrospective review showed that CPAP improved ESS similarly in OSA and TECSA patients.[106] Furthermore, a study of mixed etiology CSA patients, most with TECSA, found similar improvements in ESS score comparing ASV with other PAP modes.[107] Moreover, a randomized, prospective trial found no difference in ESS score improvement with ASV relative to CPAP despite better control of AHI on ASV.[108]

As for opioid-related CSA, there is inadequate evidence to suggest any PAP modality is superior.[109,110] A case series of 4 patients reported improved ESS score with resolution of CSA on BPAP with backup rate.[111]

Phrenic nerve stimulation is being developed to treat CSA in HF. Data from a nonrandomized pilot study of 57 patients with HF and CSA showed improvement of ESS score at 6 months by 2 when baseline ESS score was less than 10 and by 4 when baseline ESS score was greater than 10.[112] More data are anticipated from the first RCT using this system for CSA.[113]

Therapies for Sleep-Related Hypoventilation

In SRH, data on treatment-related change in EDS are mainly derived from OHS subjects. It remains unclear whether improvement in EDS is owing to treatment of OSA, typically present in OHS, or treatment of SRH. OHS patients treated with noninvasive ventilation have greater ESS score reduction compared to weight loss and lifestyle modification.[114] Mechanistically, noninvasive ventilation modes such as BPAP or volume-assured pressure support should be superior to CPAP by achieving better gas exchange, but findings from several recent studies do not support this assumption. CPAP compared with BPAP or volume-assured pressure support for initial treatment of OHS resulted in no group difference in ESS at several months of follow-up.[115–117] Thus, the best PAP modality in improving EDS in OHS remains unclear.

TREATMENT RESISTANCE
Sleepiness Despite Adequate Treatment of Obstructive Sleep Apnea

This phenomenon is termed *sleepiness*, *residual sleepiness*, or *hypersomnia* despite adequately treated OSA. In addition to complaints of sleepiness, there can be persistent elevation of ESS score and short MSL on MSLT. Determining the prevalence of inadequate response to therapy is complex because there is variation in how sleepiness and adequate therapy is defined and how and whether competing causes of sleepiness are excluded. Among studies that use ESS score greater than 10 to define sleepiness, about 10% of OSA patients on CPAP have residual sleepiness,[118] although individual studies have reported rates from 6% to 55%.[119] The study with 6% prevalence excluded patients with restless legs syndrome, narcolepsy, depression, inadequate PAP therapy, and medications affecting vigilance.[120] In a much larger, more recent study by Gasa and colleagues[121] of 1047 OSA subjects that excluded patients with inadequate CPAP efficacy, inadequate adherence, or depression, 13% overall and 18.3% of those with baseline ESS score greater than 10 had residual sleepiness with CPAP. Interestingly, 5.6% of patients not initially sleepy had ESS score greater than 10 on follow-up.

Etiology of Persistent Sleepiness

The underlying mechanisms of residual sleepiness remain unclear. Intermittent nocturnal hypoxia could result in irreversible injury to brain regions that regulate sleep and wake. This finding is based on experimental studies of mice exposed to intermittent hypoxia that had persistent sleepiness after return to normoxia.[25] Clinical studies argue against this mechanism in many patients, as those with residual sleepiness are more likely to have less severe OSA including less cumulative exposure to hypoxia.[119–121] Affected patients also are younger, have higher ESS score at baseline, and report worse general health, more fatigue, and more PAP side effects.[121] Other predictors of residual sleepiness include comorbid diabetes, hypothyroidism, heart disease, neurologic disorders, mood disorders, and other sleep disorders, especially insufficient sleep.[119,120] This finding is supported by a cross-sectional telephone interview of a representative sample that showed a large number of disease and medication factors associated with moderate-to-severe excessive sleepiness.[122] As discussed earlier, obesity may independently cause sleepiness, and this mechanism may be at play in some patients with persistent sleepiness.[36,123]

The role of inadequately treated OSA both in terms of efficacy of CPAP and adequacy of adherence must be considered. A study of 61 patients titrated on CPAP using conventional methods found that 25% of patients had residual sleep apnea (AHI >10) while using CPAP, and these patients tended to have higher ESS scores. Periodic breathing was often present in this subset.[124] The role of adherence is highlighted by Gasa and colleagues,[121] who found reduction of residual sleepiness from 18.5% to 8.7% comparing patients using CPAP ≤4 to greater than 6 hours per night, respectively. PSG parameters seen in those with residual sleepiness include lower percentage of N3, higher periodic limb movement (PLM) index, shorter MSL on MSLT, and more sleep onset rapid eye movement periods (without meeting criteria for narcolepsy without cataplexy).[125] More recently, discovery of endogenous, positive allosteric modulators of γ-aminobutyric acid type A (GABA$_A$) receptors in the cerebrospinal fluid of primary hypersomnia patients, some of whom have concurrent OSA as a secondary diagnosis, may point to another potential mechanism for residual sleepiness.[126] Lastly, a recent MRI study of brain white matter in 29 male subjects found extensive changes in a group of OSA patients with residual sleepiness compared with a matched nonsleepy group despite high levels of CPAP adherence in both groups.[127] It is unknown why the white matter changes occurred.

Management of Persistent Sleepiness

In patients with persistent sleepiness, effective PAP therapy must be verified. A data download offers information regarding adherence, efficacy, and leak. Even though adequate adherence is defined by some as use of PAP ≥70% of nights for ≥4 hours nightly, this level of use is insufficient to adequately reduce exposure to OSA for many patients. Weaver and colleagues[66] found a linear dose-response relationship between increasing use and achieving normal levels of objective and subjective daytime sleepiness, which plateaued at up to 7 hours of use. Based on this information and logic, patient adherence should optimally include all time spent asleep with lesser levels of adherence introducing the possibility that continued exposure to OSA is a potential contributor to residual sleepiness.

With regard to inadequate efficacy, residual AHI reported by PAP machines may not always be accurate. Various studies have found both overreporting and underreporting of AHI by PAP devices with APAP modes mainly implicated.[128–130] Additionally, introduction of pressure relief features to promote adherence may adversely affect adequate therapy, especially with CPAP.[131] The patient and bed partner should be queried with regard to signs and symptoms of inadequate efficacy, including persistence of snoring, observed irregular breathing, and difficulty breathing. An initial or repeat manual titration study should be performed if clinical suspicion warrants. Ultimately, the intrusive nature of PAP therapy itself may be the cause of sleep disruption, as those with residual sleepiness tend to complain of more PAP side effects including leak, mask discomfort, aerophagia, and claustrophobia.[132] Excessive mask or oral leak can cause arousals. Thus, any PAP interface issues should be addressed to ensure that this is not a cause of persistent sleepiness.

In addition to confirming effective PAP therapy, attention should be paid to thoroughly evaluating and treating non-OSA causes of sleepiness. Patient reported sleep-wake times supplemented by hours and pattern of use on PAP download can be helpful in assessing insufficient sleep syndrome and circadian rhythm disorders. Presuming good PAP adherence, hours of use is an estimate of time in bed that can assist in assessing if an adequate amount of time is reserved for sleep. Persistent concerns regarding circadian rhythm disorders and adequacy of sleep duration can be assessed with actigraphy. Other sleep disorders such as central hypersomnia, restless leg syndrome, and PLM disorder should be considered. Efforts should be made to treat contributing comorbid diseases such as a trial of alerting antidepressants in depression, thyroid hormone replacement in hypothyroidism, discontinuation of sedating medications including alcohol, and initiation of an exercise regimen. Select laboratory tests are recommended to evaluate treatable etiologies. (See laboratory evaluation subheading under patient evaluation section.)

Pharmacotherapy should be the last step in treatment of clinically significant residual sleepiness after exhaustive evaluation has not identified another cause to which an intervention can be targeted. Worldwide, caffeine is the most commonly used nonprescription stimulant. Two similarly conducted studies comparing caffeine, 600 mg; dextroamphetamine, 20 mg; modafinil, 400 mg; and placebo effects on alertness measured by psychomotor vigilance testing after an extended period of sleep deprivation found similar improvement in all 3 drug groups.[133,134] However, this dose of caffeine is 6 times higher than what is available from a standard cup of coffee, resulting in higher rates of subjective side effects.[133] Other prescription stimulants that have long been used in clinical practice include various forms of amphetamines and methylphenidate. These medications are recommended for treatment of central hypersomnias, although efficacy should be weighed against cardiovascular and gastrointestinal side effects, and risks of tolerance and addiction.[135] Neither have a labeled indication for residual sleepiness in treated OSA because of lack of studies. Currently, modafinil and armodafinil (an enantiomer of modafinil) are the only medications approved for this issue. Several recent meta-analyses using pooled data from greater than 1000 patients comparing either modafinil or armodafinil with placebo showed statistically significant ESS score reduction by 2 to 3 and MSL extension on MWT by 2 to 3 minutes.[136–139] Overall, side effects, most commonly headaches, were well tolerated and none were serious. There are no efficacy studies comparing modafinil and armodafinil for this indication. In light of recent discovery of abnormal endogenous potentiation of cerebrospinal fluid $GABA_A$ receptors in primary hypersomnia patients, negative $GABA_A$ modulators have been used with success, although this therapy is considered experimental. A recent retrospective review of 153 patients found that 20 of 35 patients with OSA with hypersomnolence treated with transdermal or sublingual flumazenil had improved sleepiness.[140] Novel drug development remains underway, such as those involving the orexin/hypocretin system and histamine H_3 receptor inverse agonist aimed at primary hypersomnia, but could hold promise in OSA with persistent sleepiness.[141,142]

EVALUATION OF OUTCOMES AND LONG-TERM RECOMMENDATIONS

The Apnea Positive Pressure Long-term Efficacy Study (APPLES) found that CPAP was effective in reducing EDS measured by ESS and MWT compared with sham CPAP at 6 months.[143,144] Other studies have also found long-term reduction in ESS score from baseline with CPAP, MAD, or upper airway surgery treatment.[145,146] In OSA patients, long-term reduction in EDS with CPAP may be greater in whites, younger age groups, women, and those with moderate-to-severe OSA.[143,147]

Because OSA is a chronic condition that typically persists through a patient's lifetime with age-related worsening, lifelong treatment and monitoring are necessary. After initiation of therapy, patients should be followed up long term with assessment of EDS at each encounter.[148] This follow-up is typically done by assessment of symptom improvement or comparative measurement using the ESS. Objective measures such as MSLT or MWT are not recommended unless there is concern for central hypersomnia in the setting of persistent sleepiness despite adequate treatment or specifically requested by licensing authorities.

For patients on PAP therapy, equipment maintenance and data monitoring should occur periodically to ensure adequate adherence and efficacy. Efficacy of non-PAP therapy should be confirmed with a sleep study in any patient with moderate-to-severe OSA or mild OSA with persistent EDS. Attention to the interval development of any comorbid conditions (eg, weight gain or HF) that could affect treatment effectiveness or alter baseline SRBD is important. A repeat PSG should be pursued for any patient in whom there is clinical suspicion that a new form of SRBD has developed or to reconfirm adequate therapy when there is recurrence of EDS. In some individuals that successfully achieve significant and sustained weight loss along with resolution of EDS, treatment may be discontinued after careful evaluation.

SUMMARY

SRBD consist of different forms of respiratory conditions occurring during sleep with OSA being the most prevalent. EDS is a well-recognized symptom in OSA, but many patients lack this complaint even when significant respiratory abnormality is present. Whether EDS is independently associated with other forms of SRBD is unclear. The underlying mechanism of EDS in OSA remains unclear. Several effective treatments are available for OSA. PAP demonstrates the most robust effect on improving EDS and is considered first-line therapy. For those intolerant of PAP, MAD is considered second-line therapy, although other forms of therapy can also alleviate EDS. In patients with persistent sleepiness despite adequately treated OSA, potential causes should be evaluated and dealt with before initiating stimulants. Routine follow-up is recommended to ensure long-term success. Further research is needed with regard to OSA-related EDS including defining the mechanisms that link OSA to EDS, identifying the causes of persistent sleepiness despite therapy, and developing more effective and tolerable therapies for OSA and persistent sleepiness. Furthermore, studies on the relationship of EDS with other types of SRBD are warranted.

REFERENCES

1. American Academy of Sleep Medicine. International classification of sleep disorders. 3rd edition. Darien (IL): American Academy of Sleep Medicine; 2014.
2. Arand D, Bonnet M, Hurwitz T, et al. The clinical use of the MSLT and MWT. Sleep 2005;28(1):123–44.
3. Mulgrew AT, Ryan CF, Fleetham JA, et al. The impact of obstructive sleep apnea and daytime sleepiness on work limitation. Sleep Med 2007; 9(1):42–53.
4. Uehli K, Mehta AJ, Miedinger D, et al. Sleep problems and work injuries: a systematic review and meta-analysis. Sleep Med Rev 2014;18(1):61–73.
5. Swanson LM, Arnedt JT, Rosekind MR, et al. Sleep disorders and work performance: findings from the 2008 National Sleep Foundation Sleep in America poll. J Sleep Res 2011;20(3):487–94.
6. Sleep in America 2009 poll highlights & key findings. National Sleep Foundation. 2009. Available at: https://sleepfoundation.org/sites/default/files/2009%20POLL%20HIGHLIGHTS.pdf. Accessed November 11, 2016.
7. Johns MW. A new method for measuring daytime sleepiness: the Epworth sleepiness scale. Sleep 1991;14(6):540–5.
8. Littner MR, Kushida C, Wise M, et al. Practice parameters for the clinical use of the multiple sleep latency test and the maintenance of wakefulness test. Sleep 2005;28(1):113–21.
9. Young T, Palta M, Dempsey J, et al. The occurrence of sleep-disordered breathing among middle-aged adults. N Engl J Med 1993;328(17): 1230–5.
10. Punjabi NM. The epidemiology of adult obstructive sleep apnea. Proc Am Thorac Soc 2008; 5(2):136–43.
11. Heinzer R, Vat S, Marques-Vidal P, et al. Prevalence of sleep-disordered breathing in the general population: the HypnoLaus study. Lancet Respir Med 2015;3(4):310–8.
12. Young T, Peppard PE, Gottlieb DJ. Epidemiology of obstructive sleep apnea: a population health perspective. Am J Respir Crit Care Med 2002; 165(9):1217–39.
13. Yayan J, Rasche K. Absence of typical symptoms and comorbidities in patients with central sleep apnea. Adv Exp Med Biol 2015;873:15–23.
14. Donovan LM, Kapur VK. Prevalence and characteristics of central compared to obstructive sleep apnea: analyses from the Sleep Heart Health Study cohort. Sleep 2016;39(7):1353–9.
15. Correa D, Farney RJ, Chung F, et al. Chronic opioid use and central sleep apnea: a review of the prevalence, mechanisms, and perioperative considerations. Anesth Analg 2015;120(6):1273–85.
16. Nigam G, Pathak C, Riaz M. A systematic review on prevalence and risk factors associated with treatment-emergent central sleep apnea. Ann Thorac Med 2016;11(3):202–10.
17. Grimm W, Hildebrandt O, Neil C, et al. Excessive daytime sleepiness and central sleep apnea in patients with stable heart failure. Int J Cardiol 2014; 176(3):1447–8.
18. Albuquerque FN, Calvin AD, Sert Kuniyoshi FH, et al. Sleep-disordered breathing and excessive daytime sleepiness in patients with atrial fibrillation. Chest 2012;141(4):967–73.
19. Perez de Llano LA, Golpe R, Ortiz Piquer M, et al. Short-term and long-term effects of nasal intermittent positive pressure ventilation in patients with obesity-hypoventilation syndrome. Chest 2005; 128(2):587–94.
20. Bingol Z, Pihtili A, Cagatay P, et al. Clinical predictors of obesity hypoventilation syndrome in obese subjects with obstructive sleep apnea. Respir Care 2015;60(5):666–72.
21. Akashiba T, Akahoshi T, Kawahara S, et al. Clinical characteristics of obesity-hypoventilation syndrome in Japan: a multi-center study. Intern Med 2006; 45(20):1121–5.
22. Basoglu OK, Tasbakan MS. Comparison of clinical characteristics in patients with obesity hypoventilation syndrome and obese obstructive sleep apnea syndrome: a case-control study. Clin Respir J 2014;8(2):167–74.
23. Wang D, Piper AJ, Yee BJ, et al. Hypercapnia is a key correlate of EEG activation and daytime sleepiness in hypercapnic sleep disordered breathing patients. J Clin Sleep Med 2014; 10(5):517–22.

24. Chouri-Pontarollo N, Borel JC, Tamisier R, et al. Impaired objective daytime vigilance in obesity-hypoventilation syndrome: impact of noninvasive ventilation. Chest 2007;131(1):148–55.

25. Veasey SC, Davis CW, Fenik P, et al. Long-term intermittent hypoxia in mice: protracted hypersomnolence with oxidative injury to sleep-wake brain regions. Sleep 2004;27(2):194–201.

26. Zhan G, Fenik P, Practico D, et al. Inducible nitric oxide synthase in long-term intermittent hypoxia: hypersomnolence and brain injury. Am J Respir Crit Care Med 2005;171(12):1414–20.

27. Dusak A, Ursavas A, Hakyemez B, et al. Correlation between hippocampal volume and excessive daytime sleepiness in obstructive sleep apnea syndrome. Eur Rev Med Pharmacol Sci 2013;17(9): 1198–204.

28. Sforza E, Celle S, Saint-Martin M, et al. Hippocampus volume and subjective sleepiness in older people with sleep-disordered breathing: a preliminary report. J Sleep Res 2016;25(2): 190–3.

29. Baril AA, Gagnon K, Arbour C, et al. Regional cerebral blood flow during wakeful rest in older subjects with mild to severe obstructive sleep apnea. Sleep 2015;38(9):1439–49.

30. Chen YC, Chen TW, Su MC, et al. Whole genome DNA methylation analysis of obstructive sleep apnea: IL1R2, NPR2, AR, SP140 methylation and clinical phenotype. Sleep 2016;39(4):743–55.

31. Castiglioni P, Lombardi C, Cortelli P, et al. Why excessive sleepiness may persist in OSA patients receiving adequate CPAP treatment. Eur Respir J 2012;39(1):226–7.

32. Pigeon WR, Sateia MJ, Ferguson RJ. Distinguishing between excessive daytime sleepiness and fatigue: toward improved detection and treatment. J Psychosom Res 2003;54(1):61–9.

33. Hirshkowitz M. Fatigue, sleepiness, and safety definitions, assessment, methodology. Sleep Med Clin 2013;8:183–9.

34. Chervin RD. Sleepiness, fatigue, tiredness, and lack of energy in obstructive sleep apnea. Chest 2000;118(2):372–9.

35. Kapur VK, Baldwin CM, Resnick HE, et al. Sleepiness in patients with moderate to severe sleep-disordered breathing. Sleep 2005;28(4):472–7.

36. Panossian LA, Veasey SC. Daytime sleepiness in obesity: mechanisms beyond obstructive sleep apnea—a review. Sleep 2012;35(5):605–15.

37. Sforza E, Pichot V, Martin MS, et al. Prevalence and determinants of subjective sleepiness in healthy elderly with unrecognized obstructive sleep apnea. Sleep Med 2015;16(8):981–6.

38. Johns MW. Sensitivity and specificity of the multiple sleep latency test (MSLT), the maintenance of wakefulness test and the Epworth sleepiness scale: failure of the MSLT as a gold standard. J Sleep Res 2000;9(1):5–11.

39. Chervin RD, Aldrich MS, Pickett R, et al. Comparison of the results of the Epworth sleepiness scale and the multiple sleep latency test. J Psychosom Res 1997;42(2):145–55.

40. Cai SJ, Chen R, Zhang YL, et al. Correlation of Epworth sleepiness scale with multiple sleep latency test and its diagnostic accuracy in assessing excessive daytime sleepiness in patients with obstructive sleep apnea hypopnea syndrome. Chin Med J (Engl) 2013;126(17):3245–50.

41. Gottlieb DJ, Whitney CW, Bonekat WH, et al. Relation of sleepiness to respiratory disturbance index: the Sleep Heart Health Study. Am J Respir Crit Care Med 1999;159(2):502–7.

42. Furuta H, Kaneda R, Kosaka K, et al. Epworth sleepiness scale and sleep studies in patients with obstructive sleep apnea syndrome. Psychiatry Clin Neurosci 1999;53(2):301–2.

43. Chervin RD, Aldrich MS. The Epworth sleepiness scale may not reflect objective measures of sleepiness or sleep apnea. Neurology 1999;52(1):125–31.

44. Fong SY, Ho CK, Wing YK. Comparing MSLT and ESS in the measurement of excessive daytime sleepiness in obstructive sleep apnoea syndrome. J Psychosom Res 2005;58(1):55–60.

45. Sullivan SS, Kushida CA. Multiple sleep latency test and maintenance of wakefulness test. Chest 2008;134(4):854–61.

46. Bonnet MH, Arand DL. Impact of motivation on multiple sleep latency test and maintenance of wakefulness test measurements. J Clin Sleep Med 2005;1(4):386–90.

47. Wise MS. Objective measures of sleepiness and wakefulness: application to the real world? J Clin Neurophysiol 2006;23(1):39–49.

48. Bonnet MH. ACNS clinical controversy: MSLT and MWT have limited clinical utility. J Clin Neurophysiol 2006;23(1):50–8.

49. Beydoun MA, Gamaldo AA, Canas JA, et al. Serum nutritional biomarkers and their associations with sleep among US adults in recent national surveys. PLoS One 2014;9(8):e103490.

50. Bertisch SM, Sillau S, de Boer IH, et al. 25-hydroxyvitamin D concentration and sleep duration and continuity: multi-Ethnic Study of Atherosclerosis. Sleep 2015;38(8):1305–11.

51. McCarty DE, Reddy A, Keigley Q, et al. Vitamin D, race, and excessive daytime sleepiness. J Clin Sleep Med 2012;8(6):693–7.

52. Yamada N. Treatment of recurrent hypersomnia with methylcobalamin (vitamin B12): a case report. Psychiatry Clin Neurosci 1995;49(5–6):305–7.

53. MaCarty DE. Resolution of hypersomnia following identification and treatment of vitamin D deficiency. J Clin Sleep Med 2010;6(6):605–8.

54. Johnson K, Sattari M. Vitamin D deficiency and fatigue: an unusual presentation. Springerplus 2015; 4:584.

55. Chervin RD, Aldrich MS. Characteristics of apneas and hypopneas during sleep and relation to excessive daytime sleepiness. Sleep 1998;21(8):799–806.

56. Punjabi NM, Bandeen-Roche K, Marx JJ, et al. The association between daytime sleepiness and sleep-disordered breathing in NREM and REM sleep. Sleep 2002;25(3):307–14.

57. Chen R, Xiong KP, Lian YX, et al. Daytime sleepiness and its determining factors in Chinese obstructive sleep apnea patients. Sleep Breath 2011;15(1):129–35.

58. Sun Y, Ning Y, Huang L, et al. Polysomnographic characteristics of daytime sleepiness in obstructive sleep apnea syndrome. Sleep Breath 2012;16(2): 375–81.

59. Mediano O, Barcelo A, de la Pena M, et al. Daytime sleepiness and polysomnographic variables in sleep apnoea patients. Eur Respir J 2007;30(1):110–3.

60. Corlateanu A, Pylchenko S, Sircu V, et al. Predictors of daytime sleepiness in patients with obstructive sleep apnea. Pneumologia 2015;64(4):21–5.

61. Wang Q, Zhang C, Jia P, et al. The association between the phenotype of excessive daytime sleepiness and blood pressure in patients with obstructive sleep apnea-hypopnea syndrome. Int J Med Sci 2014;11(7):713–20.

62. Oksenberg A, Arons E, Nasser K, et al. Severe obstructive sleep apnea: sleepy versus nonsleepy patients. Laryngoscope 2010;120(3):643–8.

63. Seneviratne U, Puvanendran K. Excessive daytime sleepiness in obstructive sleep apnea: prevalence, severity, and predictors. Sleep Med 2004;5(4): 339–43.

64. Roure N, Gomez S, Mediano O, et al. Daytime sleepiness and polysomnography in obstructive sleep apnea patients. Sleep Med 2008;9(7):727–31.

65. Giles TL, Lasserson TJ, Smith BH, et al. Continuous positive airways pressure for obstructive sleep apnoea in adults. Cochrane Database Syst Rev 2006;(3):CD001106.

66. Weaver TE, Maislin G, Dinges DF, et al. Relationship between hours of CPAP use and achieving normal levels of sleepiness and daily functioning. Sleep 2007;30(6):711–9.

67. Weaver TE, Mancini C, Maislin G, et al. Continuous positive airway pressure treatment of sleepy patients with milder obstructive sleep apnea: results of the CPAP Apnea Trial North American Program (CATNAP) randomized clinical trial. Am J Respir Crit Care Med 2012;186(7):677–83.

68. Xu T, Li T, Wei D, et al. Effect of automatic versus fixed continuous positive airway pressure for the treatment of obstructive sleep apnea: an up-to-date meta-analysis. Sleep Breath 2012;16(4):1017–26.

69. Ayas NT, Patel SR, Malhotra A, et al. Auto-titrating versus standard continuous positive airway pressure for the treatment of obstructive sleep apnea: results of a meta-analysis. Sleep 2004;27(2):249–53.

70. Ip S, D'Ambrosio C, Patel K, et al. Auto-titrating versus fixed continuous positive airway pressure for the treatment of obstructive sleep apnea: a systematic review with meta-analysis. Syst Rev 2012;1:20.

71. Gay PC, Herold DL, Olson EJ. A randomized, double-blind clinical trial comparing continuous positive airway pressure with a novel bilevel pressure system for treatment of sleep apnea syndrome. Sleep 2003;26(7):864–9.

72. Kushida CA, Berry RB, Blau A, et al. Positive airway pressure initiation: a randomized controlled trial to assess the impact of therapy mode and titration process on efficacy, adherence, and outcomes. Sleep 2011;34(8):1083–92.

73. Smith I, Lasserson TJ. Pressure modification for improving usage of continuous positive airway pressure machines in adults with obstructive sleep apnoea. Cochrane Database Syst Rev 2009;(4): CD003531.

74. Sharples LD, Clutterbuck-James AL, Glover MJ, et al. Meta-analysis of randomized controlled trials of oral mandibular advancement devices and continuous positive airway pressure for obstructive sleep apnoea-hypopnoea. Sleep Med Rev 2016; 27:108–24.

75. Ramar K, Dort LC, Katz SG, et al. Clinical practice guideline for the treatment of obstructive sleep apnea and snoring with oral appliance therapy: an update for 2015. J Clin Sleep Med 2015;11(7): 773–827.

76. Serra-Torres S, Bellot-Arcis C, Montiel-Company JM, et al. Effectiveness of mandibular advancement appliances in treating obstructive sleep apnea syndrome: a systematic review. Laryngoscope 2016; 126(2):507–14.

77. Lazard DS, Blumen M, Levy P, et al. The tongue-retaining device: efficacy and side effects in obstructive sleep apnea syndrome. J Clin Sleep Med 2009;5(5):431–8.

78. Heidsieck DS, de Ruiter MH, de Lange J. Management of obstructive sleep apnea in edentulous patients: an overview of the literature. Sleep Breath 2016;20(1):395–404.

79. Caples SM, Rowley JA, Prinsell JR, et al. Surgical modifications of the upper airway for obstructive sleep apnea in adults: a systematic review and meta-analysis. Sleep 2010;33(10): 1396–407.

80. Dixon JB, Schachter LM, O'Brien PE, et al. Surgical vs conventional therapy for weight loss for treatment of obstructive sleep apnea: a randomized controlled trial. JAMA 2012;308(11):1142–9.

81. Mason M, Welsh EJ, Smith I. Drug therapy for obstructive sleep apnoea in adults. Cochrane Database Syst Rev 2013;(5):CD003002.

82. Sukys-Claudino L, Moraes W, Guilleminault C, et al. Beneficial effect of donepezil on obstructive sleep apnea: a double-blind, placebo-controlled clinical trial. Sleep Med 2012;13(3):290–6.

83. Acar M, Cingi C, Sakallioglu O, et al. The effects of mometasone furoate and desloratadine in obstructive sleep apnea syndrome patients with allergic rhinitis. Am J Rhinol Allergy 2013;27(4):e113–6.

84. Barnes H, Edwards BA, Joosten SA, et al. Positional modification techniques for supine obstructive sleep apnea: a systematic review and meta-analysis. Sleep Med Rev 2016. [Epub ahead of print].

85. Iftikhar IH, Kline CE, Youngstedt SD. Effects of exercise training on sleep apnea: a meta-analysis. Lung 2014;192(1):175–84.

86. Aiello KD, Caughey WG, Nelluri B, et al. Effect of exercise training on sleep apnea: a systematic review and meta-analysis. Respir Med 2016;116: 85–92.

87. Araghi MH, Chen YF, Jagielski A, et al. Effectiveness of lifestyle interventions on obstructive sleep apnea (OSA): systematic review and meta-analysis. Sleep 2013;36(10):1553–62.

88. Berry RB, Kryger MH, Massie CA. A novel nasal expiratory positive airway pressure (EPAP) device for the treatment of obstructive sleep apnea: a randomized controlled trial. Sleep 2011;34(4):479–85.

89. Riaz M, Certal V, Nigam G, et al. Nasal expiratory positive airway pressure devices (Provent) for OSA: a systematic review and meta-analysis. Sleep Disord 2015;2015:734798.

90. Strollo PJ, Soose RJ, Maurer JT, et al. Upper-airway stimulation for obstructive sleep apnea. N Engl J Med 2014;370(2):139–49.

91. Woodson BT, Soose RJ, Gillespie MB, et al. Three-year outcomes of cranial nerve stimulation for obstructive sleep apnea: the STAR trial. Otolaryngol Head Neck Surg 2016;154(1):181–8.

92. Certal VF, Zaghi S, Riaz M, et al. Hypoglossal nerve stimulation in the treatment of obstructive sleep apnea: a systematic review and meta-analysis. Laryngoscope 2015;125(5):1254–64.

93. Camacho M, Certal V, Abdullatif J, et al. Myofunctional therapy for treat obstructive sleep apnea: a systematic review and meta-analysis. Sleep 2015; 38(5):669–75.

94. Verma RK, Johnson J Jr, Goyal M, et al. Oropharyngeal exercises in the treatment of obstructive sleep apnoea: our experience. Sleep Breath 2016;20(4): 1193–201.

95. Diaferia G, Santos-Silva R, Truksinas E, et al. Myofunctional therapy improves adherence to continuous positive airway pressure treatment. Sleep Breath 2017;21(2):387–95.

96. Ieto V, Kayamori F, Montes MI, et al. Effects of oropharyngeal exercises on snoring: a randomized trial. Chest 2015;148(3):683–91.

97. Ravesloot MJ, van Maanen JP, Dun L, et al. The undervalued potential of positional therapy in position-dependent snoring and obstructive sleep apnea-a review of the literature. Sleep Breath 2013;17(1):39–49.

98. Charakorn N, Hirunwiwatkul P, Chirakalwasan N, et al. The effects of topical nasal steroids on continuous positive airway pressure compliance in patients with obstructive sleep apnea: a systematic review and meta-analysis. Sleep Breath 2016; 21(1):3–8.

99. Camacho M, Riaz M, Capasso R, et al. The effect of nasal surgery on continuous positive airway pressure device use and therapeutic treatment pressures: a systematic review and meta-analysis. Sleep 2015;38(2):279–86.

100. El-Solh AA, Moitheennazima B, Akinnusi ME, et al. Combined oral appliance and positive airway pressure therapy for obstructive sleep apnea: a pilot study. Sleep Breath 2011;15(2):203–8.

101. Wu X, Fu C, Zhang S, et al. Adaptive servoventilation improves cardiac dysfunction and prognosis in heart failure patients with sleep-disordered breathing: a meta-analysis. Clin Respir J 2015. [Epub ahead of print].

102. Cowie MR, Woehrle H, Wegscheider K, et al. Adaptive servo-ventilation for central sleep apnea in systolic heart failure. N Engl J Med 2015;373(12): 1095–105.

103. Yang H, Sawyer AM. The effect of adaptive servo ventilation (ASV) on objective and subjective outcomes in Cheyne-Stokes respiration (CSR) with central sleep apnea (CSA) in heart failure (HF): a systematic review. Heart Lung 2016;45(3):199–211.

104. Edwards BA, Malhotra A, Sands SA. Adapting our approach to treatment-emergent central sleep apnea. Sleep 2013;36(8):1121–2.

105. Su M, Zhang X, Huang M, et al. Adaptive pressure support servoventilation: a novel treatment for residual sleepiness associated with central sleep apnea events. Sleep Breath 2011;15(4):695–9.

106. Pusalavidyasagar SS, Olson EJ, Gay PC, et al. Treatment of complex sleep apnea syndrome: a retrospective comparative review. Sleep Med 2006;7(6):474–9.

107. Correia S, Martins V, Sousa L, et al. Clinical impact of adaptive servoventilation compared to other ventilator modes in patients with treatment-emergent sleep apnea, central sleep apnea, and Cheyne-Stokes respiration. Rev Port Pneumol (2006) 2015;21(3):132–7.

108. Morgenthaler TI, Kuzniar TJ, Wolfe LF, et al. The complex sleep apnea resolution study: a prospective randomized controlled trial of continuous

positive airway pressure versus adaptive servoventilation therapy. Sleep 2014;37(5):927–34.

109. Aurora RN, Chowdhuri S, Ramar K, et al. The treatment of central sleep apnea syndromes in adults: practice parameters with an evidence-based literature review and meta-analysis. Sleep 2012;35(1):17–40.

110. Reddy R, Adamo D, Kufel T, et al. Treatment of opioid-related central sleep apnea with positive airway pressure: a systematic review. J Opioid Manag 2014;10(1):57–62.

111. Alattar MA, Scharf SM. Opioid-associated central sleep apnea: a case series. Sleep Breath 2009; 13(2):201–6.

112. Abraham WT, Jagielski D, Oldenburg O, et al. Phrenic nerve stimulation for the treatment of central sleep apnea. JACC Heart Fail 2015;3(5):360–9.

113. Costanzo MR, Augostini R, Goldberg LR, et al. Design of the remede System pivotal trial: a prospective, randomized study in the use of respiratory rhythm management to treat central sleep apnea. J Card Fail 2015;21(11):892–902.

114. Masa JF, Corral J, Caballero C, et al. Non-invasive ventilation in obesity hypoventilation syndrome without severe obstructive sleep apnoea. Thorax 2016;71(10):899–906.

115. Howard ME, Piper AJ, Stevens B, et al. A randomized controlled trial of CPAP versus non-invasive ventilation for initial treatment of obesity hypoventilation syndrome. Thorax 2017; 72(5):337–44.

116. Piper AJ, Wang D, Yee BJ, et al. Randomized trial of CPAP vs bilevel support in the treatment of obesity hypoventilation syndrome without severe nocturnal desaturation. Thorax 2008;63(5):395–401.

117. Masa JF, Corral J, Alonso ML, et al. Efficacy of different treatment alternatives for obesity hypoventilation syndrome. Pickwick Study. Am J Respir Crit Care Med 2015;192(1):86–95.

118. Launois SH, Tamisier R, Levy P, et al. On treatment but still sleepy: cause and management of residual sleepiness in obstructive sleep apnea. Curr Opin Pulm Med 2013;19(6):601–8.

119. Koutsourelakis I, Perraki E, Economou NT, et al. Predictors of residual sleepiness in adequately treated obstructive sleep apnoea patients. Eur Respir J 2009;34(3):687–93.

120. Pepin JL, Viot-Blanc V, Escourrou P, et al. Prevalence of residual excessive sleepiness in CPAP-treated sleep apnoea patients: the French multicenter study. Eur Respir J 2009;33(5):1062–7.

121. Gasa M, Tamisier R, Launois SH, et al. Residual sleepiness in sleep apnea patients treated by continuous positive airway pressure. J Sleep Res 2013;22(4):389–97.

122. Ohayon MM. Determining the level of sleepiness in the American population and its correlates. J Psychiatr Res 2012;46(4):422–7.

123. Slater G, Pengo MF, Kosky C, et al. Obesity as an independent predictor of subjective excessive daytime sleepiness. Respir Med 2013;107(2):305–9.

124. Mulgrew AT, Lawati NA, Ayas NT, et al. Residual sleep apnea on polysomnography after 3 months of CPAP therapy: clinical implications, predictors, and patterns. Sleep Med 2010;11(2):119–25.

125. Vernet C, Redolfi S, Attali V, et al. Residual sleepiness in obstructive sleep apnoea: phenotype and related symptoms. Eur Respir J 2011;38(1):98–105.

126. Rye DB, Bliwise DL, Parker K, et al. Modulation of vigilance in the primary hypersomnias by endogenous enhancement of GABAA receptors. Sci Transl Med 2012;4(161):161ra151.

127. Xiong Y, Zhou XJ, Nisi RA, et al. Brain white matter changes in CPAP-treated obstructive sleep apnea patients with residual sleepiness. J Magn Reson Imaging 2017;45(5):1371–8.

128. Denotti AL, Wong KK, Dungan GC 2nd, et al. Residual sleep-disordered breathing during autotitrating continuous positive airway pressure therapy. Eur Respir J 2012;39(6):1391–7.

129. Zhu K, Roisman G, Aouf S, et al. All APAPs are not equivalent for the treatment of sleep disordered breathing: a bench evaluation of eleven commercially available devices. J Clin Sleep Med 2015; 11(7):725–34.

130. Stepnowsky C, Zamora T, Barker R, et al. Accuracy of positive airway pressure device-measured apneas and hypopneas: role in treatment followup. Sleep Disord 2013;2013:314589.

131. Zhu K, Aouf S, Roisman G, et al. Pressure-relief features of fixed and autotitrating continuous positive airway pressure may impair their efficacy: evaluation with a respiratory bench model. J Clin Sleep Med 2016;12(3):385–92.

132. Tippin J, Aksan N, Dawson J, et al. Sleep remains disturbed in patients with obstructive sleep apnea treated with positive airway pressure: a three-month cohort study using continuous actigraphy. Sleep Med 2016;24:24–31.

133. Killgore WD, Rupp TL, Grugle NL, et al. Effects of dextroamphetamine, caffeine and modafinil on psychomotor vigilance test performance after 44 h of continuous wakefulness. J Sleep Res 2008; 17(3):309–21.

134. Wesensten NJ, Killgore WD, Balkin TJ. Performance and alertness effects of caffeine, dextroamphetamine, and modafinil during sleep deprivation. J Sleep Res 2005;14(3):255–66.

135. Morganthaler TI, Kapur VK, Brown T, et al. Practice parameters for the treatment of narcolepsy and other hypersomnias of central origin. Sleep 2007; 30(12):1705–11.

136. Sukhal S, Khalid M, Tulaimat A. Effect of wakefulness-promoting agents on sleepiness in patients with sleep apnea treated with CPAP: a

meta-analysis. J Clin Sleep Med 2015;11(10): 1179–86.

137. Avellar AB, Carvalho LB, Prado GF, et al. Pharmacotherapy for residual excessive sleepiness and cognition in CPAP-treated patients with obstructive sleep apnea syndrome: a systematic review and meta-analysis. Sleep Med Rev 2016;30:97–107.

138. Kuan YC, Wu D, Huang KW, et al. Effects of modafinil and armodafinil in patients with obstructive sleep apnea: a meta-analysis of randomized controlled trials. Clin Ther 2016;38(4):874–88.

139. Chapman JL, Vakulin A, Hedner J, et al. Modafinil/armodafinil in obstructive sleep apnoea: a systematic review and meta-analysis. Eur Respir J 2016; 47(5):1420–8.

140. Trotti LM, Saini P, Koola C, et al. Flumazenil for the treatment of refractory hypersomnolence: clinical experience with 153 patients. J Clin Sleep Med 2016;12(10):1389–94.

141. Heifetz A, Bodkin MJ, Blggin PC. Discovery of the first selective, nonpeptidic orexin 2 receptor agonists. J Med Chem 2015;58(20):7928–30.

142. Dauvilliers Y, Bassetti C, Lammers GJ, et al. Pltolisant versus placebo or modafinil in patients with narcolepsy: a double-blind, randomized trial. Lancet Neurol 2013;12(11):1068–75.

143. Batool-Anwar S, Goodwin JL, Kushida CA, et al. Impact of continuous positive airway pressure (CPAP) on quality of life in patients with obstructive sleep apnea (OSA). J Sleep Res 2016;25(6):731–8.

144. Kushida CA, Nichols DA, Holmes TH, et al. Effects of continuous positive airway pressure on neurocognitive function in obstructive sleep apnea patients: the Apnea Positive Pressure Long-term Efficacy Study (APPLES). Sleep 2012;35(12):1593–602.

145. Woods CM, Gunawardena I, Chia M, et al. Long-term quality-of-life outcomes following treatment for adult obstructive sleep apnoea: comparison of upper airway surgery, continuous positive airway pressure and mandibular advancement splints. Clin Otolaryngol 2016;41(6):762–70.

146. Huang Z, Liu Z, Luo Q, et al. Long-term effects of continuous positive airway pressure on blood pressure and prognosis in hypertensive patients with coronary heart disease and obstructive sleep apnea: a randomized controlled trial. Am J Hypertens 2015;28(3):300–6.

147. Walia HK, Griffith SD, Thompson NR, et al. Impact of sleep-disordered breathing treatment on patient reported outcomes in a clinic-based cohort of hypertensive patients. J Clin Sleep Med 2016; 12(10):1357–64.

148. Epstein LJ, Kristo D, Strollo PJ Jr, et al. Clinical guideline for the evaluation, management and long-term care of obstructive sleep apnea in adults. J Clin Sleep Med 2009;5(3):263–76.

Drug-Induced Hypersomnolence

J.F. Pagel, MS, MD

KEYWORDS

- Hypnotics • Sedatives • Somnolence • Side effects • MVA • Drug • Medication

KEY POINTS

- Drug-induced hypersomnolence is involved in at least one-third of deaths from motor vehicular accidents.
- Drug-induced sleepiness is among the most commonly reported effects and/or side effects of pharmacologic agents.
- Hypnotics demonstrate minimal next-day sleepiness in clinical testing.
- Sedatives induce next-day somnolence in a significant percentage of those individuals using the drug.

Many drugs induce sedation. Drug-induced hypersomnolence has significant negative personal and social effects, including an involvement in approximately one-third of motor vehicular accident (MVA) deaths.[1] Drugs of abuse most often induce hypersomnolence as a direct effect (ethanol, cannabis, opiates), or by potentiating sleep disturbances known to induce daytime sleepiness such as sleep apnea (ethanol, opiates) and chronic sleep deprivation (amphetamines). Drug-induced sleepiness is among the most commonly reported effect and/or side effect of pharmacologic agents.[2] Sedating prescription medications are generally classified as (1) hypnotics, which are short-acting agents clinically used to induce sleep with minimal effects on waking performance, (2) sedatives, which are agents that diminish arousal, and commonly produce sedation that affects both wake and sleep, and (3) agents used clinically for other purposes that produce sedation as a side effect. These categories are not concrete. Primarily as based on the vagaries of somnolence testing, some drugs meet criteria for multiple categories.

EPIDEMIOLOGY

Sleepiness is estimated to cause 20% of motorway accidents with the National Highway Traffic Safety Administration estimating that drowsy driving was responsible for 72,000 crashes, 44,000 injuries, and 800 deaths in 2013.[3] This is a particular problem in the United States, which compared with 20 other countries with high motor vehicle use, has the highest rate of crash deaths per 100,000 population (10.3).[4] Among nearly 150,000 adults aged at least 18 years or older in 19 states and the District of Columbia, 4% report that they have fallen asleep while driving at least once in the previous 30 days.[5] Daytime sleepiness has been demonstrated to contribute significantly to impairment in all domains of the Medical Outcomes Study Short Form (36-item) Health Survey, affecting an individual's ability to gain or maintain employment.[6]

It is somewhat unclear as to the degree drug sedation contributes to MVAs. The effects of drugs of abuse have received the most study. In 2014, there were 9967 people killed in alcohol-impaired driving crashes, accounting for 31% of

No commercial or financial conflicts of interest for the last 8 years.
No funding sources.
Rocky Mountain Sleep Disorders Center, Southern Colorado Family Medicine Residency Program, Department of Family Medicine, University of Colorado School of Medicine, PO Box 3065, Pueblo, CO 81005, USA
E-mail address: pueo34@earthlink.net

Sleep Med Clin 12 (2017) 383–393
http://dx.doi.org/10.1016/j.jsmc.2017.03.011
1556-407X/17/© 2017 Elsevier Inc. All rights reserved.

all traffic-related deaths in the United States.[7] Drugs other than alcohol are involved in 16% of motor vehicle crashes.[8] The medications known to increase the risk of sleepiness-related crashes include benzodiazepine anxiolytics, long-acting sedative/hypnotics, sedating antihistamines (H1 class), and tricyclic antidepressants.[9–13] The risks are higher with higher drug doses and for people taking more than 1 sedating drug simultaneously.[14] Because a high percentage of the population uses drugs of abuse as well as medications for underlying illness, the use of multiple sedating drugs use has increasingly become a problem. In 1993, about 1 in 8 drivers were using more than 1 drug, but by 2010, it was closer to 1 in 5. The number of drivers dying in MVAs with 3 or more sedating drugs in their system increased from 11.5% to 21.5% during this period. Among drivers who tested positive for any drug, 48% also tested positive for alcohol.[15]

METHODOLOGIC CONSIDERATIONS

Actual assessment of daytime somnolence is confused by both commonly applied terminology and techniques of assessment. The terminology describing daytime sleepiness, generally considered to be "the subjective state of sleep need," is poorly defined, interchangeably including such contextual terminology as drowsiness, languor, inertness, fatigue, and sluggishness.[16] In most clinical trials, somnolence is usually addressed with a 1-item question as to reported drug-induced sleepiness. Clinically, sleepiness is most commonly assessed using questionnaires. Some studies suggest that more than 50% of the general adult medical clinic population report an Epworth scale of greater than 10 (moderate sleepiness on this scale).[17] However, such subjective reports do not necessarily reflect the results of other forms of testing.[18] The effects of sleepiness on daytime performance is also assessed by tests of complex reaction and coordination, and by tests that assess complex behavioral tasks likely to be affected by sleepiness (ie, tests of driving performance).[19] Performance measures are susceptible to non–task-related influences of motivation, distraction, and comprehension of instructions, with specific components of performance tests also demonstrating variable effects. Daytime sleepiness can also be assessed physiologically using either the Multiple Sleep Latency Test or the Maintenance of Wakefulness Test, modified polysomnographic evaluations assessing sleep onset latency across a series of wake time nap periods. Unfortunately, in assessing sleepiness, the results of questionnaire rating tests, performance tests, and physiologic tests do not always correlate.[16] Newer tests using neurophysiologic measures and PET scanning have also been applied in the attempt to assess the impacts of pharmacologic interventions on brain function.[20] Epidemiologically, it has been difficult to correlate any test results with real-world data for MVAs and MVA-associated mortality.[21] When sedative medication dosages are increased beyond dosages that produce drowsiness, other types of mental impairment become apparent, suggesting that drowsiness and cognitive impairment are manifestations of the same pharmacologic effect.[22]

Pharmacologic data such as drug effect half-life and drug elimination have proven useful in addressing the cognitive effects for some sedating agents. For other agents, such as the short-acting gamma-aminobutyric acid (GABA) hypnotics, this approach has proven far less useful, particularly after agents that have been adopted into widespread general use. Reports of next-day daytime sleepiness and an increased propensity for MVAs may extend well outside drug half-life parameters.[23] Despite this overlap in effects, hypnotic drugs are significantly less likely than either sedative agents or agents producing sedation as a side effect to induce significant levels of daytime sleepiness as determined by questionnaires, performance tests, polysomnography-based testing, and accident data.

SEDATING DRUGS OF ABUSE

Ethanol is the most widely used drug with sedative effects.[24] Ethanol has a high level of use and well-described negative social and driving effects. Ethanol-induced cognitive effects extend well beyond the drugs tendency to induce somnolence. Negative effects on cognitive performance while driving has documented dose dependence beginning at legal doses with the fatal odds ratio calculated at 1.75 per 0.02% increase in blood alcohol concentration.[25] Because of its sedating effects, individuals with chronic insomnia often develop problems with alcohol use (up to 22% in some studies).[26] Chronic use can produce sleep disturbance and deprivation.[27] Ethanol, a noted respiratory suppressant, can be lethal in overdose, particularly when used with other respiratory-suppressant agents. A moderate level of chronic alcohol use is known to increase the level and severity of breathing disturbance in individuals with sleep apnea.[28]

Cannabis (tetrahydrocannabinol is its most psychoactive compound) can induce daytime sleepiness and cause serious driving impairment, especially at higher blood levels. Testing has been limited as to its effects by legal constraints, and the results of performance testing have been mixed.[29] In the United States, 13% of nighttime, weekend drivers have marijuana in their system. Between 4% and 14% of drivers who sustain injury or die in traffic accidents test positive for cannabis.[30] Although not nearly as great a risk factor for driving as alcohol, marijuana may nearly double the risk of having a vehicle collision.[31] In the United States, marijuana users are about 25% more likely to be involved in an MVA than drivers with no evidence of marijuana use.[32]

Opiate use and abuse is at historically high levels in the United States. Opiate overdose deaths, including both prescribed pain relievers and heroin, hit record levels in 2014, with a 14% increase in just 1 year.[33] Opiates can induce daytime sleepiness, and exacerbate apnea severity. Approximately 30% of individuals on methadone maintenance therapy develop significant central sleep apnea.[34] Sedation and cognitive impairment are common side effects of opiates.[35] Combinations of opiates and other central nervous system (CNS) depressant drugs such as barbiturates, benzodiazepines, antidepressants, and antipsychotics may have additive effects on sedation.

Although amphetamines can be used to treat daytime sleepiness, when used on a chronic basis, they can induce sleep disruption and sleep deprivation. Methamphetamine users may present clinically with somnolence after periods of bingeing. As based on drug testing of MVAs resulting in significant injuries or death, positive results involving stimulants have decreased by 40% since 2005.[8] However, amphetamines of abuse such as methamphetamine have a very short half-life (drug testing may be negative when conducted during somnolent periods after bingeing).

HYPNOTICS

Hypnotics are sleep-inducing drugs, medications specifically designed to induce somnolence and sleep directly after intake, affecting cognitive performance during this period, while inducing minimal next-day sleepiness. Among the first hypnotics, an agent still in use, is chloral hydrate—the original "Mickey Finn" slipped into the drinks of unsuspecting marks for the purposes of criminal activity. Unfortunately, this medication is difficult and dangerous to use because the potentially fatal dose is quite close to the therapeutic dose. In the years leading up to the1970s, rapidly acting barbiturates were commonly used for their hypnotic effects. Unfortunately, these medications, also drugs of abuse, had a significant danger of overdose and contributed to an era defined in part by

deaths owing to overdoses of sleeping pills. These medications and similar barbiturate-like medications (methaqualone, glutethimide, ethchorovynol, and methyprylon) have limited availability and are rarely used owing to limited efficacy, cognitive effects, potential for abuse, and lethal toxicity associated with overdose.[36,37] Today their primary therapeutic uses include executions and facilitated euthanasia.[38]

Most hypnotics affect GABA—the primary negative neurotransmitter active in the human CNS. In the 1970s, benzodiazepines (GABA agonists) with minimal overdose danger and less potential for abuse were first marketed as hypnotics. Some of these agents had an extremely short duration of action (eg, triazolem [Halcion]). Although this agent induced minimal next-day somnolence, use was associated with daytime memory impairment, particularly at higher dosages.[12,39] In the 1990s, newer agents were developed and marketed that had selective effects on GABA receptors, including zolpidem (Ambien), zaleplon (Sonata), eszapaclone (Estorra), and indiplon. Although these agents were less likely to have deleterious side effects than most over-the-counter treatments for insomnia, with increased use, more side effects including next-day effects on driving were reported, particularly for higher doses of zolpidem.[40,41] In many cases, MVAs occurred in the period of somnolence and cognitive impairment during the first few hours after ingestion. These drugs produce initial somnolence and cognitive impairment, with psychomotor test performance returning to normal outside the pharmacologically effective life of the agent (3–11 hours as based on the half-life).[42] At higher doses, these agents can exhibit benzodiazepine-like effects. Some individuals, particularly the elderly, report idiosyncratic reactions of persistent daytime somnolence, memory loss, or next-day sedation after the nighttime use of hypnotics.[42] For the agents listed in **Table 1**, such reports were forthcoming only after the drugs became generic and widely used in clinical practice.

Melatonin is a neural hormone effective in resetting circadian rhythms of sleep and body core temperature through its actions on the suprachiasmatic nucleus.[42] Melatonin can act as a hypnotic and is a useful adjunct to treatment in individuals with circadian disturbance. Prescription synthetic analogs of melatonin such as ramelteon are available. The impact of this agent on next-day performance is generally considered to be minimal. Next-day psychomotor test results may not be affected, although 1 study demonstrated significant effects on next-day deviation of lateral position in driving tests.[43] Sleep tendency and

Table 1
Hypnotics and associated next-day sleepiness

Drug and Class	Half-Life (h)	Next-day Sleepiness Clinical Trials and Case Reports	Next-day Effects on Performance and Driving Tests	Reported Association With MVAs	Toxicity and/or Significant Side Effects
Short-acting GABA agonist					
Triazolam	1–2	Placebo equivalent	None reported	Anecdotal after generic release	Antegrade amnesia
GABA-selective agents					
Zaleplon	1	Placebo equivalent	Equivalent to norms 3.25 h after ingestion	Epidemiologic after generic release	[a]
Indiplon	1.5	Placebo equivalent	None reported	Minimal (not widely used)	[a]
Zolpidem	1.5	Placebo equivalent	Multiple studies with variable results; equivalent to norms 6.25 h after ingestion	Epidemiologic after generic release (worst for agents in this class)	Symptomatic parasomnias
Eszopiclone	6	Placebo equivalent	Possible in the elderly at higher doses (>2 mg)	Minimal reports	[a]
Melatonin agonists					
Generic	1.5	Placebo equivalent	None reported	Anecdotal and epidemiologic	Neuroendocrine side effects
Ramelteon	0.8–1.9	Placebo equivalent	In 1 of 4 studies driving performance compromised	Minimal (not widely used)	Neuroendocrine side effects

None reported is based on the results of literature search including PubMed and Google.
Abbreviations: GABA, gamma-aminobutyric acid; MVAs, motor vehicle accidents.
[a] Minimal data exist for an agent that is not in widespread use as a hypnotic.
Data from Refs. [2,12,36,37,39–44,54]

reduced sleep latency is affected from 1.75 to 4.75 hours after ingestion.[44] Reported next-day sleepiness associated with hypnotic use is summarized in **Table 1**.

SEDATIVES

Sedative drugs, although often used to induce sleep, are also used to induce calming and reduce arousal during waking. Historically, this category included the opiates, particularly laudanum—a tincture of opium that mixed with water or wine was used as a soporific even for crying infants. Most drugs exert their sedative effect by selectively affecting neurotransmitters and neuromodulators.[45] Multiple factors and systems are involved, with no single chemical neurotransmitter identified as necessary or sufficient for modulating sleep and wakefulness. Sedative drugs can exert primary effects either at the neurotransmitter GABA, or at sedating neuromodulators (amitriptyline, serotonin, or dopamine). Others potentiate sedation by antagonizing one of the widely dispersed central activating neuromodulators, namely, epinephrine, norepinephrine, histamine, adenosine, and orexin.

Fifty years ago, longer acting benzodiazepines, particularly diazepam (Valium) preempted the role of opiates in sedation. Some of these agents had active breakdown products that produced an extraordinarily long active half-life (>11 days).[12,36] The prolonged effect is one of waking calming and sedation, associated with increased auto accidents and falls with hip fractures. Medium half-life agents, including alprazolam, temazepam, clonidine, and lorazepam, affect next-day performance tests. The use of these agents may be associated with an increased level of next-day MVAs.[14]

Other agents induce sedation by affecting the neuromodulators acetylcholine, dopamine, and serotonin. Most of these agents are classified as sedating antidepressants. Sedating antidepressants include the tricyclics (amitriptyline, imipramine, nortriptyline, etc) and tetracyclics (trazadone and mirtazapine). Among the selective serotonin reuptake inhibitors, paroxetine can induce mild sedation. The use of sedating antidepressants has been associated with declines in daytime performance, driving test performance, and an increased potential for involvement in MVAs.[46] Both tricyclic and tetracyclic antidepressants are widely used as a hypnotics despite significant next-day sedation.[47] Dopaminergic agents, especially pramipexole, can induce significant somnolence as well as sleep attacks in some individuals.[48]

Many patients suffering from chronic insomnia are hyperaroused, unable to fall asleep even after minimal sleep the night before. Sedating medications are used to treat this hyperarousal by antagonizing the wake-producing neuromodulating systems: epinephrine, norepinephrine, histamine, adenosine, and orexin. Both prescription and over-the-counter agents are marketed for sedative effects produced pharmacologically by antagonizing orexin, histamine, and norepinephrine.

Antihistamines and antipsychotics induce sedation based on their antihistaminic effects. Over-the-counter sleeping pills contain sedating H-1 antihistamines, usually diphenhydramine, hydroxyzine, or triprolidine. These agents induce sedation with acute use, and often induce increased daytime sleepiness and cognitive impairment persisting into the day after nighttime use.[49] In comparative studies, driving performance at 2.5 hours after administration of 50 mg of diphenhydramine is worse than in individuals with a blood alcohol concentration of 0.1%—the level of legal intoxication in most states.[50] Nighttime drug use can produces drowsiness severe enough to affect next-day performance and driving tests.[20,22] Sedation is infrequent with H2 antagonists (eg, cimetidine, ranitidine, famotidine, and nizatidine), but somnolence as a side effect is reproducible in susceptible individuals.[51] Sedation is a common side effect of the traditional antipsychotics, with chlorpromazine and thioridazine somewhat more sedating than haloperidol. Clinical studies have shown a high incidence of persistent sedation with clozapine (46%), with less frequent reports of sedation with risperidone, olanzapine, sertindole, and quetiapine. The sedation associated with these agents is most likely associated with their known effects on histaminic receptors.[2]

Doxepin, a sedating psychotropic agent with pronounced histamine (H1) receptor antagonism exerts at least part of its effects by antagonizing orexin.[52] Survexant is an oxexin antagonist designed to lower waking arousal. Currently, it is being heavily marketed as a hypnotic. As based on performance and driving tests, this agent is known to produce a dose-related next-day increase in somnolence and severe somnolence for all age groupings tested.[53] As for the hypnotic class, the effects of these drugs on reported MVAs, MVA-associated deaths, and the incidence of more unusual side effects often becomes apparent only after these drugs become generic and are adopted into widespread clinical use. Sedative drug effects on daytime sleepiness are summarized in **Table 2**.

Table 2
Sedatives, drug classes, neurotransmitter effects, side effects, and associated next-day sleepiness

Class (Drug) [Neuromodulator Effected]	Half-life	Next-day Sleepiness Clinical Trials	Next-day Effects on Performance and Driving Tests	Reported Association with MVAs	Toxicity and/or Significant Side Effects
Antidepressants					
Tricyclics (amitriptyline, etc) [serotonin]	10–20 h	Significant	Significant with minimal study	Anecdotally noted, minimally studied	Anticholinergic, suicide
Tetracyclics (trazadone, mirtazapine) [serotonin]	Trazadone (8 h) Mirtazapin 20–40 h	Significant	Significant with minimal study	Anecdotally noted, minimally studied	Suicide
H1 antihistamines diphenhydramine, hydroxyzine, triprolidine) [histamine]	2–12 h	Significant	Significant, multiple studies	Significant	Confusion (black box warning for the elderly)
Antipsychotics					
Olanzapine [histamine]	6–8 h	Significant	Significant with minimal study	Anecdotally noted, minimally studied	Potentially persistent extrapyramidal side effects
Doxepin [histamine, orexin]	1/2–15 h (dose based) 5-wk active metabolite	Significant	Significant with minimal study	Anecdotally noted, minimally studied	Potentially persistent extrapyramidal side effects
GABA agonists					
Medium half-life benzodiazepines (estalolam, clonazepam, temazepam, etc) [GABA]	7–10 h	Significant	Significant, multiple studies	Significant, multiple studies	Disinhibition
Long half-life benzodiazepines (flurazepam, diazepam, etc) [GABA]	≤11 d	Significant	Significant, multiple studies	Significant, multiple studies	Disinhibition falls in the elderly
Orexin antagonists (suvorexant) [orexin]	10–22 h	Significant	Significant	Unknown new agent	Unknown new agent

Significant compared with placebo or drugs with known waking somnolence effects such as zopiclone.
Abbreviations: GABA, gamma-aminobutyric acid; MVAs, motor vehicle accidents.
Data from Refs.[2,10–14,16,20,22,36,37,40,46,47,49–54]

OTHER AGENTS INDUCING DAYTIME SEDATION

Among antihypertensive agents in wide use, the complaints of tiredness, fatigue, and daytime sleepiness are commonly associated with drugs having antagonistic effects at the norepinephrine neuroreceptor. The complaints of tiredness, fatigue, and daytime sleepiness (2.0%–4.3%) associated with beta-blocker use may occur secondary to disturbed sleep or direct action of the drug. Beta-blocking drugs with vasodilating properties (eg, carvedilol, labetalol) are also associated with reported fatigue and somnolence (3%–11%). Sedation is the most common side reported for the alpha-2 agonists clonidine and methyldopa (30%–75%).[54] Alpha-1 antagonists (eg, terazosin, prazosin) are sometimes associated with transient sedation. Prazosin, a norepinephrine antagonist, has shown value in treating the insomnia associated with posttraumatic stress disorder nightmares.[55] Clonidine has proven usefulness in treating the agitation and insomnia that results from using amphetamines to treat attention deficit hyperactivity disorder in pediatric patients.[56]

Sedation is among the most common side effects of antiepileptic drugs reported at levels of 70% with phenobarbital, 42% with carbamazepine and valproate, and in 33% of patients using phenytoin and primidone.[57] Sedation is reported at levels of 15% to 27% for topiramate and at levels of 5% to 10% in the clinical trials for gabapentin, lamotrigine, vigabatrin, and zonisamide. The neurochemical basis for the sedation induced by many of these agents remains poorly defined, except for those agents know to have GABA agonist effects (eg, gabapentin, phenobarbital).[58] Some drugs may act by glutamate antagonism, and others by having direct effects on CNS electophysiology.[59] In individuals being treated with such medications for seizure disorders, the clinical differential between medication effects and sedation secondary to recurrent seizures can be difficult to determine.[60]

Gamma-hydroxybutyrate is an interesting GABA agonist agent with a very short half-life. It is recommended that this drug be taken while sitting or lying down, because the acute effect of precipitating deep sleep may cause some patients to fall. The use of this agent to treat cataplexy in patients with the diagnosis of narcolepsy induces increased alertness in the day after use.[61]

Almost all drugs with CNS activity induce sleepiness as a side effect in some patients. The sedative side effects of some of these agents are clinically used in specific situations. However, sleepiness is a common and often unwanted side effect for many types of prescription medications, including commonly used antitussives, skeletal muscle relaxants, antiemetics, antidiarrhea agents, and genitourinary smooth muscle relaxants (**Table 3**). These sedative side effects can limit the use of these agents in patients in which the level of persistent daytime sleepiness affects waking. All sedating agents can contribute to an increased risk for MVAs.

DISCUSSION

Drug-induced hypersomnolence is a considerable problem. Drug-induced daytime sleepiness contributes significantly to waking impairment with primary negative health effects on motor vehicle operation. Focus in the United States has been to indemnify the use drugs of abuse, making the use ethanol and cannabis while driving illegal and potentially a path to incarceration. Australia, the United Kingdom, and the European Union, while addressing the negative impact of drugs of abuse on driving, are now focusing more closely on the social and legal implications of the use and prescription of sedating medications. The marketing, prescription, and use of sedating medication has significant legal implications.[62] In Australia, pharmacists working with industry are involved in attempts to label all potentially sedating medications to foster awareness and individual self-responsibility among drivers.[63] In Europe, "Driving licenses shall not be issued to, or renewed for, applicants or drivers who regularly use psychotropic substances, in whatever form, which can hamper the ability to drive safely where the quantities absorbed are such as to have an adverse effect on driving. This shall apply to all other medicinal products or combinations of medicinal products which affect the ability to drive (ie, it is illegal to drive while taking sedative medication)."[64] In the United States, the country with the highest rate of crash deaths, there has been limited legal, medical, industry, pharmacologic, or medical association focus on the sedative effects of prescription medications on driving.[4] Medications with significant sedating effects, even those known to negatively affect driving test performance, are marketed directly to consumers without addressing effects on motor vehicle operation. Today, the most commonly used agent for sleep induction is one with low efficacy, high levels of associated waking sedation, and proven negative effects on driving performance. Despite such known effects, this agent (diphenhydramine) is rarely part of drug testing conducted after MVAs. One logic for the development of driverless cars is the increasing use of multiple sedating medications and the

Table 3
Other prescription medication inducing daytime sleepiness as a side effect

Medication Class	Neurochemical Basis for Sleepiness
Antiparkinsonian agents	Dopamine receptor agonists
Antimuscarinic/antispasmotic	Varied effects
Skeletal muscle relaxants	Varied effects
Alpha-adrenergics blocking agents	Alpha-1 adrenergic antagonists
Beta-adrenergic blocking agents	Beta adrenergic antagonists
Gamma-hydroxy-butyrate	GABA agonist
Opiate agonists	Opioid receptor agonists (general CNS depression)
Opiate partial agonists	Opioid receptor agonists (general CNS depression)
Anticonvulsants	
Barbiturates	GABA agonist
Benzodiazepines	GABA agonist
Hydantoins	Electrophysiologic?
Succinimides	Electrophysiologic?
Other antidepressants	
MAOI	Norepinephrine, 5HT and dopamine
SSRI	5HT uptake inhibition
Agents with mixed effects	5HT, dopamine, and norepinephrine
Other antipsychotics	Dopamine receptor blockage, varied effects on histaminic, cholinergic and alpha adrenergic receptors
Barbiturates	GABA agonist
Other benzodiazepines	GABA agonist
Anxiolytics, miscellaneous sedative and hypnotics	GABA agonist, varied effects
Antitussives	General?
Antidiarrhea agents	Opioid, general?
Antiemetics	Antihistamine and varied effects
Genitourinary smooth muscle relaxants	General?

Abbreviations: 5HT, 5-hydroxytryptamine; CNS, central nervous system; GABA, gamma-aminobutyric acid; MAOI, monoamine oxide inhibitor; SSRI, selective serotonin reuptake inhibitor.
Data from Refs.[2,11,34–36,38,40,46–48,50,54,57,59]

resultant increase in MVAs among American drivers.[65]

Currently, there is considerable confusion in the medical and pharmaceutical fields, as well as the associated regulatory agencies as to how to approach the medications that induce somnolence. All drugs known to induce daytime sleepiness and affect waking function tend to be classified in the global category of sedative-hypnotics, a category that includes drugs with minimal side effects, low toxicity, and idiosyncratic reports of daytime sleepiness, as well as agents that have high toxicity and negatively affects waking performance for a high percentage of the individuals using the agent. Pharmacologically, dissimilar agents acting on the CNS in very different ways have been put into the same category, so that what is known as to drug actions and pharmacodynamics no longer logically applies to this category of medications. This conflation of drug categorization has produced considerable confusion among both the practitioners and the patients involved in the selection of a sedating agent for use.

It would seem quite reasonable, as in this article, to reinstitute an older classification system for these agents, classifying somnolence-inducing agents into the separated but intertwined categories of hypnotics, sedatives, and agents used off-label for their sedative effects. The hypnotics include those low toxicity drugs designed to induce sleep and have minimal effects on next-day waking performance (see **Table 1**). Idiosyncratic reports of next-day sleepiness occur with drugs classified as hypnotics, but the level of next-day sedation induced by these agents in clinical trials and pharmaceutical double-blind studies is comparable with the level of sedation induced by placebos. Agents classified as sedatives can be used as hypnotics, but they will also induce waking sedation in a significant percentage of those individuals using the drug (see **Table 2**). The prescriber, the pharmacy, and the direct to consumer marketing for these agents should be expected to inform the user of these drugs of their potential negative effects on waking performance and driving. Practitioners, pharmacists, and users need to be aware of the many other agents that induce sedation as a side effect (see **Table 3**) as well as their potential sedating interaction with commonly used drugs of abuse (ethanol and cannabis). The use of these medications for sleep induction should be considered off label.

SUMMARY

Many drugs of abuse, over-the-counter preparations, and prescription medications induce daytime hypersomnolence. Such hypersomnolence, whether self-induced or induced by commission, has significant individual and social cost. Despite the health and potential legal implications, outside of the intoxication and somnolence induced by drugs of self-abuse and their noted effects on driving, the diagnosis of drug-induced hypersomnolence is rarely made or the potential consequences addressed. This paper advocates and presents the logic for the reinstitution of a classification system for somnolence-inducing agents into the categories of hypnotics, sedatives, and drugs that induce sedation as a side effect to their use.

REFERENCES

1. Tefft BC. AAA foundation for traffic safety. Prevalence of motor vehicle crashes involving drowsy drivers, United States, 2009 – 2013. Washington, DC: AAA Foundation for Traffic Safety; 2014.
2. Pagel JF. Medications that induce sleepiness. In: Lee-Chiong T, editor. Sleep a comprehensive handbook. Hoboken (NJ): Wiley and Sons; 2006. p. 175–82.
3. National Highway Traffic Safety Administration. Research on drowsy driving. Available at: https://www.nhtsa.gov/risky-driving/drowsy-driving. Accessed October 20, 2015.
4. Sauber-Schatz EK, Ederer DJ, Dellinger AM, et al. Vital signs: motor vehicle injury prevention — United States and 19 comparison countries. MMWR Morb Mortal Wkly Rep 2016;65(26):672–7.
5. Wheaton AG, Chapman DP, Presley-Cantrell LR, et al. Drowsy driving – 19 states and the District of Columbia, 2009-2010. MMWR Morb Mortal Wkly Rep 2013;61:1033.
6. Sforza E, De Saint Hilaire Z, Pelissolo A, et al. Personality, anxiety and mood traits in patients with sleep-related breathing disorders: effect of reduced daytime alertness. Sleep Med 2002;3:139–45.
7. Department of Transportation (US), National Highway Traffic Safety Administration (NHTSA). Traffic Safety Facts 2014 data: alcohol-impaired driving. Washington, DC: NHTSA; 2015. Available at. http://www-nrd.nhtsa.dot.gov/Pubs/812231.pdf.
8. Berning A, Compton R, Wochinger K. Results of the 2013–2014 National Roadside Survey of alcohol and drug use by drivers. Washington, DC: NHTSA; 2015 (DOT HS 812 118).
9. Ceutel C. Risk of traffic accident injury after a prescription for a benzodiazepine. Ann Epidemiol 1995;5(3):239–44.
10. Gengo F, Manning C. A review of the effects of antihistamines on mental processes related to automobile driving. J Allergy Clin Immunol 1990;86:1034–9.
11. Leveille SG, Buchner DM, Koepsell TD, et al. Psychoactive medications and injurious motor vehicle collisions involving older drivers. Epidemiology 1994;5:591–8.
12. Ray WA, Griffen MR, Downey W. Benzodiazepines of long and short elimination half life and the risk of hip fracture. JAMA 1989;262:3303–7.
13. Van Laar M, van Willigenburg AP, Volkerts ER. Acute and subchronic effects of nefazodone and imipramine on highway driving, cognitive functions, and daytime sleepiness in healthy adult and elderly subjects. J Clin Psychopharmacol 1995;15(1):30–40.
14. Ray WA, Fought RL, Decker MD, et al. Psychoactive drugs and the risk of injurious motor vehicle crashes in elderly drivers. Am J Epidemiol 1992;136:873–83.
15. Disney L, Pelkey S, Wipperman M, et al. Drug testing and drug-involved driving of fatally injured drivers in the United States: 2005–2009. 2011. Available at: http://www.whitehouse.gov/ondcp/drugged-driving. Accessed November 10, 2016.
16. Buysse DJ. Drugs affecting sleep sleepiness and performance. In: Monk TM, editor. Sleep sleepiness and performance. West Sussex (United Kingdom): John Wiley & Sons; 1991. p. 4–31.
17. Alattar M, Harrington JJ, Mitchell CM, et al. Sleep problems in primary care: a North Carolina family Practice Research Network (NC-FP-RN) study. J Am Board if Fam Med 2007;20(4):365–74.
18. Roehrs T, Carskadon MA, Dement WC, et al. Daytime sleepiness and alertness. In: Kryger M, Roth T, Dement B, editors. Principles and practice of sleep medicine. Philadelphia: W.B. Saunders and Co; 2000.
19. Pivik RT. The several qualities of sleepiness. In: Monk TM, editor. Psychophysiological considerations in sleep sleepiness and performance. West

Sussex (United Kingdom): John Wiley & Sons; 1991. p. 3–38.

20. Zhang D, Tashiro M, Shibuya K, et al. Next-day residual sedative effect after nighttime administration of an over-the-counter antihistamine sleep aid, diphenhydramine, measured by positron emission tomography. J Clin Psychopharmacol 2010;6:694–701.

21. Gevins A, Smith M, McEvoy L. Tracking the cognitive pharmacodynamics of psychoactive substances with combinations of behavioral and neurophysiological measures. Neuropsychopharmacology 2002;26: 27–39.

22. Gango F, Gabos C, Miller J. The pharmacodynamics of diphenhydramine-induced drowsiness and changes in mental performance. Clin Pharm Ther 1989;45(1):15–21.

23. Verster J, Volkerts E, Olivier B, et al. Zolpidem and traffic safety—the importance of treatment compliance. Curr Drug Saf 2007;2(3):220–6.

24. Breslau N, Roth T, Rosenthal L, et al. Sleep disturbance and psychiatric disorders: a longitudinal epidemiological study of young adults. Biol Psychiatr 1996;39:411–8.

25. Taylor B, Pelam J. The relationship between alcohol consumption and fatal motor vehicle injury: high risk at low alcohol levels. Alcohol Clin Exp Res 2012; 36(10):1827–34.

26. Sateia MJ, Doghramji K, Hauri PJ, et al. Evaluation of chronic insomnia. Sleep 2000;23:243–314.

27. Stein M, Friedmann P. Disturbed sleep and its relationship to alcohol use. Subst Abus 2005;26(1):1–13.

28. Scanlan MF, Roebuck T, Little PJ, et al. Effect of moderate alcohol upon obstructive sleep apnoea. Eur Respir J 2000;16(5):909–13.

29. Hartman RL, Huestis MA. Cannabis effects on driving skills. Clin Chem 2013;59(3):478–92.

30. Elvik R. Risk of road accident associated with the use of drugs: a systematic review and meta-analysis of evidence from epidemiological studies. Accid Anal Prev 2013;60:254–67.

31. Sewell R, Poling J, Sofuoglu M. The effect of cannabis compared with alcohol on driving. Am J Addict 2009;18(3):185–93.

32. Compton RP, Berning A. Traffic safety facts research note: drugs and alcohol crash risk. Washington, DC: NHTSA; 2015. Available at: http://www.nhtsa.gov/staticfiles/nti/pdf/812117-Drug_and_Alcohol_Crash_Risk.pdf.

33. CDC's Morbidity and Mortality Weekly Report. 2015. Available at: www.cdc.gov/mmwr/index2015.html. Accessed November 18, 2016.

34. Wang D, Teichtahl H. Opioids, sleep architecture and sleep disordered breathing. Sleep Med Rev 2007;11(1):35–46.

35. Hayes B, Klein-Schwartz W, Barrueto F. Polypharmacy and the geriatric patient. Clin Geriatr Med 2007;23(2):371–90.

36. Pagel JF. Sleep disorders and insomnia. Am Fam Physician 1978;17:165–9.

37. Pagel JF. Medication effects on sleep. In: Pandi-Perumal S, Ruoti R, Kramer M, editors. Sleep and psychosomatic medicine. Andover, Hampshire (UK): Informa Ltd; 2007. p. 109–24.

38. Lossignol D. Euthanasia: medications and medical procedures. Rev Med Brux 2008;29:435–40.

39. Roehrs T, Carskadon MA, Dement WC, et al. Daytime sleepiness and alertness. In: Kryger M, Roth T, Dement W, editors. Principles and practice of sleep medicine. 3rd edition. Philadelphia: Saunders Company; 2000. p. 43–53.

40. Pagel JF, Parnes B. Medications for the treatment of sleep disorders: an overview. Prim Care Companion J Clin Psychiatry 2001;3(3):118–25.

41. Verster JC, Volkerts ER, Schreuder AH, et al. Residual effects of middle-of-the-night administration of zaleplon and zolpidem on driving ability, memory functions, and psychomotor performance. J Clin Psychopharmacol 2002;22:576–83.

42. Paul MA, Gray G, Kenny G, et al. Impact of melatonin, zaleplon, zopiclone, and temazepam on psychomotor performance. Aviat Space Environ Med 2003;74:1263–70.

43. Mets MA, de Vries JM, de Senerpont Domis LM, et al. Next-day effects of ramelteon (8 mg), zopiclone (7.5 mg), and placebo on highway driving performance, memory functioning, psychomotor performance, and mood in healthy adult subjects. Sleep 2011;34(10):1327–34.

44. Stone BM, Turner C, Mills SL, et al. Hypnotic activity of melatonin. Sleep 2000;23(5):663–70.

45. Schwartz JH. Neurotransmitters. In: Kandel ER, Schwartz JH, Jessell TM, editors. Principles of neural science. 4th edition. New York: McGraw Hill; 2000. p. 280–97.

46. Volz HP, Sturm Y. Antidepressant drugs and psychomotor performance. Neuropsychobiology 1995;31: 146–55.

47. Settle EC. Antidepressant drugs: disturbing and potentially dangerous adverse effects. J Clin Psychiatry 1998;59(S16):25–9.

48. Micalief J, Rey M, Eusebio A, et al. Antiparkinsonism drug-induced sleepiness: a double-blind placebo-controlled study of L-dopa, bromocriptine and pramipexole in healthy subjects. Br J Clin Pharm 2009;87(3):333–40.

49. O'Hanlon JF, Ramaekers JG. Antihistamine effects on actual driving performance in a standard driving test: a summary of Dutch experience. 1989-94. Allergy 1995;50:234–42.

50. Wiler J, Bloomfield J, Woodworth G, et al. Effects of fexofenadine, diphenhydramine, and alcohol on driving performance: a randomized, placebo-controlled trial in the Iowa driving simulator. Ann Intern Med 2000;132:354–63.

51. White JM, Rumbold GR. Behavioural effects of histamine and its antagonists: a review. Psychopharmacology (Berl) 1988;95(1):1–14.

52. Krystal AD, Durrnace HH, Scharf M, et al. Efficacy and safety of doxepin 1 mg and 3 mg in a 12 week sleep laboratory and outpatient trial of elderly subjects with chronic primary insomnia. Sleep 2013;33:1553–61.

53. Farkus R. Suvorexant safety and efficacy—FDA. 2013. Available at: www.fda.gov/downloads/.../UCM354215.pdf. Accessed November 20, 2016.

54. AHFS drug information. Bethesda (MD): American Society of Health-System Pharmacists; 2003.

55. Raskind MA, Peskind ER, Kanter ED, et al. Reduction of nightmares and other PTSD symptoms in combat veterans by prazosin: a placebo-controlled study. Am J Psychiatry 2003;160(2):371–3.

56. Pagel JF, Kram G. Insomnia: differential diagnosis and current treatment approach. In: Monti JM, Pandi-Perumal SR, Mohler H, editors. GABA and sleep – molecular, functional and clinical aspects. Basel (Switzerland): Springer; 2010. p. 363–82.

57. Schweitzer PK, Muehlbach MJ, Walsh JK. Medical Drugs affecting sleep, sleepiness and performance. Am J Geriatr Psychiatry 2003;11:205–13.

58. Westbrook G. Seizures and epilepsy. In: Kandel ER, Schwartz JH, Jessell TM, editors. Principles of neural science. 4th edition. New York: McGraw-Hill; 2000. p. 199–935.

59. Pagel JF. Pharmacologic Alterations of sleep and dream: a clinical framework for utilizing the electrophysiological and sleep stage effects of psychoactive medications. Hum Psychopharmacology 1996; 11:217–23.

60. Manni R, Tartara A. Evaluation of sleepiness in epilepsy. Clin Neurophysiol 2000;111(Suppl 2):S111–4.

61. Mamelak M, Escriu JM, Stokan O. The effects of gamma-hydroxybutyrate on sleep. Biol Psychiatry 1977;12(2):273–88.

62. Jones C, Dorrian J, Rajaratnam S. Fatigue and the criminal law. Ind Health 2005;43:63–70.

63. Nicholas R, Lee N, Roche A. Pharmaceutical drug misuse in Australia: complex problems, balanced responses. National Centre for Education and Training on Addiction (NCETA). Adelaide (Australia): Flinders University; 2011. ISBN: 978 1 876897 39 0.

64. European Monitoring Center for Drugs and Drug Addiction (EMCDDA | Legal approaches to drugs and driving. Annex III of Council Directive 91/439/EEC of 29 July 1991 on driving licenses. Available at: www.eur-lex.europa.eu. Accessed November 21, 2016.

65. Lipson H, Kurman M. Driverless: intelligent cars and the road ahead. Cambridge (MA): MIT Press; 2016.

Depression and Hypersomnia
A Complex Association

Régis Lopez, MD, PhD[a,b,c,*], Lucie Barateau, MD[a,b,c],
Elisa Evangelista, MD[a,b], Yves Dauvilliers, MD, PhD[a,b,c,*]

KEYWORDS

- Hypersomnolence • Sleepiness • Hypersomnia • Mood • Depression

KEY POINTS

- Hypersomnolence in depression is commonly considered a consequence of the disorder, in line with disturbances in monoamine activity. However, associated factors may contribute to hypersomnolence in patients with depression.
- Depressive symptoms and hypersomnolence are often associated with complex and often bidirectional interactions.
- Although depressive symptoms are common in patients with central hypersomnia, the formal diagnosis of a major depressive episode requires a structured evaluation to avoid frequent clinical overlap between the 2 conditions.
- Ideally, the management of both depressive symptoms in central hypersomnias and hypersomnolence in depressive disorders requires a collaboration between sleep specialists and psychiatrists.

INTRODUCTION

Depression and hypersomnia are 2 conditions linked in a complex and bidirectional manner. Excessive daytime sleepiness (EDS) is a common complaint among patients suffering from depression. On the other hand, patients with central hypersomnia, such as narcolepsy type 1 (NT1) or type 2 (NT2), and idiopathic hypersomnia (IH), often present depressive symptoms, probably due to their chronic and disabling condition, but also potentially due to an intrinsic predisposition in NT1. The aims of this review are to focus on the following: (1) the definition and prevalence of hypersomnolence as a pathologic condition; (2) the frequency, pathophysiology, and practical assessment of depression in central hypersomnia

disorders; and (3) hypersomnolence in depressive disorders.

EPIDEMIOLOGY AND NOSOGRAPHIC CONSIDERATION

The definition of hypersomnolence and its frequency remain problematic. The terms "hypersomnia," "hypersomnolence," "somnolence," "excessive somnolence," and "excessive daytime sleepiness" (EDS) were often used interchangeably in literature, leading to high heterogeneity in the results with thus potential for bias.[1]

The Diagnostic and Statistical Manual of Mental Disorders, fifth edition (DSM-5) recently introduced the concept of "hypersomnolence disorder," a syndrome that associates excessive daytime or

[a] National Reference Center for Orphan Disease, Narcolepsy and Hypersomnia, Sleep disorder Unit, Gui de Chauliac hospital, 80 avenue Augustin Fliche, Montpellier F-34000, France; [b] Inserm U1061, Montpellier F-34000, France; [c] University of Montpellier, Montpellier F-34000, France
* Corresponding author. National Reference Center for Orphan Disease, Narcolepsy and Hypersomnia, Sleep disorder Unit, Gui de Chauliac hospital, 80 avenue Augustin Fliche, Montpellier F-34000, France.
E-mail addresses: r-lopez@chu-montpellier.fr (R.L.); y-dauvilliers@chu-montpellier.fr (Y.D.)

Sleep Med Clin 12 (2017) 395–405
http://dx.doi.org/10.1016/j.jsmc.2017.03.016
1556-407X/17/© 2017 Elsevier Inc. All rights reserved.

nighttime sleep, impaired vigilance, and/or sleep inertia, not due to narcolepsy, disturbed nighttime sleep, circadian rhythm disorder, or a substance that can be associated, but not entirely explained, by a medical or mental disorder.[2] The diagnostic criteria of the hypersomnolence disorder may overlap with those of IH in the third edition of the International Classification of Sleep Disorders, third edition.[3] In this latter classification, the terms "hypersomnia" and "central disorders of hypersomnolence" are used to label specific sleep disorders such as narcolepsy but also when associated or due to various medical, psychiatric, or environmental (insufficient sleep, substance use) conditions. In the DSM-5, the term "hypersomnia" was also used, in reference to a symptom, for example, a symptom criteria for mood disorders.[2]

Hypersomnolence needs currently to be defined as a clinical syndrome characterized by the occurrence of 3 major symptoms, being potentially associated, with large variability regarding severity among patients: (1) an excessive quantity of nighttime and/or daytime sleep; (2) an alteration in the quality of arousal defined by an incapacity to maintain a satisfactory level of vigilance during the day; and (3) sleep inertia,[4] defined by major difficulties in waking up in the morning or after a nap with frequent reentries in sleep, reduced vigilance, and impaired performance, lasting few minutes to hours.

The frequency of an excessive duration of nighttime sleep (>9 hours) is 8.4% in the general population, with a higher prevalence in women than in men (9.2% vs 7.6%), and with a large age effect (decreasing until 65 years of age and increasing thereafter).[5,6] Excessive nighttime sleep is associated with significant daytime consequences in 1.6%.[6] In addition, some studies highlighted its association with increased risk of developing cardiovascular,[7,8] neurodegenerative disorders, and even with a higher risk of mortality.[9] The inability to maintain satisfactory alertness during the day, or having at least 2 sleep attacks 3 days per week, for at least 3 months is seen in 4.7% of the general population.[6] Because of the lack of standardized definition of sleep inertia,[4] there are no robust data on its prevalence; however, a large recent study reported a nonrestorative prolonged sleep episode in 1.2% of the general population.[6] The latter 3 symptoms were often associated together, and with numerous medical and psychiatric disorders, and the use of psychotropic medication. After the exclusion of these comorbid conditions, the prevalence of the hypersomnolence disorder is estimated at 1.5%.[6]

To avoid potential confusion in terminology in this review, the terms "central hypersomnia" refers to a specific sleep disorder and "hypersomnolence" refers to the complaints of either excessive nighttime or daytime sleep, unsatisfactory alertness, and sleep inertia that can be associated with environmental, medical, or psychiatric conditions.

DEPRESSIVE SYMPTOMS IN CENTRAL HYPERSOMNIAS

Central hypersomnias are rare and disabling sleep abnormalities that include NT1, NT2, and IH. NT1 is characterized by hypersomnolence and cataplexy, frequently associated with hypnagogic hallucinations, sleep paralysis, and disturbed nighttime sleep.[10,11] IH and NT2 are 2 other central hypersomnias mainly characterized by hypersomnolence, but without pathognomonic symptom, with unclear prevalence and often unstable disease course.[12,13]

Assessing Depressive Symptoms in Central Hypersomnias

The assessment of depressive symptoms in central hypersomnias warrants specific clinical considerations. According to the DSM-5, the diagnosis of major depression requires sad mood and/or anhedonia plus 4 of the following symptoms: suicidal ideation, fatigue, weight or appetite change, psychomotor agitation or slowing, feelings of excessive guilt, cognitive and sleep complaints.[2] Accordingly, hypersomnolence could be one of the symptom criteria for major depression. Furthermore, central hypersomnias are frequently associated with fatigue, cognitive alterations such as inattention and risk-taking behavior, with feelings of being lazy, slow, or with motor hyperactivity,[14–17] and with increased weight gain and appetite, especially in NT1.[18] Overall, 5 out of 9 symptom criteria for major depression are shared with central hypersomnia, resulting in a clinical overlap between the 2 conditions. Then, screening questionnaires for depression, such as the Beck Depression Inventory,[19] being largely administrated in patients with central hypersomnia, should be used with caution because of the risk of false positive results. For example, one case-control study found depressive symptoms in one-third of narcolepsy patients, whereas no significant difference was found between patients and controls regarding the formal mood disorder diagnosis.[20] To date, no questionnaire has been validated to assess the presence or the severity of depressive symptoms in patients with central hypersomnia specifically. Instead, a structured clinical interview remains essential to conduct an optimal evaluation of depressive symptoms in these conditions. Another challenging issue concerns depression as an exclusion criterion for the diagnosis of IH.

However, a potential overlap has been suggested between hypersomnia associated with depression and IH with some depressive symptoms.[21]

Frequency of Depressive Symptoms in Central Hypersomnias

NT1 has been frequently associated with a high level of psychiatric comorbidities,[18] including mood, anxiety, attention deficit hyperactivity,[17] eating,[22] and rarely, psychotic disorders.[23] Comorbidity between hypersomnia disorders and mood symptoms, particularly depression, has been frequently reported in both clinical setting and the general population.

Several studies found a high prevalence of depressive symptoms in NT1,[24–29] ranging from 15% to 37%, with a relative stability within a 5-year follow-up in one study.[30] A large cross-sectional narcolepsy study found that depressive symptoms (using self-reported assessment) were associated with greater alterations in quality of life, higher EDS, and the occurrence of rapid eye movement (REM) dysregulation-related symptoms, such as cataplexy, hypnagogic hallucinations, or sleep paralysis.[31] Interestingly, similar associations were found in the general population between sleep paralysis, sleep-related hallucinations, and depressive symptoms.[32,33] In IH, depressive symptoms were reported in 15% to 25% of patients in clinical-based samples.[21,31,34,35] No study was specifically designed to assess depressive symptoms or diagnosis in patients with NT2.

Pathophysiologic Hypotheses

The causal relationship between depressive symptoms and central hypersomnia remains unclear, with potential for a multifactorial origin. First, patients with narcolepsy or IH often report poor academic and work performances, and a higher incidence of car, work, and house accidents.[36] Their hypersomnolence may also affect social and familial functioning with frequent poor tolerance by family members concerning the lengthy time they spend in bed or the need to sleep instead of recreational activities. These consequences lead to large alterations of the quality of life and may contribute to depressive feelings, symptoms, and then a disorder.[37]

Second, the frequent occurrence of depressive symptoms may also rely on the neurobiological mechanisms of central hypersomnias. NT1 is the unique human model of chronic hypocretin-1 (Hcrt-1)/orexin-A deficiency.[10] Hcrt-1 neurons arise in the lateral hypothalamus and project widely through the brain with a dense innervation of structures involved in the regulation of physiologic processes frequently disturbed in depression, such as arousal, motivation, food intake, sexual behavior, cognitive processes, and stress response.[33] Hypocretin has been implicated in the modulation of monoamine systems, which are major actors in the pathophysiology of mood disorders. The results of several preclinical studies suggested a pathophysiologic link between hypocretin and depression, with changes in the activity of hypocretin signaling pathways being associated with depression-like behaviors. It was suggested that the balance of hypocretin action, either on the Hcrtr-1 or on the Hcrtr-2 receptor, produces an antidepressant or pro-depressant-like effect, depending on the receptor subtype activated.[21]

Management of Depression in Central Hypersomnias

The management of depressive symptoms in central hypersomnias is challenging, especially in NT1. In the Harmony study, narcoleptic patients treated with both stimulants and anticataplectic drugs (mainly serotonergic and noradrenergic antidepressants) had more depressive symptoms compared with those treated with stimulants alone.[31] These results highlighted that the antidepressant effects differ from their anticataplectic effects, the latter being usually reached more rapidly and at lower doses than with antidepressant therapeutic doses.[34–36] Clinicians should be aware that antidepressants at doses prescribed for cataplexy management might be not effective to treat depressive symptoms in narcolepsy. The optimal management of comorbid mood disorder in narcolepsy should associate antidepressants at sufficient doses and supportive psychotherapeutic interventions. Furthermore, sodium oxybate, a first-line anticataplectic treatment, may induce or worsen depressive symptoms.[37,38] Its initiation thus required careful screening of baseline depressive symptoms and suicidality.[39]

HYPERSOMNOLENCE IN DEPRESSIVE DISORDERS

Depression is seen in various psychiatric diseases, including major depressive disorder (MDD), bipolar disorder (BD), and seasonal affective disorder (SAD). A high frequency of EDS, prolonged nocturnal sleep, and sleep inertia has been reported in these conditions.

Assessing Hypersomnolence in Depressive Disorders

Most studies in clinical psychiatric settings assessed hypersomnolence by 1 or 2 questions only ("*How long do you sleep at night?*", "*Do you feel sleepy during the day*" and so forth). However, several validated subjective and objective tests can be used to quantify the severity of hypersomnolence.

The Epworth Sleepiness Scale assesses the sleep propensity and its consequences in 8 situations of the daily life during the past month.[40] Other simple questionnaires, such as the Stanford Sleepiness Scale or the Karolinska Sleepiness Scale, can be used to estimate the vigilance at a given time.[41,42] Sleep diary is a useful tool to characterize the reported nighttime and daytime sleep duration over several days or weeks. It may help the clinician to distinguish excessive sleep duration and clinophilia by differentiating the time in bed and the total sleep time reported. However, these responses may depend on the subject's perceptual experience. Sleep diaries are also helpful to rule out sleep deprivation and sleep-delayed phase syndrome in the context of hypersomnolence. The Sleep Inertia Questionnaire was recently developed to assess sleep inertia in the context of depression with satisfactory psychometric properties.[43]

All these subjective tools provide interesting results but with large discrepancies with those obtained with objective assessments. The latter tests include wrist actigraphy, polysomnography (PSG), the multiple sleep latency test (MSLT), the maintenance of wakefulness test (MWT), and forced-awakening nap protocols. The actigraphy is a noninvasive method monitoring the rest/activity cycles that provides an estimation of the total sleep time.[44] It may be useful in assessing extended nocturnal sleep in patients with hypersomnolence. Although it is well accepted and less expensive than polysomnographic assessments, actigraphy may overestimate sleep and underestimate wakefulness during the day.[45] The PSG is the gold-standard objective measure of the nocturnal sleep, providing detailed information such as time in bed, sleep-onset latency, REM sleep onset latency, total sleep time, sleep efficiency, and percentages of sleep stages. The PSG is performed during the major nighttime sleep period, thus being not designed to assess the extended sleep duration. In contrast, continuous 24h-PSG recordings or longer ad libitum sleep-wake protocols may quantify the long nocturnal and diurnal total sleep time. However, these tests, often used to diagnose IH, still lack standardized procedures and normative values stratified by age and gender.[46]

The MSLT is the most widely used objective test in clinical practice and is often considered the "gold standard" for the objective diagnosis of EDS.[47] It measures the propensity to fall asleep during the day under soporific conditions. The subject, lying down on a bed, follows a standardized protocol over 5 sessions between 9:00 AM and 5:00 PM with the instructions of trying to fall asleep.[48] The main outcome measure of the MSLT is the mean sleep latency that corresponds to the average time taken to fall asleep in the 5 tests. Mean sleep latencies shorter than 8 minutes are considered abnormal. The MWT is another widely used neurophysiologic test that measures the capacity to remain awake during the day.[49] The subject, seated in a chair in dim-light conditions, follows a standardized protocol for 4 sessions between 10:00 AM and 4:00 PM, with instructions of remaining awake for as long as possible. Several thresholds for the mean sleep latency have been proposed varying from 19 minutes (the most widely accepted) to 33 minutes (threshold to minimize accident risk) or even 40 minutes (no falling asleep, the most conservative threshold).[48] The MWT is often used to measure the effectiveness of stimulant treatments in central hypersomnias.

Unfortunately, few standardized objective tests exist to assess sleep inertia. One of these tests measures the P300 latencies using an auditory evoked potentials protocol during a forced awakening after nap.[50] One study suggested that this measure may distinguish psychiatric from neurologic forms of hypersomnia.[51]

The Frequency of Hypersomnolence in Depressive Disorders

The complaint of hypersomnolence is very frequent in psychiatric disorders and especially in mood disorders. However, its frequency in mood disorders remains difficult to sum up, because of various definitions of hypersomnolence and tests used among studies leading to heterogeneous findings. Here the focus is on MDD, bipolar-related diagnoses (BD), and SAD.

The frequency of hypersomnolence symptoms in MDD greatly varies across studies, with a significant age and gender effect. Hypersomnolence symptoms may include EDS, long non-refreshing naps, long nocturnal sleep time, and sleep inertia. Hypersomnolence complaints are higher in women, with a prevalence ranging from 9% in children to 76% in adults.[52] No studies investigated the increased sleep duration in MDD with a sleep diary protocol. However, in one cohort study of consecutive patients with MDD, the frequency of "increased sleep" was 24%.[53] Excessive sleep duration (>10 hours) was significantly associated with MDD in another cohort of 219 subjects from the general population. In addition, excessive sleep duration was found in 6% of MDD patients with current depression in contrast to 1.7% with remitted depression.[54] Few studies investigated hypersomnolence in MDD with objective measures such as the MSLT or continuous PSG. A recent meta-analysis revealed that MDD patients with hypersomnolence complaints evaluated with the MSLT demonstrated mean sleep latencies comparable to normative values.[55] A study comparing nighttime sleep duration over a 2-day protocol in psychiatric hypersomnia (mainly MDD patients) and in IH revealed that only 14% of psychiatric hypersomnia slept more than 9 hours, with a lower sleep duration than in the IH group (7.68 vs 9.92 hours).[56] Similar results were obtained using in a 44-hour protocol, as the total sleep duration did not differ between depressive patients and controls.[34] To the authors' knowledge, no study focused on excessive sleep duration in ecological conditions with actigraphic protocols in MDD.

Hypersomnolence symptoms are also frequent in patients with both type 1 and type 2 BD, ranging from 23% to 78%.[53,57,58] One study assessing sleepiness with the MSLT in BD depressed patients with hypersomnolence complaint did not report objective daytime sleepiness.[59] Conversely, actigraphic measures revealed longer sleep durations in remitted BD patients than in controls.[60] However, none of these studies included in a recent meta-analysis reported the frequency of the excessive sleep duration (>9 or even 10 hours).[61] A recent study evaluated both subjective and objective dimensions of hypersomnolence in a large clinical sample of euthymic BD patients that showed that excessive sleep and impaired vigilance are 2 distinct clinical features of hypersomnolence in BD.[62] Again, in this study, the complaint of excessive sleep duration was not confirmed with actigraphic measures. The investigators also found that excessive sleepiness predicted relapse to mania.[62] In the same way, another study found that subjective hypersomnolence in the euthymic period predicts the risk of future depressive symptoms.[63]

Hypersomnolence is one of the major features of SAD, with frequencies varying from 67% to 76%.[52] Again, most of these studies did not use validated subjective or objective tests to assess the hypersomnolence, thus leading to doubtful findings with a general tendency to overestimate the sleep problems using self-reports only.[64–66]

Despite a high heterogeneity of the definitions and the assessment methods, the frequency of hypersomnolence appears to be high in depressive disorders. Moreover, the hypersomnolence seems associated with a poorer prognosis, resistance to treatment, increased risk for relapse, and a functional impairment.

Pathophysiologic Hypotheses

Hypersomnolence in depression is commonly considered a consequence of the disorder, in line with disturbances in monoamine activity.[67] However, several associated factors may contribute to hypersomnolence in patients with depression.

First, most of the psychotropic drugs usually prescribed in mood disorders may be responsible for hypersomnolence. They included antidepressants, hypnotic and anxiolytic benzodiazepines, but also mood stabilizers, and antihistaminic and antipsychotic drugs. Evening or night intake of sedative drugs may cause increased sleep duration and sleep inertia, whereas a daytime prescription may worsen the daytime sleepiness propensity. From an individual point of view, ascertaining the relationship between the current use of sedative drugs and the occurrence of hypersomnolence symptoms is challenging because of the involvement of various parameters such as dose effects, between drugs interactions, intrinsic susceptibility, pharmacogenetics, and renal or liver metabolisms.

Hypersomnolence may also relate to nocturnal sleep disturbances. Several cross-sectional studies consistently found impairments in the sleep architecture with decreased slow-wave sleep duration and increased REM sleep pressure. Among mood disorders, MDD was associated with the most severe sleep continuity with both non-REM and REM sleep instability. REM sleep characteristics (ie, REM latency, density, and duration) are often altered in major depression that may relate to an increased central cholinergic activity and sensitivity. Interestingly, such REM sleep disturbances have also been found in relatives of patients with MDD, with no personal history of psychiatric illness.[68]

The complaint of hypersomnolence may also relate to the presence of an underlying sleep disorder such as obstructive sleep apnea syndrome (OSAS). In presence of nocturnal symptoms (snoring, nocturia, heavy night sweats, increased salivation at night, periods of silence followed by gasps reported by the bed partner, restless sleep at night, multiple arousals, and so forth) and daytime complaints (EDS, morning headaches, cognitive impairment, irritability, and reduce sexual drive), an OSAS should be suspected. Sleep-related breathing disorders can be screened with simple tools such as the STOP-BANG or the Berlin questionnaire[69–71] and formally diagnosed with respiratory polygraphy, a technique that can be performed in ambulatory or in hospitalized patients. A high frequency of OSAS has been found in patients with MDD (36.3%) or BD (24.5%).[72] In addition, clinicians should know that OSAS may represent a potential cause for psychotropic drug resistance in the context of mood disorders.[73] The nature of the link between OSAS and mood disorders is multifactorial, with overweight and metabolic syndrome frequently seen in this population. Moreover, potential adverse events of their medications such as benzodiazepines, opioids, and antipsychotic agents may exist with direct effects on either airway obstruction or central breathing control during sleep.[74]

The underlying mechanisms of association between hypersomnolence and mood disorders may also differ according to the different depressive phenotypes. Some studies found that circadian rhythm disruption is a major feature in BD, even in drug-naive patients and independently of mood status,[75] but with more frequent biological alterations in depressed than in euthymic patients. Delayed sleep phase syndrome (DSPS) is characterized by delayed habitual sleep-wake timing, usually greater than 2 hours, relative to conventional or socially acceptable timing.[76] Affected individuals complain of difficulty falling asleep and arising at the required times, and frequently experience daytime hypersomnolence, especially in the first hours of the day. Clinical investigations together with daily profiles of melatonin levels and cortisol indicated a frequent DSPS in the BP population.[77] In a study using a constant routine procedure controlling for light exposure and exogenous circadian cues, individuals with SAD displayed a significantly delayed temperature rhythm compared with controls.[78] These results are further supported by a general improvement with morning bright light in individuals with SAD and hypersomnia.[79] Some investigators proposed that a diminished sensitivity to corticotropin-releasing hormone might play a role in atypical depression, a condition that frequently associates depressive symptoms, hypersomnolence, hyperphagia, and leaden weakness.[80]

Management of Hypersomnolence in Mood Disorders

The first objective in treating hypersomnolence in depressed patients is to obtain a symptomatic remission. Unfortunately, sleepiness is often encountered as a residual symptom among MDD or BD patients who have remitted from depressive symptoms following optimal treatment. Addressing residual sleepiness in euthymic patients is thus challenging. Management options may include lowering the dose of psychotropic drugs, switching to a shorter-acting medication, prescribing a sedative drug in the evening instead of morning, or using antidepressant or mood stabilizer medications that are less likely to exacerbate hypersomnolence. **Table 1** provides a nonexhaustive list of antidepressant medications with their preferential sedative/neutral/stimulant profile and main characteristics. However, in one study, up to 70% of depressed patients with hypersomnolence had persistent complaints of EDS or prolonged nocturnal sleep despite remission of mood symptoms with the nonsedative antidepressant fluoxetine.[81]

A careful clinical examination of the phenotype of hypersomnolence and its associated symptoms may lead to specific therapeutic interventions (**Fig. 1**). Moderate sleep-related breathing disturbances might be improved with dietetic measures for weight loss, lowering the dose, or switching sedative medications. In the case of severe OSAS, a treatment with continuous positive airway pressure or oral appliance is required. Chronotherapeutic interventions such as sleep hygiene and psychological therapies that target circadian misalignment may improve DSPS and hypersomnolence. Adjunctive melatonin or melatonin agonist treatments showed some promising results in BDs.[82] Furthermore, hypersomnolence can be reduced with bright light or dawn simulation therapy, with good response in almost half of patients with SAD.[83]

The cooccurrence of a central hypersomnia disorder (ie, IH, narcolepsy) has to be considered when the strategies mentioned above failed to resolve hypersomnolence, when the patient was severely sleepy, or when the patient reported cataplexy-like symptoms. In such conditions, patients should be referred for a PSG and MSLT assessment in a reference center for central hypersomnias.[84,85] A withdrawal of all psychotropic drugs needs to be discussed before the PSG-MSLT; however, some patients are unwilling to stop or cannot stop due to a severe underlying psychiatric condition. In doubtful clinical cases of NT1, a biomarker diagnostic approach such as HLA DQB1*0602 typing and CSF Hcrt-1 level measurement may be helpful.[10,85]

Finally, in the case of unsuccessful therapeutic interventions and negative investigation outcomes, the off-label use of adjunctive psychostimulant should be considered, even if their prescriptions are not well codified. The use of stimulant (ie, modafinil, methylphenidate, amphetamine) should be used with caution because of an increased risk for psychotic symptoms with high-dose stimulants

Table 1
Main antidepressant medications with their preferential sedative/neutral/stimulant profile and some practical considerations

Sedation Profile	Antidepressant	Therapeutic Class	Practical Considerations
Sedative	Moclobemide	MAOI	High risk for drug interactions Weight gain
	Amitryptyline, clomipramine	TCA	Weight gain
	Mirtazapine	NaSSA	Sedative at low doses (15 mg/d) Weight gain
	Trazodone,	SARI	Approved for insomnia in some countries
	Agomelatine	Melatonergic	Evening administration only
	Paroxetine	SSRI	Withdrawal syndrome Weight gain
Neutral	Fluvoxamine	SSRI	Less risk of sexual side effects
	Citalopram, escitalopram	SSRI	Balanced antidepressants
	Sertraline	SSRI	Approved in children in some countries
	Tianeptine	SSRE	Potential risk for abuse
	Fluoxetine	SSRI	Most stimulant SSRI
	Venlafaxine, duloxetine	SNRI	Widely used anticataplectic antidepressants
	Protriptyline, nortriptyline	TCA	Most stimulant TCAs
	Reboxetine, viloxazine	NRI	Moderate antidepressant effects
Stimulant	Bupropion, Atomoxetine	NDRI	Stimulant antidepressants also used for the treatment of ADHD

Abbreviations: ADHD, attention-deficit/hyperactivity disorder; MAOI, monoamine oxidase inhibitors; NaSSA, noradrenergic and specific serotonergic antidepressants; NDRI, norepinephrine and dopamine reuptake inhibitors; NRI, norepinephrine reuptake inhibitors; SARI, serotonin antagonist and reuptake inhibitors; SNRI, serotonin and norepinephrine reuptake inhibitors; SSRE, selective serotonin reuptake enhancer; SSRI, selective serotonin reuptake inhibitors; TCA, tricyclic antidepressants.

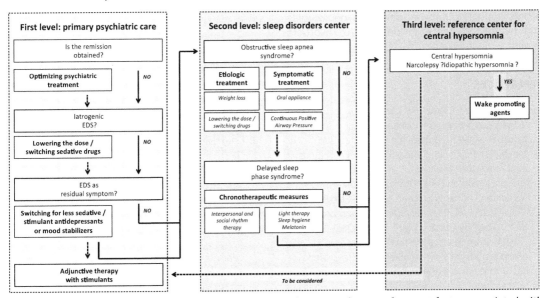

Fig. 1. Diagnostic and therapeutic algorithm to rule out and manage the most frequent factors associated with hypersomnolence in psychiatric disorders.

and the hypothetical increased risk of manic/hypomanic switch in BD patients. However, there is no clear evidence of such a risk in BD patients treated with stimulants as add-on to mood stabilizers, and no study could detect an increased risk for mood switch in such condition.[86–88] The first-in-class histamine-3-receptor inverse agonist pitolisant has recently been approved for the treatment of EDS in narcolepsy by the French and European drug authorities.[89,90] Furthermore, preclinical data indicated that histamine 3 antagonists might alleviate depressive symptoms via a hippocampal-dependent mechanism.[91] Its good benefit-risk ratio provides a promising potential therapy for patients with hypersomnolence and depressive disorders.[72]

SUMMARY

Despite a high frequency of depressive symptoms in central hypersomnia, the formal diagnosis of a major depressive episode requires a structured evaluation to avoid frequent clinical overlap between the 2 conditions. Furthermore, no evidence supports that patients with both major depression and hypersomnolence complaints had abnormal increased daytime sleep propensity or total sleep duration. The complaint of EDS and prolonged nocturnal sleep time seem related to other symptoms, such as apathy, decreased energy, or psychomotor slowdown inherent of the depressive state, rather than an objective hypersomnolence. Clinicians should be aware of practical considerations when treating hypersomnolence in mood disorders and depression in central hypersomnias. The optimal assessment and management of both depressive symptoms in central hypersomnias and hypersomnolence in depressive disorders require a close collaboration between sleep specialists and psychiatrists.

REFERENCES

1. Dauvilliers Y, Lopez R, Lecendreux M. French consensus. Hypersomnolence: evaluation and diagnosis. Rev Neurol (Paris) 2017;173(1):19–24.
2. American Psychiatric Association. The diagnostic and statistical manual of mental disorders. 5th edition. Arlington (VA): APA; 2013 (DSM-5).
3. American Academy of Sleep Medicine. International classification of sleep disorders. 3rd edition. Darien (IL): AASM Resource Library; 2014 (ICSD-3).
4. Trotti L. Waking up is the hardest thing I do all day: sleep inertia and sleep drunkenness. Sleep Med Rev 2016. http://dx.doi.org/10.1016/j.smrv.2016.08.005.
5. Ohayon MM, Reynolds CF, Dauvilliers Y. Excessive sleep duration and quality of life. Ann Neurol 2013; 73(6):785–94.
6. Ohayon MM, Dauvilliers Y, Reynolds CF. Operational definitions and algorithms for excessive sleepiness in the general population: implications for DSM-5 nosology. Arch Gen Psychiatry 2012;69(1):71–9.
7. Cappuccio FP, Cooper D, D'Elia L, et al. Sleep duration predicts cardiovascular outcomes: a systematic review and meta-analysis of prospective studies. Eur Heart J 2011;32(12):1484–92.
8. Heslop P, Smith GD, Metcalfe C, et al. Sleep duration and mortality: the effect of short or long sleep duration on cardiovascular and all-cause mortality in working men and women. Sleep Med 2002;3(4):305–14.
9. Liu T, Xu C, Rota M, et al. Sleep duration and risk of all-cause mortality: a flexible, non-linear, meta-regression of 40 prospective cohort studies. Sleep Med Rev 2017;32:28–36.
10. Dauvilliers Y, Arnulf I, Mignot E. Narcolepsy with cataplexy. Lancet 2007;369(9560):499–511.
11. Scammell TE. Narcolepsy. N Engl J Med 2015; 373(27):2654–62.
12. Baumann CR, Mignot E, Lammers GJ, et al. Challenges in diagnosing narcolepsy without cataplexy: a consensus statement. Sleep 2014;37(6):1035–42.
13. Billiard M, Sonka K. Idiopathic hypersomnia. Sleep Med Rev 2016;29:23–33.
14. Beck AT, Ward CH, Mendelson M, et al. An inventory for measuring depression. Arch Gen Psychiatry 1961;4:561–71.
15. Fortuyn HD, Lappenschaar MA, Furer JW, et al. Anxiety and mood disorders in narcolepsy: a case–control study. Gen Hosp Psychiatry 2010; 32(1):49–56.
16. Ohayon MM. Narcolepsy is complicated by high medical and psychiatric comorbidities: a comparison with the general population. Sleep Med 2013; 14(6):488–92.
17. Lecendreux M, Lavault S, Lopez R, et al. Attention-deficit/hyperactivity disorder (ADHD) symptoms in pediatric narcolepsy: a cross-sectional study. Sleep 2015;38(8):1285–95.
18. van Holst RJ, van der Cruijsen L, van Mierlo P, et al. Aberrant food choices after satiation in human orexin-deficient narcolepsy type 1. Sleep 2016; 39(11):1951–9.
19. Dauvilliers Y, Gaig C, Barateau L, et al. Absence of NMDA receptor antibodies in the rare association between type 1 narcolepsy and psychosis. Sci Rep 2016;6:25230.
20. Roy A. Psychiatric aspects of narcolepsy. Br J Psychiatry 1976;128(6):562–5.
21. Scott MM, Marcus JN, Pettersen A, et al. Hcrtr1 and 2 signaling differentially regulates depression-like behaviors. Behav Brain Res 2011;222(2):289–94.
22. Kales A, Soldatos CR, Bixler EO, et al. Narcolepsy-cataplexy: II. Psychosocial consequences and associated psychopathology. Arch Neurol 1982; 39(3):169–71.

23. Krishnan RR, Volow MR, Miller PP, et al. Narcolepsy: preliminary retrospective study of psychiatric and psychosocial aspects. Am J Psychiatry 1984; 141(3):428–31.

24. Mosko S, Zetin M, Glen S, et al. Self-reported depressive symptomatology, mood ratings, and treatment outcome in sleep disorders patients. J Clin Psychol 1989;45(1):51–60.

25. Vignatelli L, D'Alessandro R, Mosconi P, et al. Health-related quality of life in Italian patients with narcolepsy: the SF-36 health survey. Sleep Med 2004;5(5):467–75.

26. Dodel R, Peter H, Spottke A, et al. Health-related quality of life in patients with narcolepsy. Sleep Med 2007;8(7):733–41.

27. Vignatelli L, Plazzi G, Peschechera F, et al. A 5-year prospective cohort study on health-related quality of life in patients with narcolepsy. Sleep Med 2011; 12(1):19–23.

28. Dauvilliers Y, Paquereau J, Bastuji H, et al. Psychological health in central hypersomnias: the French Harmony Study. J Neurol Neurosurg Psychiatry 2009;80(6):636–41.

29. Billiard M, Partinen M, Roth T, et al. Sleep and psychiatric disorders. J Psychosom Res 1994; 38(Suppl 1):1–2.

30. Dolenc L, Besset A, Billiard M. Hypersomnia in association with dysthymia in comparison with idiopathic hypersomnia and normal controls. Pflugers Arch 1996;431:R303–4.

31. Roth B, Nevsimalova S. Depresssion in narcolepsy and hypersommia. Schweiz Arch Neurol Neurochir Psychiatr 1974;116(2):291–300.

32. Pizza F, Jaussent I, Lopez R, et al. Car crashes and central disorders of hypersomnolence: a French study. PLoS One 2015;10(6):e0129386.

33. Sakurai T. The neural circuit of orexin (hypocretin): maintaining sleep and wakefulness. Nat Rev Neurosci 2007;8(3):171–81.

34. Billiard M, Bassetti C, Dauvilliers Y, et al. EFNS guidelines on management of narcolepsy. Eur J Neurol 2006;13(10):1035–48.

35. Thorpy MJ, Dauvilliers Y. Clinical and practical considerations in the pharmacologic management of narcolepsy. Sleep Med 2015;16(1):9–18.

36. Lopez R, Dauvilliers Y. Pharmacotherapy options for cataplexy. Expert Opin Pharmacother 2013;14(7): 895–903.

37. Ortega-Albás JJ, López-Bernabé R, García ALS, et al. Suicidal ideation secondary to sodium oxybate. J Neuropsychiatry Clin Neurosci 2010;22(3). 352r.e26–352.e26.

38. Rossetti AO, Heinzer RC, Tafti M, et al. Rapid occurrence of depression following addition of sodium oxybate to modafinil. Sleep Med 2010;11(5):500–1.

39. Barateau L, Lopez R, Dauvilliers Y. Treatment options for narcolepsy. CNS Drugs 2016;30(5):369–79.

40. Johns M. A new method for measuring daytime sleepiness: the Epworth Sleepiness Scale. Sleep 1991;14(6):540–5.

41. Kaida K, Takahashi M, Akerstedt T, et al. Validation of the Karolinska sleepiness scale against performance and EEG variables. Clin Neurophysiol 2006; 117(7):1574–81.

42. Hoddes E, Zarcone V, Dement W. Development and use of Stanford Sleepiness Scale (SSS). Psychophysiology. New York: Cambridge Univ Press; 1972. p. 150.

43. Kanady JC, Harvey AG. Development and validation of the Sleep Inertia Questionnaire (SIQ) and assessment of sleep inertia in analogue and clinical depression. Cognit Ther Res 2015;39(5):601–12.

44. Martin JL, Hakim A. Wrist actigraphy. Chest 2011; 139(6):1514–27.

45. Ancoli-Israel S, Cole R, Alessi C, et al. The role of actigraphy in the study of sleep and circadian rhythms. Sleep 2003;26(3):342–92.

46. Vernet C, Arnulf I. Idiopathic hypersomnia with and without long sleep time: a controlled series of 75 patients. Sleep 2009;32(6):753–9.

47. Carskadon MA, Dement WC, Mitler MM, et al. Guidelines for the multiple sleep latency test (MSLT): a standard measure of sleepiness. Sleep 1986;9(4):519–24.

48. Littner M, Kushida C, Wise M, et al. Practice parameters for clinical use of the multiple sleep latency test and the maintenance of wakefulness test. Sleep 2005;28(1):113–21.

49. Mitler MM, Gujavarty KS, Browman CP. Maintenance of wakefulness test: a polysomnographic technique for evaluating treatment efficacy in patients with excessive somnolence. Electroencephalogr Clin Neurophysiol 1982;53(6):658–61.

50. Bastuji H, Perrin F, Garcia-Larrea L. Event-related potentials during forced awakening: a tool for the study of acute sleep inertia. J Sleep Res 2003; 12(3):189–206.

51. Peter-Derex L, Perrin F, Petitjean T, et al. Discriminating neurological from psychiatric hypersomnia using the forced awakening test. Neurophysiol Clin 2013;43(3):171–9.

52. Kaplan KA, Harvey AG. Hypersomnia across mood disorders: a review and synthesis. Sleep Med Rev 2009;13(4):275–85.

53. Akiskal HS, Benazzi F. Atypical depression: a variant of bipolar II or a bridge between unipolar and bipolar II? J Affect Disord 2005;84(2):209–17.

54. van Mill JG, Hoogendijk WJG, Vogelzangs N, et al. Insomnia and sleep duration in a large cohort of patients with major depressive disorder and anxiety disorders. J Clin Psychiatry 2010;71(3):239.

55. Plante DT. Sleep propensity in psychiatric hypersomnolence: a systematic review and meta-analysis of multiple sleep latency test findings. Sleep Med Rev 2017;31:48–57.

56. Billiard M, Dolenc L, Aldaz C, et al. Hypersomnia associated with mood disorders: a new perspective. J Psychosom Res 1994;38:41–7.

57. Detre T, Himmelhoch J, Swartzburg M, et al. Hypersomnia and manic-depressive disease. Am J Psychiatry 1972;128(10):1303–5.

58. Casper RC, Redmond DE, Katz MM, et al. Somatic symptoms in primary affective disorder: presence and relationship to the classification of depression. Arch Gen Psychiatry 1985;42(11):1098–104.

59. Nofzinger EA, Thase ME, Reynolds CF, et al. Hypersomnia in bipolar depression: a comparison with narcolepsy using the multiple sleep latency test. Am J Psychiatry 1991;148(9):1177–81.

60. Millar A, Espie CA, Scott J. The sleep of remitted bipolar outpatients: a controlled naturalistic study using actigraphy. J Affect Disord 2004;80(2): 145–53.

61. Geoffroy PA, Scott J, Boudebesse C, et al. Sleep in patients with remitted bipolar disorders: a meta-analysis of actigraphy studies. Acta Psychiatr Scand 2015;131(2):89–99.

62. Kaplan KA, McGlinchey EL, Soehner A, et al. Hypersomnia subtypes, sleep and relapse in bipolar disorder. Psychol Med 2015;45(08):1751–63.

63. Kaplan KA, Gruber J, Eidelman P, et al. Hypersomnia in inter-episode bipolar disorder: does it have prognostic significance? J Affect Disord 2011; 132(3):438–44.

64. Terman M, Amira L, Terman JD, et al. Predictors of response and nonresponse to light treatment for winter depression. Am J Psychiatry 1996;153(11): 1423.

65. Sadovnick AD. Depressive symptoms and family history in seasonal and nonseasonal mood disorders. Am J Psychiatry 1993;150:443–8.

66. Winkler D, Willeit M, Praschak-Rieder N, et al. Changes of clinical pattern in seasonal affective disorder (SAD) over time in a German-speaking sample. Eur Arch Psychiatry Clin Neurosci 2002; 252(2):54–62.

67. Staner L. Comorbidity of insomnia and depression. Sleep Med Rev 2010;14(1):35–46.

68. Rao U, Hammen CL, Poland RE. Risk markers for depression in adolescents: sleep and HPA measures. Neuropsychopharmacology 2009;34(8):1936–45.

69. Netzer NC, Stoohs RA, Netzer CM, et al. Using the Berlin questionnaire to identify patients at risk for the sleep apnea syndrome. Ann Intern Med 1999; 131(7):485–91.

70. Chung F, Yegneswaran B, Liao P, et al. STOP questionnaire: a tool to screen patients for obstructive sleep apnea. Anesthesiology 2008;108(5):812–21.

71. Heinzer R, Vat S, Marques-Vidal P, et al. Prevalence of sleep-disordered breathing in the general population: the HypnoLaus study. Lancet Respir Med 2015; 3(4):310–8.

72. Stubbs B, Vancampfort D, Veronese N, et al. The prevalence and predictors of obstructive sleep apnea in major depressive disorder, bipolar disorder and schizophrenia: a systematic review and meta-analysis. J Affect Disord 2016;197:259–67.

73. Plante DT, Winkelman JW. Sleep disturbance in bipolar disorder: therapeutic implications. Am J Psychiatry 2008;165(7):830–43.

74. Rishi MA, Shetty M, Wolff A, et al. Atypical antipsychotic medications are independently associated with severe obstructive sleep apnea. Clin Neuropharmacol 2010;33(3):109–13.

75. Geoffroy P, Boudebesse C, Bellivier F, et al. Sleep in remitted bipolar disorder: a naturalistic case-control study using actigraphy. J Affect Disord 2014;158:1–7.

76. Lack LC, Wright HR, Bootzin RR. Delayed sleep-phase disorder. Sleep Med Clin 2009;4(2):229–39.

77. Melo MC, Abreu RL, Neto VB, et al. Chronotype and circadian rhythm in bipolar disorder: a systematic review. Sleep Med Rev 2016. http://dx.doi.org/10.1016/j.smrv.2016.06.007.

78. Avery DH, Dahl K, Savage MV, et al. Circadian temperature and cortisol rhythms during a constant routine are phase-delayed in hypersomnic winter depression. Biol Psychiatry 1997;41(11):1109–23.

79. Avery DH, Kouri ME, Monaghan K, et al. Is dawn simulation effective in ameliorating the difficulty awakening in seasonal affective disorder associated with hypersomnia? J Affect Disord 2002;69(1):231–6.

80. Gold PW, Licinio J, Wong M, et al. Corticotropin releasing hormone in the pathophysiology of melancholic and atypical depression and in the mechanism of action of antidepressant drugs. Ann N Y Acad Sci 1995;771(1):716–29.

81. Worthington J, Fava M, Davidson K, et al. Patterns of improvement in depressive symptoms with fluoxetine treatment. Psychopharmacol Bull 1995;31(2):223–6.

82. Geoffroy PA, Etain B, Micoulaud Franchi J, et al. Melatonin and melatonin agonists as adjunctive treatments in bipolar disorders. Curr Pharm Des 2015;21(23):3352–8.

83. Danilenko KV, Ivanova IA. Dawn simulation vs. bright light in seasonal affective disorder: treatment effects and subjective preference. J Affect Disord 2015; 180:87–9.

84. Leu-Semenescu S, Quera-Salva MA, Dauvilliers Y. French consensus. Idiopathic hypersomnia: investigations and follow-up. Rev Neurol (Paris) 2017; 173(1):32–7.

85. Monaca C, Franco P, Philip P, et al. French consensus. Type 1 and type 2 narcolepsy: investigations and follow-up. Rev Neurol (Paris) 2017;173(1):25–31.

86. Calabrese JR, Ketter TA, Youakim JM, et al. Adjunctive armodafinil for major depressive episodes associated with bipolar I disorder: a randomized, multicenter, double-blind, placebo-controlled,

proof-of-concept study. J Clin Psychiatry 2010; 71(10):1363–70.

87. Frye MA, Grunze H, Suppes T, et al. A placebo-controlled evaluation of adjunctive modafinil in the treatment of bipolar depression. Am J Psychiatry 2007;164(8):1242–9.

88. Auger RR, Goodman SH, Silber MH, et al. Risks of high-dose stimulants in the treatment of disorders of excessive somnolence: a case-control study. Sleep 2005;28(6):667–72.

89. Dauvilliers Y, Bassetti C, Lammers GJ, et al. Pitolisant versus placebo or modafinil in patients with narcolepsy: a double-blind, randomised trial. Lancet Neurol 2013;12(11):1068–75.

90. Szakacs Z, Dauvilliers Y, Mikhaylov V, et al. Safety and efficacy of pitolisant on cataplexy in patients with narcolepsy: a randomised, double-blind, placebo-controlled trial. Lancet Neurol 2017;16(3): 200–7.

91. Femenía T, Magara S, DuPont CM, et al. Hippocampal-dependent antidepressant action of the H3 receptor antagonist clobenpropit in a rat model of depression. Int J Neuropsychopharmacol 2015; 18(9) [pii:pyv032].

Sleepiness in Children
An Update

Gustavo Antonio Moreira, MD, PhD[a,b,*], Marcia Pradella-Hallinan, MD, PhD[a]

KEYWORDS

- Sleepiness • Daytime somnolence • Children • Narcolepsy • Obstructive sleep apnea
- Sleep deprivation

KEY POINTS

- Sleepiness in children has increased in the last decades as a consequences of sleep habits changes and diminished sleep duration.
- Chronic pain, movement disorder, and sleep-disordered breathing in children impair sleep quality and predispose to daytime sleepiness.
- Many questionnaire have been validated to evaluate sleep problems in children and are an important tools to evaluate subjective sleepiness.
- Children with central hypersomnia or circadian rhythm disorders have significant daytime problems and impairment of daytime functioning.

Sleep is essential for children's learning, memory processes, school performance, and general well-being.[1] Sleep deprivation and fragmented sleep are the main mechanism that leads to daytime sleepiness in children.[2] Evaluation of sleepiness in this age group is quite challenging owing to the age-dependent maturation of the central nervous system. As age progresses, time spent sleeping is reduced and the polyphasic sleep pattern of preschool children matures to an exclusive nocturnal monophasic sleep in older children. This may, in part, explain why the evaluation of sleepiness in children is taxing. Many tools have been developed to evaluate sleep in a pediatric age group, however, a limited number of questionnaires have been fully validated to comprehend sleepiness in children.[3]

PREVALENCE OF SLEEPINESS IN CHILDREN

A survey of 1413 Swedish children aged 6 to 11 years highlighted a prevalence of 4% prevalence rate of daytime sleepiness. In this age group, there were no differences between boys and girls. A Korean study validated the School Sleep Habits Survey for a sample of 1457 schoolchildren aged 9 to 19 years. They found that 6.6% of the respondents admitted to daytime sleepiness being a major problem. As grade levels increased from the 5th to 12th grade, so did the prevalence of daytime sleepiness. Sleep duration decreased by approximately 3 hours on school nights from grades 5 to 12. The authors noted that sleepiness was slightly more prevalent in girls than boys. The increasing prevalence of daytime sleepiness with advancing grade level in children and adolescents is further corroborated by other studies.[4,5] In a study of 535 Brazilian adolescents, daytime sleepiness increased from 10 to 17 years of age. Students from private schools had higher sleepiness scores than students from public schools. More than 2 hours of sleep debt, measured as the difference of the mean sleep duration between school night and weekend nights, was present in 39% of these adolescents.[4]

Disclosure Statement: The authors have nothing to disclose.
[a] Department of Psychobiology, Universidade Federal de São Paulo, Rua Napoleão de Barros, 925, São Paulo, São Paulo 04024-002, Brazil; [b] Department of Pediatrics, Universidade Federal de São Paulo, Rua Botucatu, 598, São Paulo, São Paulo 04023-062, Brazil.
* Corresponding author. Rua Napoleão de Barros, 925, São Paulo, São Paulo 04024-002, Brazil.
E-mail address: gustavo_a_moreira@hotmail.com

Sleep Med Clin 12 (2017) 407–413
http://dx.doi.org/10.1016/j.jsmc.2017.03.013
1556-407X/17/© 2017 Elsevier Inc. All rights reserved.

EFFECTS OF SLEEP DEPRIVATION

In the last few decades, the time adults, adolescents and children have spent sleeping has decreased. This change in habits is mainly owing to the overwhelming use of electricity. Currently, artificial light and electronic gadgets have invaded the lives of humans, day and night. Many studies have showed that increases in screen time have reduced the duration of sleep in children.[6] It is not surprising that these reductions of sleep duration have daytime consequences, such as sleepiness, behavior problems, cognitive deficits, poor school performance, inflammation, and metabolic dysfunction.[1,2,7–9] A recent systematic review demonstrated a consistent correlation of screen time with reduced sleep duration.[6] The authors suggested that the reduction in sleep time can be associated with biological, psychological, and environmental factors. The 2013 International Sleep Poll reported that 7% to 21% of adults in the United States, Germany, the United Kingdom, Canada, Mexico, and Japan sleep fewer than 6 hours per night on work days.[10] The 2011 Sleep in America Poll reported that about 60% of adolescents in the United States receive less than 8 hours of sleep on school nights. In the same report, 90% of 13 to 18 years olds had at least 1 electronic device (TV, laptop, cell phone, tablet, video game, and/or music player) in their bedroom.[11] With the ubiquitous presence of media items in a child's or an adolescent's bedroom, screen time is hypothesized to be a cause of insufficient and low-quality sleep, operating through several mechanisms. The first is time displacement. With more time spent in front of screens, less time is naturally available for sleep. Second, psychological and physiologic arousals owing to the content of the media and social interaction may also interfere with the ability to fall and stay asleep. Finally, there is the effect of light on both circadian rhythm and general alertness. The effect in the circadian rhythm is mainly owing to light suppression of melatonin secretion.[6]

Recent reviews have shown that sleep quantity and quality in children correlates with levels of daytime sleepiness.[12–14] Sleep quality and sleep duration may be seen as 2 separate sleep domains. Although these sleep domains overlap to some extent, qualitative differences do exist between them. Sleep quality refers to the subjective indices of how sleep is experienced, including the feeling of feeling rested when waking up and experiencing satisfaction with sleep. Sleep duration, on the other hand, is a more objective sleep domain, namely, the actual time during which the individual is asleep. Correlations between children and adolescents' sleep duration and sleep quality are low or not significant, supporting the idea that sleep quality and sleep duration represent 2 separate sleep domains. In fact, the strength of association of sleep quantity and sleep duration with sleepiness may vary by student age and sex; 1 recent metaanalysis of sleep and school functioning reported that studies of younger children, particularly those that enrolled more boys, tended to show the greatest effects.[14]

Poor sleep quality owing to pain,[15] periodic limb movement,[16] and sleep-disordered breathing[17] may also lead to sleepiness in children.[18] Obstructive sleep apnea (OSA) is a sleep disorder characterized by repetitive upper airway obstruction during sleep, leading to hypoxemia, hypercapnia, fragmented sleep, and daytime symptoms.[17] Although daytime somnolence in children with OSA is not as significant as when seen in adults,[19] studies have shown that OSA in children aged 5 to 12 years has been linked to poor classroom grades, sleepiness, inattention, hyperactivity, oppositional behavior, and mood deregulation.[20] Further evidence that links pediatric OSA and sleepiness is the fact that treatment with adenotonsillectomy[21,22] or positive airway pressure[23] improves daytime behavior, sleepiness, and quality of life. Restless leg syndrome and period limb movements disorder may also lead to sleep fragmentation and, consequently, daytime dysfunction. Cross-sectional studies have shown associations of restless leg syndrome and period limb movements disorder with hyperactivity, impulsivity, attention, and daytime sleepiness.[16,24,25] Currently, there is no evidence that intervention for movement disorders in children may improve these symptoms.

ASSESSMENT OF SLEEPINESS

There are a few tools for the assessment of sleep duration and sleepiness in children. Approximately 57 pediatric sleep questionnaires were developed to evaluate sleep problems in children and/or adolescents. Only a few underwent a thorough validation process.[3] The questionnaires evaluate sleep environment and settling down periods, sleep behavior, sleep habits, circadian typology, emotional well-being, scholastic achievement, and sleepiness. Assessment of sleepiness represented whole or part of the questionnaires (**Table 1**). These tools look to age differences in sleep patterns, split into infants, preschoolers, school-age children, and adolescents. The age range varies from 2 to 18 years, although most of them focus on adolescents. The Epworth Sleepiness Scale, a well-known scale used in adults, was modified in 2 items to be more applicable to

Table 1
Subjective tools for evaluation sleepiness in children and adolescents

	Scale	Age Range (y)	Questions Concerning Sleepiness
Bruni et al,[26] 1996	Sleep Disturbances Scale for Children	6.5–15.3	5/26
Chervin et al,[28] 2000	Pediatric Sleep Questionnaire	2–18	4/22
Luginbuehl et al,[27] 2008	Sleep Disorder Inventory for Children (child version)	2–10	3/25
Luginbuehl et al,[27] 2008	Sleep Disorder Inventory for Children (adolescent version)	11–18	5/25
Melendres et al,[18] 2004	Modified Epworth Sleepiness Scale	2–16	8/8
Spilsbury et al,[29] 2007	Cleveland Adolescent Sleepiness Questionnaire	11–17	16/16
Drake et al,[13] 2003	Pediatric Daytime Sleepiness Scale	11–15	8/8

children. Although the modified Epworth Sleepiness Scale scores were statistically higher in children with OSA than in controls, the scale fails to demonstrate differences between patients with primary snoring and OSA.[18] The Pediatric Daytime Sleepiness Scale is a self-report scale developed for children and adolescents aged 11 to 18 years. Eight questions on a 5-step Likert scale were selected from an initial 32 questions, based on factor analysis and internal consistency. Pediatric daytime sleepiness scores was higher in children and adolescents who reported low school achievement, high rates of absenteeism, low school enjoyment, low total sleep time, and frequent illness.[13] Three well-validated and common questionnaires for sleep problems in a wide pediatric age range highlighted many aspects of sleep problems, and some of these questions evaluate sleepiness.[26–28] The Pediatric Sleep Questionnaire and the Modified Epworth Sleepiness Scale had recently shown, in a randomized, controlled trial, statistically significant improvement in sleepiness scores after adenotonsillectomy.[30]

Objective evaluation of sleepiness using the Multiple Sleep Latency Test (MSLT) can be performed in children older than 5 years. MSLT measures the speed of falling asleep. A faster sleep onset indicates a greater level of sleepiness.[31,32] During an MSLT, subjects are asked to fall asleep while lying in bed in a dark and quiet room during five 20-minute periods spaced at 2-hour intervals. If sleep occurs during this time period, it is allowed for only 15 minutes. If no sleep occurs, lights are turned on after the 20-minute test and the subject has to get out of bed and stay awake until the next testing period. A nocturnal polysomnography is recommended to rule out other sleep disorders

and ensure that the child is not sleep deprived. Prepubertal children are less likely to fall asleep during the MSLT than older adolescents, suggesting that the standard protocol may underestimate mild degrees of sleepiness.[33,34] To address this concern, some researchers have modified the standard protocol by using 30-minute nap opportunities instead of 20 minutes.[19,35] In children with suspected sleep-disordered breathing, they demonstrated that daytime sleepiness is associated with the degree of obesity, severity of OSA, and tumor necrosis factor-α levels.[19,35] Adenotonsillectomy improves the degree of sleepiness measured with MSLT and tumor necrosis factor-α levels.[35,36] MSLT, preceded by nocturnal polysomnography, is indicated in children as a part of the evaluation for suspected narcolepsy. The American Academy of Sleep Medicine stated that there is sufficient evidence to use MSLT diagnose narcolepsy in children older than 5 years, and report it as a standard recommendation.[32]

Additional studies when daytime sleepiness and decrease of alertness in children or adolescents become a serious concern are recommended. Below, we refer to the more frequently discussed conditions associated with daytime sleepiness for these age groups.

NARCOLEPSY

Narcolepsy is a disorder of central origin characterized by recurrent attacks of irresistible daytime sleepiness. The characteristic picture of narcolepsy encompasses a tetrad of symptoms that includes excessive daytime sleepiness, sleep paralysis, hypnagogic/hypnopompic hallucinations, and cataplexy; fragmented nocturnal sleep tends also to occur. The prevalence of narcolepsy is

0.02% in the world general population. About 30% of narcoleptic patients exhibit its initial symptoms during childhood and in 16% of these cases, narcolepsy begins before the age of 10 years. Narcolepsy is probably underestimated because of the high rate of misdiagnosis. The incidence is approximately 1.37 per 100,000 person-years.[37–40]

The disease affects both males and females and the etiopathogenesis remains unknown. Recently, the involvements of the hypocretin-1 and hypocretin-2 pathways have shed new light on the disorder. These neurotransmitters produce exclusively from the lateral hypothalamus, playing a major role in wakefulness and REM sleep physiology.[37,39] The revised *International Classification of Sleep Disorders, 3rd edition* (ICSD-3) divides the disease into narcolepsy type 1 (N1), which is characterized by excessive daytime sleepiness and cataplexy associated with hypocretin-1 deficiency. The close association with HLA DQB10602 haplotype together with the role of environmental triggers such as H1N1 influenza virus infection or vaccination, streptococcus β-hemolyticus infection, and low or undetectable hypocretin-1 levels in the cerebrospinal fluid support the hypothesis of an autoimmune etiology.[37,38,41,42]

Children with N1 may present with a peculiar cataplexy phenotype, characterized by persistent hypotonia with prominent facial involvement known as cataplectic facies and by hyperkinetic movements that occurs associated to emotional or strong stimulation by sounds, fright, or tickling. This pediatric phenotype progressively changes to the adult phenotype of cataplexy, with muscle weakness evoked by emotions. Frequently, childhood also shows behavioral abnormalities and psychiatric disorders, encompassing depressive feelings, hyperactive or aggressive behavior, and even psychotic features. The association with obesity and precocious puberty strikingly suggests that N1 arising in prepubertal children may reflect a wide hypothalamic dysfunction probably owing to hypocretin neuronal loss. Children with N1 phenotypes need specific evaluation and management, especially regarding behavioral and metabolic features. N1 is indeed a lifelong disorder with a devastating impact on quality of life, especially when arising at a developmental age. Targeted school programs, and juridical and psychological supports are all essential for patients and families.[38,39]

Diagnostic criteria are based on clinical, nocturnal polysomnography, and MSLT findings that are specific for children.[43] Narcolepsy type 2 is characterized by excessive daytime sleepiness without cataplexy and hypocretin deficiency, and is diagnosed based on patients' complaints and polysomnographic evidence in the absence of other causes of daytime sleepiness.[41]

The secondary or symptomatic form of narcolepsy is owing to a medical condition. This includes brain tumors, brain trauma, some diseases such as sarcoidosis, Niemann–Pick type C, demyelinating disorders, and stroke resulting in damage to the hypocretin pathways.[37–39,43]

IDIOPATHIC HYPERSOMNIA WITH OR WITHOUT PROLONGED SLEEP TIME

The condition is characterized by excessive daytime sleepiness that extends over several months. Nocturnal sleep may have prolonged duration (12–14 hours) or be in the normal range. Diurnal naps generally are prolonged (3–4 hours) but unrefreshing. After a sleep period, it is not infrequent that children present with confusion on awakening and sleep drunkenness, associated with automatic and complex behavior. Microsleeps (1–4 seconds) may be recorded during the day.[44] The prevalence is however not well established. It may begin in the midteens and seems to be more common in women than in men. Polysomnography and MSLT recordings show short sleep latency with increased or normal total sleep time. Sleep architecture is normal but it may have an increase in NREM stage 3 in the second half of the night. Daytime sleep shows mainly NREM episodes and the latency is always less than 10 minutes.[45,46]

The most important consequences are poor academic performance. Treatment consists of the use of stimulants and, more recently, L-carnitine alone or in association with stimulants was introduced and seems to have beneficial effect.[46,47] When off medication, children with excessive daytime sleepiness were more likely to get hit or nearly hit by traffic than a group of children matched by age, sex, race, and household income.[48]

RECURRENT HYPERSOMNIAS
Klein-Levin Syndrome

Klein-Levin syndrome is characterized by recurrent episodes of hypersomnolence that are frequently associated with hyperphagia and hypersexual behaviors. The episodes may last 1 or 2 days or several weeks and are characterized by spending an overly long time in bed (16–18 hours). During this period, the patient sometimes can get up, eat, and go to the restroom. A change in personality, behavior, and psychological mood is frequently seen and also a stuporous appearance can be noticed.[49,50]

It is a rare condition, 3 times more frequent in males than females and starts during adolescence. The pathophysiology is not conclusive, but some studies highlighted diffuse brain hypoperfusion (more pronounced in the thalamic and frontotemporal areas), viral and autoimmune causative factors based on the frequent report of flulike symptoms at onset. The most frequent precipitating factor (70%) is the presence of inflammatory lesions in the thalamus, diencephalon, and midbrain on postmortem neuropathology, suggesting a viral infection, increased frequency of the human leukocyte antigen DQB1*0201 allele, and, in a few cases, abnormalities in serotonin and dopamine metabolism, suggesting a neurotransmitter imbalance in the serotonergic or dopaminergic pathway. There are also some patients who started with somnolence after a head trauma.[49,50] Polysomnography and MSLT are not required for diagnostic reasons. There is no treatment consensus. Lithium may be beneficial to reduce relapses, and modafinil may reduce duration of episodes. Recently, clarithromycin was also suggested as a treatment, but the effectiveness of this drug needs to be studied in more patients.[51]

Menstrual-Related Hypersomnia

There is an association of hypersomnolence periods with menstruation. Patients experienced longer sleep nocturnal duration and daytime sleepiness. Polysomnography shows shortened sleep latency and normal architecture. A good response with anovulatory agents reinforces the suspicion of a hormonal origin of the condition.[52,53]

Hypersomnia Associated with Behaviorally Induced Insufficient Sleep

Sleep deprivation in children and adolescents is considered a health concern. In the last century, children decreased sleep duration and now they are sleeping about 1 hour less compared with 100 years ago.[11,54] Studies with sleep deprivation have shown the importance and necessity of having adequate sleep quality and duration.[2] For children, it is believed, and easily seen in clinical practice, that sleep influences physical growth, emotional stability, behavior, and cognitive function, including memory consolidation. Studies have shown that insufficient sleep is associated with fatigue, attention problems, learning difficulties, impulse control, and organizational skills poverty. In children and adolescents, short sleep is associated with overweight and obesity, higher caloric intake derived from fat and lower caloric intake from carbohydrates, and insulin resistance.[55,56]

The medical literature from the last 50 years shows that concepts of modernity have been associated with overstimulation that predisposes children not getting the sleep that they need. Recently, the influence of electronic media including video games, cell phones, and the Internet were implicated in increased night-time activity and affected sleep patterns of not only in adults, but also in children and adolescents. Strategies to reduce sleep deprivation are necessary to prevent damages during developmental ages and to promote a better quality of sleep for all.[4,55,56]

Hypersomnia Associated with Circadian Rhythm Disorder

Delayed sleep phase syndrome is a circadian rhythm disorder characterized by a constitutional inability to anticipate sleep and a tendency to fall asleep at progressively later times at night. Because sleep-onset time is often as late as 1 to 3 AM, children and adolescents with this disorder are often sleep deprived on school nights and are consequently sleepy during the daytime.[57] Although delayed sleep phase syndrome has its peak incidence during adolescence, many children already have symptoms in prepubertal years. If allowed to sleep uninterrupted, as happens on weekends or holidays, the individual may sleep until noon and feel refreshed. There is no qualitative or quantitative abnormality in sleep. Sleep onset and offset are simply at socially inappropriate times and lead to daytime sleepiness when the patient has to conform to the societal norms for attending school or work. Complaints of difficulty of sleeping early at night are viewed as insomnia. In the morning, patients manifest chronic hypersomnia. Being late or absent to school becomes a serious problem. Delayed sleep phase syndrome is related to a dysfunction of the suprachiasmatic nucleus, which is our circadian timekeeper. Patients show a delay in the timing of release of melatonin (a sleep-inducing hormone), and in reaching the nadir of the core body temperature, which corresponds with the time that a person is likely to be most sleepy.[58] Delayed sleep phase syndrome may be associated with certain polymorphisms in the PER3 circadian gene.[59] Treatment consists of keeping a rigid morning wake up time 7 days a week, early exposure to bright sunlight for 30 minutes immediately on awakening in the morning, and oral melatonin before the desired bedtime.[60]

REFERENCES

1. Beebe DW. Cognitive, behavioral, and functional consequences of inadequate sleep in children

and adolescents. Pediatr Clin North Am 2011; 58(3):649–65.

2. Beebe DW, Rose D, Amin R. Attention, learning, and arousal of experimentally sleep-restricted adolescents in a simulated classroom. J Adolesc Health 2010;47(5):523–5.

3. Spruyt K, Gozal D. Pediatric sleep questionnaires as diagnostic or epidemiological tools: a review of currently available instruments. Sleep Med Rev 2011;15(1):19–32.

4. de Souza Vilela T, Bittencourt LR, Tufik S, et al. Factors influencing excessive daytime sleepiness in adolescents. J Pediatr (Rio J) 2016;92(2):149–55.

5. Ohayon MM, Roberts RE, Zulley J, et al. Prevalence and patterns of problematic sleep among older adolescents. J Am Acad Child Adolesc Psychiatry 2000;39(12):1549–56.

6. Hale L, Guan S. Screen time and sleep among school-aged children and adolescents: a systematic literature review. Sleep Med Rev 2015;21:50–8.

7. Magee L, Hale L. Longitudinal associations between sleep duration and subsequent weight gain: a systematic review. Sleep Med Rev 2012; 16(3):231–41.

8. Koren D, O'Sullivan KL, Mokhlesi B. Metabolic and glycemic sequelae of sleep disturbances in children and adults. Curr Diab Rep 2015;15(1):562.

9. Kim J, Hakim F, Kheirandish-Gozal L, et al. Inflammatory pathways in children with insufficient or disordered sleep. Respir Physiol Neurobiol 2011; 178(3):465–74.

10. 2013 International bedroom poll. National Sleep Foundation. Available at: https://sleepfoundation.org/sites/default/files/RPT495a.pdf. Accessed September 03, 2013.

11. 2011 Sleep in America poll. National Sleep Foundation. Available at: http://sleepfoundation.org/sites/default/files/sleepinamericapoll/SIAP_2011_Summary_of_Findings.pdf. Accessed March 11, 2011.

12. Dewald JF, Meijer AM, Oort FJ, et al. The influence of sleep quality, sleep duration and sleepiness on school performance in children and adolescents: a meta-analytic review. Sleep Med Rev 2010;14(3): 179–89.

13. Drake C, Nickel C, Burduvali E, et al. The pediatric daytime sleepiness scale (PDSS): sleep habits and school outcomes in middle-school children. Sleep 2003;26(4):455–8.

14. Fallone G, Owens JA, Deane J. Sleepiness in children and adolescents: clinical implications. Sleep Med Rev 2002;6(4):287–306.

15. Valrie CR, Bromberg MH, Palermo T, et al. A systematic review of sleep in pediatric pain populations. J Dev Behav Pediatr 2013;34(2):120–8.

16. O'Brien LM. The neurocognitive effects of sleep disruption in children and adolescents. Child Adolesc Psychiatr Clin N Am 2009;18(4):813–23.

17. Marcus CL, Brooks LJ, Draper KA, et al. Diagnosis and management of childhood obstructive sleep apnea syndrome. Pediatrics 2012;130(3):576–84.

18. Melendres MC, Lutz JM, Rubin ED, et al. Daytime sleepiness and hyperactivity in children with suspected sleep-disordered breathing. Pediatrics 2004;114(3):768–75.

19. Gozal D, Wang M, Pope DW Jr. Objective sleepiness measures in pediatric obstructive sleep apnea. Pediatrics 2001;108(3):693–7.

20. Beebe DW. Neurobehavioral morbidity associated with disordered breathing during sleep in children: a comprehensive review. Sleep 2006;29(9): 1115–34.

21. Marcus CL, Moore RH, Rosen CL, et al. A randomized trial of adenotonsillectomy for childhood sleep apnea. N Engl J Med 2013;368(25): 2366–76.

22. Venekamp RP, Hearne BJ, Chandrasekharan D, et al. Tonsillectomy or adenotonsillectomy versus non-surgical management for obstructive sleep-disordered breathing in children. Cochrane Database Syst Rev 2015;(10):CD011165.

23. Marcus CL, Radcliffe J, Konstantinopoulou S, et al. Effects of positive airway pressure therapy on neurobehavioral outcomes in children with obstructive sleep apnea. Am J Respir Crit Care Med 2012; 185(9):998–1003.

24. Rogers VE, Marcus CL, Jawad AF, et al. Periodic limb movements and disrupted sleep in children with sickle cell disease. Sleep 2011;34(7): 899–908.

25. Turkdogan D, Bekiroglu N, Zaimoglu S. A prevalence study of restless legs syndrome in Turkish children and adolescents. Sleep Med 2011;12(4):315–21.

26. Bruni O, Ottaviano S, Guidetti V, et al. The Sleep disturbance scale for children (SDSC). Construction and validation of an instrument to evaluate sleep disturbances in childhood and adolescence. J Sleep Res 1996;5(4):251–61.

27. Luginbuehl M, Bradley-Klug KL, Ferron J, et al. Pediatric sleep disorders: validation of the sleep disorders inventory for students. Sch Psych Rev 2008; 37(3):409–31.

28. Chervin RD, Hedger K, Dillon JE, et al. Pediatric sleep questionnaire (PSQ): validity and reliability of scales for sleep-disordered breathing, snoring, sleepiness, and behavioral problems. Sleep Med 2000;1(1):21–32.

29. Spilsbury JC, Drotar D, Rosen CL, et al. The Cleveland adolescent sleepiness questionnaire: a new measure to assess excessive daytime sleepiness in adolescents. J Clin Sleep Med 2007;3(6):603–12.

30. Paruthi S, Buchanan P, Weng J, et al. Effect of adenotonsillectomy on parent-reported sleepiness in children with obstructive sleep apnea. Sleep 2016; 39(11):2005–12.

31. Millman RP. Excessive sleepiness in adolescents and young adults: causes, consequences, and treatment strategies. Pediatrics 2005;115(6): 1774–86.

32. Aurora RN, Lamm CI, Zak RS, et al. Practice parameters for the non-respiratory indications for polysomnography and Multiple Sleep Latency Testing for children. Sleep 2012;35(11):1467–73.

33. Carskadon MA, Dement WC. Multiple Sleep Latency Tests during the constant routine. Sleep 1992;15(5): 396–9.

34. Carskadon MA, Harvey K, Duke P, et al. Pubertal changes in daytime sleepiness. Sleep 1980;2(4): 453–60.

35. Gozal D, Serpero LD, Kheirandish-Gozal L, et al. Sleep measures and morning plasma TNF-alpha levels in children with sleep-disordered breathing. Sleep 2010;33(3):319–25.

36. Chervin RD, Ruzicka DL, Giordani BJ, et al. Sleep-disordered breathing, behavior, and cognition in children before and after adenotonsillectomy. Pediatrics 2006;117(4):e769–78.

37. Coelho FMS, Aloe F, Moreira GA, et al. Narcolepsy in childhood and adolescence. Sleep Sci 2012;5(4): 139–44.

38. Rocca FL, Pizza F, Ricci E, et al. Narcolepsy during childhood: an update. Neuropediatrics 2015;46(3): 181–98.

39. Kacar Bayram A, Per H, Ismailogullari S, et al. Efficiency of a combination of pharmacological treatment and nondrug interventions in childhood narcolepsy. Neuropediatrics 2016;47(6):380–7.

40. Coelho FM, Pradella-Hallinan M, Pedrazzoli M, et al. Traditional biomarkers in narcolepsy: experience of a Brazilian sleep centre. Arq Neuropsiquiatr 2010; 68(5):712–5.

41. American Academy of Sleep Medicine. International classification of sleep disorders (ICSD-3). 3rd edition. Darien (IL): American Academy of Sleep Medicine; 2014.

42. Lopes DA, Coelho FM, Pradella-Hallinan M, et al. Infancy narcolepsy: streptococcus infection as a causal factor. Sleep Sci 2015;8(1):49–52.

43. Marcus CL, Trescher WH, Halbower AC, et al. Secondary narcolepsy in children with brain tumors. Sleep 2002;25(4):435–9.

44. Bassetti C, Aldrich MS. Idiopathic hypersomnia. A series of 42 patients. Brain 1997;120(Pt 8):1423–35.

45. Vernet C, Arnulf I. Idiopathic hypersomnia with and without long sleep time: a controlled series of 75 patients. Sleep 2009;32(6):753–9.

46. Ali M, Auger RR, Slocumb NL, et al. Idiopathic hypersomnia: clinical features and response to treatment. J Clin Sleep Med 2009;5(6):562–8.

47. Miyagawa T, Kawamura H, Obuchi M, et al. Effects of oral L-carnitine administration in narcolepsy patients: a randomized, double-blind, cross-over and placebo-controlled trial. PLoS One 2013;8(1): e53707.

48. Avis KT, Gamble KL, Schwebel DC. Does excessive daytime sleepiness affect children's pedestrian safety? Sleep 2014;37(2):283–7.

49. Arnulf I, Zeitzer JM, File J, et al. Kleine-Levin syndrome: a systematic review of 186 cases in the literature. Brain 2005;128(Pt 12):2763–76.

50. Ramdurg S. Kleine-Levin syndrome: etiology, diagnosis, and treatment. Ann Indian Acad Neurol 2010;13(4):241–6.

51. Rezvanian E, Watson NF. Kleine-Levin syndrome treated with clarithromycin. J Clin Sleep Med 2013; 9(11):1211–2.

52. Sagalés T. Outras hipersonias. In: Paiva T, Andersen ML, Tufik S, editors. O Sono e a Medicina do Sono. 1st edition. Barueri (Brazil): Editora Manole; 2014. p. 340–5.

53. Baker F. Menstrual-related hypersomnia. In: Thorpy MJ, Billiard M, editors. Sleepiness: causes, consequences and treatment. Cambridge (United Kingdom): Cambridge University Press; 2011. p. 147–9.

54. Paruthi S, Brooks LJ, D'Ambrosio C, et al. Consensus statement of the American Academy of sleep medicine on the recommended amount of sleep for healthy children: methodology and discussion. J Clin Sleep Med 2016;12(11):1549–61.

55. Pereira EF, Barbosa DG, Andrade RD, et al. Sleep and adolescence: how many hours sleep teenagers need? J Bras Psiquiatr 2015;64(1):40–4.

56. Matricciani LA, Olds TS, Blunden S, et al. Never enough sleep: a brief history of sleep recommendations for children. Pediatrics 2012; 129(3):548–56.

57. Garcia J, Rosen G, Mahowald M. Circadian rhythms and circadian rhythm disorders in children and adolescents. Semin Pediatr Neurol 2001;8(4):229–40.

58. Crowley SJ, Acebo C, Carskadon MA. Sleep, circadian rhythms, and delayed phase in adolescence. Sleep Med 2007;8(6):602–12.

59. Archer SN, Robilliard DL, Skene DJ, et al. A length polymorphism in the circadian clock gene Per3 is linked to delayed sleep phase syndrome and extreme diurnal preference. Sleep 2003;26(4): 413–5.

60. Mundey K, Benloucif S, Harsanyi K, et al. Phase-dependent treatment of delayed sleep phase syndrome with melatonin. Sleep 2005;28(10):1271–8.

Sleepiness in Adolescents

Roah A. Merdad, MD, MSc[a,b], Hammam Akil, MD[c],
Siraj Omar Wali, MBBS, FRCPC[d],*

KEYWORDS

- Adolescents • Sleepiness • Sleep deprivation • Clinical • Public health

KEY POINTS

- Sleepiness in the adolescent age group is an issue that is gaining increasing attention from researchers and clinicians as well as other stakeholders.
- Although clinical sleep disorders do affect some adolescents and warrant proper diagnosis and treatment, insufficient nighttime sleep is the main underlying cause of sleepiness in this age group.
- Points in medical history taking that may need to be explored for adolescent patients include personal habits, such as energy drink consumption and electronic media use, and environmental factors, such as parent-set bed times and school start times.
- Tackling the problem of sleepiness among adolescents may need collaboration from pediatricians and family physicians as well as public health agencies, parents, and school boards.

INTRODUCTION

Over the past decade, the issue of adolescent sleep has gained increasing attention from researchers, clinicians, parents, and the general public. Receiving sufficient and good quality sleep is integral to the optimal development, academic success, and overall well-being of adolescents. Although clinical sleep disorders affect some adolescents, sleepiness among this age group is increasingly being recognized as a public health concern, with many of its determinants lying beyond the biomedical scope of explanation. Chronic sleep loss, also termed insufficient sleep or inadequate sleep, is the main, albeit not only, cause of sleepiness during the daytime. In addition, the transition from childhood into adulthood is accompanied by many biological changes in the adolescent, and changes in the biological clock are no exception.

The consequences of sleepiness, in particular in this age group, have wide implications for mental, psychological, and physical health, as well as the academic achievement of adolescents. In this article, the authors walk the reader through an understanding of the physiologic changes in sleep-wake regulation and the circadian rhythm in the adolescent age group; the scope of the problem of sleep loss and sleepiness among adolescents; its etiologic factors, which encompass physiologic, lifestyle, and pathologic factors; its consequences; and the different approaches by which it can be addressed in clinical practice and beyond (for example, by policy changes in the educational sector). Because of the unique contributors to the epidemic of sleepiness in this age group, and because most sleepy adolescents will not present to sleep medicine physicians with their complaints, it is pertinent that the problem is presented from both a clinical and a public health perspective.

Disclosure Statement: The authors have no conflicts of interest to declare.
[a] Department of Family and Community Medicine, Faculty of Medicine, King Abdulaziz University, PO Box 80200, Jeddah 21589, Saudi Arabia; [b] Department of Community Health and Epidemiology, Faculty of Medicine, Dalhousie University, 6299 South Street, Halifax, Nova Scotia B3H 4R2, Canada; [c] Department of Pediatrics, Jeddah Maternity & Children's Hospital, Saud Al-Faisal Street, Jeddah 21423, Saudi Arabia; [d] College of Medicine, Sleep Medicine and Research Center, King Abdulaziz University Hospital, King Abdulaziz University, PO Box 80215, Jeddah 21589, Saudi Arabia
* Corresponding author.
E-mail address: sowali@kau.edu.sa

THE BIOLOGY OF SLEEP IN ADOLESCENTS

Sleep in humans is a physiologic state that recurs on a regular basis.[1] The timing of sleep is determined by the biological clock, the sleep-wake physiologic equilibrium, as well as behavioral choice.[2,3] The circadian rhythm is affected by puberty.[4] Adolescents who reach puberty experience a delay in their circadian phase.[4] Scientists have therefore argued that it is not a change in sleep requirements that occurs during the transition from childhood into adolescence, but rather a shift in melatonin peak levels to later in the evening.[5] In general, adolescents and young adults seem to have the greatest delay in their circadian rhythm compared with other age groups,[6] reaching the most extreme "lateness" of their circadian-induced sleep time at around the age of 20.[6]

It is recommended that teenagers get between 8.5 to 9.25 hours of sleep each night on a regular basis.[7] Most recently, the amount of sleep needed by children and adolescents was published in a consensus recommendation that was developed by members of the American Academy of Sleep Medicine.[8] In their recommendation, adolescents 13 to 18 years of age require 8 to 10 hours of sleep every 24 hours on a regular basis to entertain full daytime alertness and achieve optimal health.[9,10] These recommendations are comparable to those of the National Sleep Foundation.[11]

THE PREVALENCE AND CONSEQUENCES OF SLEEPINESS AMONG ADOLESCENTS
Prevalence of Sleepiness Among Adolescents

In most adolescents suffering from daytime sleepiness, chronic insufficient sleep is the underlying cause.[12] Furthermore, there seems to be a consensus that adolescents worldwide are not acquiring sufficient sleep. Hence, it is no surprise that daytime sleepiness is common among adolescents.[13–17] Studies as early as 1981 have shown the effect of sleep deprivation on the daytime tendency to fall asleep.[18] When individuals are restricted from acquiring the amount of hours required for sleep, they tend to doze off in quiet settings the following day.[18,19] Such excessive sleepiness following sleep restriction has been measured both subjectively and objectively.[18–20] The percentage of adolescents who complain from daytime sleepiness varies across surveys. This variation may be due, in part, to the measurements of "daytime sleepiness" using various questionnaires and tools, or to bona fide cross-cultural differences.[21] The reported percentages of sleepy adolescents range from approximately 25% to 84% in countries worldwide.[13–16,22] It is important to keep in mind that these figures likely include both adolescents who are sleep simply deprived, in addition to those suffering from excessive daytime sleepiness due to other causes, such as sleep disorders, medication side effects, or other chronic conditions. Hence, sleepiness is a direct manifestation, but is not limited to sleep deprivation.

Reports from various countries have shown that adolescents sleep on average of 6.4 to 7.7 hours each night,[13,22–31] with a tendency to oversleep during the weekend for more than 2 hours.[21] Three recent reviews, two of which are systematic reviews with meta-analyses, have painted a global picture of adolescent sleep habits.[21,32,33] Gradisar and colleagues[21] reported findings from 41 worldwide surveys and found that the mean school-night bed time for adolescents aged 11 to 18 years was after 10:30 PM and that approximately half (53%) were obtaining less than 8 hours of sleep each night. The second review assessed differences in sleep patterns by age, sex, and day-type on a global scale.[32] Findings suggest that as adolescents grow older, they sleep less, with a 14 minute per night decline in sleep per 1-year increase in age.[32] In addition, girls acquire, on average, more sleep than boys.[32] In the third review, secular trends in the sleep time of children and adolescents were analyzed.[33] Data from 20 countries dating from 1905 to 2008 were included. The results suggest that there has been a consistent decline in sleep duration over the years across age and sex. However, some variations across geographic regions were observed.[33] Some studies have found that adolescents with a lower socioeconomic status and from minority groups are more likely to have later bed times and fewer hours of sleep at night, compared with those from a higher socioeconomic status and from nonminority groups.[34,35]

Consequences of Sleepiness Among Adolescents

Sleepiness and sleep deprivation have been linked to a myriad of negative outcomes in adolescents.[26,36–49] Examples of some of these consequences are presented in **Box 1**. It must be noted, however, that some of the associations presented have not always been consistent, such as in the case of students with higher grades sometimes exhibiting worse sleep than those with poor grades,[48] and that bidirectional relationships, such as those between sleep duration and substance use, are sometimes present.[40]

APPROACH TO A SLEEPY ADOLESCENT
Measuring Sleepiness

It is important to differentiate sleepiness from chronic fatigue. Sleepiness is defined as an inability

<table>
<tr><td>

Box 1
Examples of negative outcomes that have been linked to sleep deprivation and daytime sleepiness in adolescents

Weight gain and obesity[18,36]

Cardiovascular diseases[37]

Headaches and abdominal pain[38]

Suicidal ideation[39]

Cigarette, alcohol, and marijuana use[40]

Drowsy driving and motor vehicle collisions[41–43]

Affected memory[44]

Deteriorated cognitive abilities (sustained attention and working function)[35]

Poor academic performance[45–47]

Weakened emotional-behavioral regulation[49]

</td><td>

Box 2
Measuring sleepiness in adolescents

Subjective measures

Generic, short questions (eg, levels of morning sleepiness, oversleeping, or frequency of daytime naps)[24]

Cleveland Adolescent Sleepiness Questionnaire[53]

Epworth Sleepiness Scale[32]

Modified Epworth Sleepiness Scale[54]

Pediatric Daytime Sleepiness Scale[55]

Objective measures

Multiple sleep latency tests[56]

Actigraphy, accompanied by a sleep log when possible[57]

</td></tr>
</table>

to maintain an alert state during the major waking episodes of the day.[50] Sleepiness is described in terms of the following: Eyelids drooping, head sagging, and short periods of sleep occurring inappropriately. Fatigue, on the other hand, is defined as a lack of physical energy and a sense of muscular exhaustion.[51] When daytime sleep occurs, it usually follows a period of rest. To assess for sleepiness, subjective and objective measures are available and can be used as indicated.

Subjective measures
Adolescents have been assessed for levels of daytime sleepiness using various questions. Often, these are generic direct questions that inquire about levels of morning sleepiness, of oversleeping or a desire to have more sleep, or the number or frequency of daytime naps.[21] Lengthier tools that have been developed to specifically measure daytime sleepiness in the population of adolescents and young adults are available. They differ in their reliability and validity. Ji and Liu[52] recently published a systematic review of subjective sleep measures for adolescents. Domain-specific scales that assess sleepiness are listed in **Box 2**.

Some have argued that the Epworth Sleepiness Scale (ESS) is not a sensitive measure of daytime sleepiness in adolescents, because the situations assessed to quantify daytime sleepiness in adults are not always applicable to adolescents.[58] In a study in 2009 assessing adolescents aged 13 to 16 years, Moore and colleagues[54] used a modified version of the ESS in which the last statement inquiring about the chance of dozing off "in a car while stopped for a few minutes in traffic" was replaced by "(while) doing homework or taking a

test." The reliability of the modified scale was equal to a Cronbach's α of 0.75. However, construct validity was not assessed.

The pediatric daytime sleepiness scale was developed to assess daytime sleepiness in individuals in middle school (11–15 years old). It is an 8-item scale that includes statements assessing the frequency of a behavior related to sleep. It is easily administered and has a Cronbach's α of 0.80.[55] Some limitations of this tool include the vagueness of some statements that can introduce confusion, and the limited age range that it can test. The tool was assessed for its clinical utility in a Chinese population and showed good psychometric properties to differentiate among the sleepiness severity associated with narcolepsy, obstructive sleep apnea (OSA), and normal subjects.[59] However, it may not be suitable as a screening tool for excessive sleepiness.[59]

The Cleveland Adolescent Sleepiness Questionnaire was introduced in 2007 as a tool to assess excessive daytime sleepiness in adolescents.[53] It is a simple and straightforward questionnaire. The tool shows good psychometric properties, in terms of both internal consistency and construct validity.[52–55,58,59]

Objective measures
Multiple sleep latency test The multiple sleep latency test (MSLT) is the most commonly used and experimentally validated objective test of daytime sleepiness. It is sensitive and reproducible.[56] The principle of MSLT is that the sleepier the subject, the faster he or she will fall asleep. The clinical protocol is based on performing polysomnography (PSG) before MSLT to objectively characterize the preceding sleep followed by five 20-minute naps at 2-hour intervals. The first nap begins 1.5

to 3 hours following the end of nocturnal sleep. The primary measures from the MSLT are the mean sleep latency and the number of sleep-onset rapid eye movement naps.[56]

Actigraphy An actigraph is a wristwatch-like device to monitor movement at night for a period of 1 to 2 weeks.[57] Actigraphy is a validated method against PSG that provides a reliable evaluation of the sleep-wake pattern in children and adults. It is characterized by its ability to capture data for several days from the home environment. Actigraphy data ideally should be interpreted together with a sleep log.[57]

Assessment of the Underlying Cause of Sleepiness

Once the presence of excessive sleepiness is established, the clinician can then move to assess the underlying cause. The causes underlying sleepiness can be broadly categorized into the following groups: sleep disorders, behavioral factors, environmental influences, medical illnesses other than sleep disorders, and medication side effects.

Mindell and Owens[60] present a symptom-based algorithm, or flowchart, to guide clinicians in the assessment of daytime sleepiness in the adolescent population (**Fig. 1**). The approach begins with assessing 3 main issues: total sleep time; severity of excessive daytime sleepiness and its impact on daytime functioning; and the presence of medical or psychiatric conditions that may be related to the sleep disturbance. From that point, the clinician can continue to refine the cause of sleepiness either by asking questions or by using more objective measures of the sleep state and patterns when indicated, until a diagnosis can be reached.[53]

History taking

An understanding of normal sleep physiology and obtaining a complete sleep history and medical background are the cornerstones for reaching the proper diagnosis of a sleep disorder or other underlying cause. Sleepiness can be assessed in terms of duration, profile of onset, frequency, severity, and night-to-night variability.[61] Bedtime routines and sleep patterns, in addition to the physical environment surrounding sleep (eg, room-sharing, noise level), have to be assessed because they may reveal environmental factors that interrupt sleep. In addition, lifestyle behaviors such as the intake of energy drinks or other sources of caffeine, and electronic use at or before bed time, may point to habits contributing to suboptimal sleep.

Screening for a sleep disorder can be conveniently performed using the BEARS acronym, which has been developed to aid the physician in comprehensively assessing for the most common sleep disorders in the pediatric and adolescent age groups.[62] Five areas pertaining to sleep are addressed (B = Bedtime issues; E = Excessive daytime sleepiness; A = Night Awakenings; R = Regularity and duration of sleep; S = Sleep-disordered breathing).[62] When a sleep disorder is suspected, nocturnal symptoms that may indicate OSA (loud snoring, sweating, choking, or gasping), periodic limb movement disorders (PLMD; restless sleep, or repetitive kicking movements), and other disorders should be elicited. Information on potential non-sleep-related medical causes should also be obtained. The clinician should also note medication or recreational drug use that may account for the presenting complaints.

Sleep log

A sleep diary in which the adolescent can log daily sleep habits can give the clinician a deeper understanding of the pattern of sleep. Information can be recorded over a week or two. The sleep log should include the following information: bed time, sleep latency, number of awakenings, rise time, nocturnal events, napping and its duration, perceived quality of sleep, and self-assessment regarding the level of alertness or sleepiness during the day.[50]

Further assessment

Given the right clinical context, the MSLT is able to diagnose disorders of hypersomnolence such as narcolepsy.[50] A sleep latency time of less than 8 minutes is generally considered abnormal and objectively supports hypersomnia. In adolescents, a mean sleep latency value of 8 to 15 minutes may be suggestive of pathologic sleepiness.[62] When unexplained sleepiness or nighttime symptoms suggestive of a sleep disorder are present, an overnight sleep study may be performed. This however does not need to be routinely done to all adolescents presenting with excessive sleepiness.

THE CAUSE OF SLEEPINESS AMONG ADOLESCENTS
Sleep Disorders

In this article, the authors do not intend to present a thorough review of the diagnosis and management of sleep disorders in adolescents, but rather to provide an overview of differential diagnoses to aid clinicians in reaching a diagnosis or provide them with an understanding of the underlying cause of sleepiness.

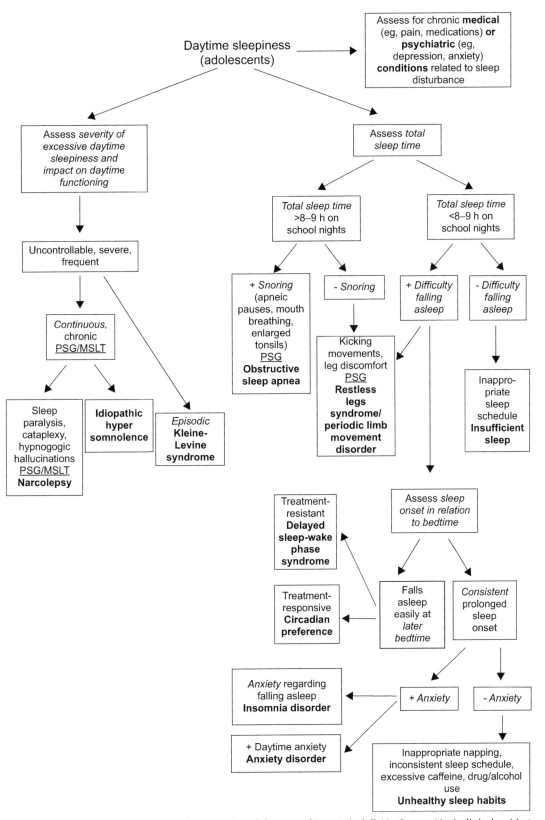

Fig. 1. A flowchart to assess daytime sleepiness in adolescents. (*From* Mindell JA, Owens JA. A clinical guide to pediatric sleep: diagnosis and management of sleep problems. Philadelphia: Lippincott Williams & Wilkins, 2015; with permission.)

Circadian rhythm disorders: mainly delayed sleep phase syndrome

Although the prevalence of delayed sleep phase syndrome (DSPS) is not well established, available data suggest that between 0.1% and 8% of the general population suffer from this condition, and that it peaks in adolescence.[61,63–65] DSPS affects both genders equally. The cardinal clinical features of DSPS are delayed bed times as well as wake times compared with usual or desired times. These features often lead to chronic sleep insufficiency and daytime sleepiness with impaired cognitive function.[66,67] Morning awakenings are difficult and associated with excessive sleep inertia.[50] The natural history of DSPS is not well known. It typically appears during adolescence and may persist into adulthood if left untreated.[50]

DSPS is a clinical diagnosis that should be suspected in individuals who complain of insomnia with difficulty falling asleep at conventional times, failure to obtain sufficient nightly sleep, difficulties with morning awakening, and prolonged sleep inertia. Such a clinical history supported by sleep logs and actigraphy is sufficient to make the diagnosis in most patients.[67] Actigraphy may replace the sleep log in patients with poor compliance or when symptoms are inconsistent with the sleep log data.[68] The salivary melatonin immunoassay needs further validation before it can be used clinically.[69]

Central disorders of hypersomnolence

Narcolepsy Although symptoms of narcolepsy start in childhood, this condition is often diagnosed during adolescence. Narcolepsy is characterized by its tetrad. The cardinal symptom is excessive daytime sleepiness, including sleep attacks during meals, talking, or sporting. Excessive daytime sleepiness usually precedes other ancillary symptoms that include cataplexy: a sudden loss of skeletal muscle tone, partial or complete, that is often precipitated by an emotion such as laughter; sleep paralysis; and hypnagogic hallucinations, vivid, dreamlike visual or auditory imagery that occurs during sleep onset.[70–74] The diagnostic evaluation of narcolepsy includes medical history and physical examination, PSG, and MSLT.

Idiopathic hypersomnia Idiopathic hypersomnia (IH) is a rare disorder of unexplained hypersomnia that affects 4 per 100,000 people. Onset usually occurs between the ages of 10 and 30 years. The condition develops over several weeks, stabilizes, and then resolves in 25% of cases. The typical history consists of nocturnal sleep that is often long (>10 hours) with prolonged and severe sleep inertia and difficult and slow wakening.

However, it may occur without a long sleep time. Naps tend to be prolonged and are not refreshing, in contrast to narcolepsy.[75]

IH is a diagnosis of exclusion. However, a firm diagnosis is necessary because long-term treatment is required. The diagnosis of exclusion is based on an overnight sleep study that is usually unremarkable, followed by MSLT that confirms hypersomnia but without REM sleep (the number of naps with REM sleep should be <2). Neuroimaging studies should be considered.[76]

Kleine-Levin syndrome Kleine-Levin syndrome is a rare disorder that is characterized by recurrent episodes of hypersomnia with a total sleep time of 12 to 20 hours per day and sustained sleep inertia. These episodes last for 1 to 2 weeks and usually recur once a year and at least every 18 months. In between episodes, the patient has normal alertness, cognitive functioning, behavior, and mood. The patient must demonstrate at least one of the following during episodes: Cognitive dysfunction, altered perception, an eating disorder (anorexia or hyperphagia), and disinhibited behavior (such as hypersexuality), which are not better explained by other sleep/medical disorders, medications, or drugs. The median age of onset is 15 years, with a range from 4 to 82 years. Spontaneous remission is common with a median disease duration of 14 years.[77]

Obstructive sleep apnea

Although the obesity epidemic is accompanied by an increase in the prevalence of OSA, adenotonsillar hypertrophy is the main cause of this disorder in the adolescent population. The cardinal symptoms of OSA are snoring and excessive daytime sleepiness. However, the latter is less obvious than in adults with OSA but may be evident upon specific questioning. Furthermore, in contrast to adults with OSA, teenagers may not snore or experience recurrent awakenings following obstructive respiratory events.[50] Other symptoms include waking up gasping for air or choking episodes. Neurobehavioral symptoms are also common and, in this age group, may include hyperactivity, irritability, distraction, and poor concentration. Other daytime symptoms may include nasal obstruction, mouth breathing, or other signs of adenotonsillar hypertrophy. Adolescents with marked adenotonsillar hypertrophy or obesity and any of these symptoms warrant a more detailed clinical evaluation that usually includes PSG.[78]

Restless leg syndrome and periodic limb movement disorder

Restless leg syndrome (RLS), also known as Willis-Ekbom disease (WED), is a common, complex, and treatable neurologic condition. RLS is characterized by an urge to move the legs that is usually accompanied by an uncomfortable or unpleasant sensation in the legs. The symptoms begin or worsen during rest or inactivity, are relieved by movement, and occur exclusively or predominantly in the evening or at night. Children with RLS or PLMD often have depressed serum ferritin levels, indicating reduced iron stores, and in such cases, the disorder may improve with iron supplementation.

In children, PLMD appears to be closely related to RLS because there is significant overlap between the 2 entities.[79–81] In population-based studies, the prevalence of RLS/WED in children and adolescents is 2% to 4%.[82–86] Furthermore, symptoms of RLS/WED start before 20 years of age in approximately 40% of adults.[87–89] Although in younger age groups, RLS/WED affects men and women equally, the female predominance observed in adults emerges in adolescence or the early twenties.[90] Leg symptoms are rarely the chief complaints in patients with RLS/WED or PLMD. The most common complaints, however, include restless sleep (86%) and disturbed sleep with sleep onset difficulty (81%) or asleep maintenance (65%).[81] Although patients may present with daytime sleepiness, excessive daytime sleepiness is not commonly reported by patients with PLMD or RLS/WED.[91]

Insufficient Sleep and Inadequate Sleep Hygiene

Insufficient sleep syndrome

A range of different terms, such as sleep deprivation, sleep restriction, insufficient sleep, inadequate sleep, short sleep duration, and sleep loss, has been used in the literature interchangeably to describe the construct "less sleep than needed."[12] Lifestyle choices, including inappropriate sleep schedules, late night electronic use, caffeine use, and daytime napping, are all contributing factors.[12]

Insufficient sleep syndrome (ISS) has been presented as a sleep disorder in the third edition of the International Classification of Sleep Disorders.[50] ISS is characterized by daily episodes of an irrepressible need to sleep or daytime lapses of sleep (ie, excessively pressing daytime sleepiness) accompanied by a short total sleep time compared with that needed for his or her age, almost every day over a period of at least 3 months. In addition to these 3 criteria, the patient usually sleeps longer when not awakened by another person or an alarm clock (eg, during vacations or on weekends); the sleep time extension is accompanied by a resolution of the sleepiness symptoms;

and finally, no better explanation for the symptoms is present, particularly by other sleep, medical, neurologic, or mental disorders, or medications and drugs.[50]

Personal habits that contribute to inadequate sleep hygiene

Personal habits have a direct and significant impact on sleep and, subsequently, daytime functioning. In 2009, Calamaro and colleagues[92] described adolescents as "living the 24/7 lifestyle" because of patterns of caffeine consumption and technology use. In the following section, the authors present personal habits that have been associated with insufficient sleep and sleepiness in adolescents.

Electronic media use Data on 13 to 21 year olds from the 2011 National Sleep Foundation's Sleep in American Poll revealed that the use of some form of technology at or before bed time was reported by almost all respondents (97%). Those with an increased frequency of technology use were more likely to wake up too early, to feel unrefreshed in the morning, and to exhibit greater daytime sleepiness.[30] Similarly, a US study found that adolescents who slept longer (8 or more hours) reported less technology use after 9 PM in comparison to those who reported sleeping less (6–8 hours and 3–5 hours).[92] Electronics associated with later bed times and shorter hours of sleep include television, computers, electronic games, and mobile phones.[93] A study showed that computer and mobile phone use in bed was associated with insomnia but not daytime sleepiness.[94] Such distinctions need to be further evaluated.

The ways in which exposure to technology before or at bed time may influence sleep are subject to investigation. In a recent study, the impact of reading from an iPad in comparison to a book for 30 minutes in bed before sleep was assessed in a group of young adults (mean age of 25 years). In the iPad group, subjective sleepiness was decreased, and there was a 30-minute delay in the electroencephalogram dynamics of slow-wave activity. However, measures of sleep onset latency and sleep timing did not differ between the 2 groups.[95]

Stimulant use including caffeine With the introduction of energy drinks to the market, caffeine use is on the increase among adolescents. This trend is reflected in academics labeling adolescents as the "Red Bull Generation" after a popular internationally available energy drink.[60] Products that contain caffeine and are used by adolescents include coffee, tea, iced tea, energy drinks, sodas, and chocolate, in addition to some forms of over-the-counter gums, candies, and medications. Reasons for caffeine consumption include accessibility, image enhancement, taste, and the desire to increase energy levels.[96] Caffeine is present in many of the products being consumed by adolescents, including carbonated beverages (sodas).[97] Reports indicate that, on average, adolescents consume approximately 50 mg of caffeine per day.[98] Knowledge about the recommended daily consumption levels of caffeine may be low among adolescents.[96] Up to a quarter of adolescents who consume caffeine in Canada exceed the Canadian maximal guidelines, based on a national study of data collected from 2007 to 2010.[98] Caffeine is associated with poor sleep in adolescents, in terms of both quantity and quality.[12] However, this relationship requires further evaluation, particularly in terms of understanding the direction of association between caffeine consumption, poor sleep, and sleepiness.[12] Experts recommend that clinicians inquire about caffeine use during clinical encounters and that education about intake and the recommended maximum daily use be provided.[60] In addition, adolescents and their parents should be aware that caffeine is an active psychoactive substance rather than a type of food.[60] Finally, caffeine should not be viewed as an alternative to a good night's sleep and that its energy and alertness-enhancing qualities are temporary and soon wear off and get replaced with negative effects on sleep and daytime sleepiness.[60]

Environmental influences that contribute to inadequate sleep hygiene

Early school start times An important factor that has been consistently linked to shorter sleep times in adolescents is early school start time.[99–101] Internationally, many schools start the first class before 8 AM. The biological sleep-wake clock runs from approximately 11 PM to 8 AM in adolescents.[99] Therefore, with early start times, students are forced to wake up against their biological needs, as students who start school between 7:30 and 8 AM would have to wake up between 6:30 and 7 AM.[99] If they were to acquire their needed 9 hours of sleep, the students would need to go to sleep before 10:30 PM.[21] Students lose as much as 2 hours of sleep per night when they return to school from summer vacation.[99] In addition, students were reported to perform better later in the day in comparison to early morning, a finding consistent with the need for longer sleep in the morning.[99]

Parental and cultural factors Researchers have evaluated the potential impact of parenting behaviors on adolescent sleep and levels of daytime sleepiness. In a recent longitudinal study, researchers found that parental monitoring and the quality of parent-adolescent relationships were associated with better sleep quality and lower levels of daytime sleepiness.[102] Similarly, among a group of 13 to 18 year olds in South Australia, those with parent-set bed times had significantly earlier bed times, acquired longer hours of sleep, and had better levels of daytime wakefulness compared with students without parent-set bed times. On weekends, when parent-set bed times were not enforced, sleep patterns ceased to differ between the 2 groups.[103] Other parental factors that may influence adolescent sleep include parental shift work and parental perceptions toward bed-sharing.[104,105]

It has also been shown that the sleep habits and behaviors of adolescents sometimes differ across cultures.[21] Gradisar and colleagues[21] have suggested that the worldwide pattern of delayed bed time and wake times is more prevalent in certain regions including Asia and Iceland, suggesting potential cultural influences. Some studies shed light on potential factors that may drive the observed cross-cultural differences. A study comparing a group of Australian adolescents to a group of adolescents from the United States found that the former group acquired, on average, 47 more minutes of sleep during school nights and that they had later school start times (8:32 AM vs 7:45 AM, respectively), were more likely to have parent-set bed times, and were less likely to be involved in extracurricular activities. All of those factors were significant mediators in the acquisition of more sleep.[100] A study from Saudi Arabia documented extreme sleep schedules, in which 10% of the studied population of high school students reported staying up all night (ie, pulling a so-called all-nighter) and acquiring their sleep during the day after returning from school.[31] Further insight and more objective assessments of such extreme sleep patterns are needed.

Chronic Medical Illnesses and Medication Side Effects

Several medical conditions may be associated with excessive daytime sleepiness, lethargy, or other related symptoms that may be challenging to distinguish from sleepiness.[106] In addition, many medications that are used in chronic diseases may also contribute to sleepiness.[107] A list of medical conditions and medications contributing to daytime sleepiness is presented in **Box 3**.

Box 3
The cause of sleepiness among adolescents

Sleep disorders[61–91,108,109]

Circadian rhythm disorders: mainly delayed sleep phase syndrome

Central disorders of hypersomnolence: Narcolepsy, idiopathic hypersomnia, Kleine-Levin syndrome

Obstructive sleep apnea

Restless leg syndrome and periodic limb movement disorder

Insufficient sleep and inadequate sleep hygiene[12,50,60,92–105]

Insufficient sleep syndrome

Personal habits that contribute to inadequate sleep hygiene: Electronic media use and stimulant use, including caffeine

Environmental influences that contribute to inadequate sleep hygiene: Early school start times, and parental and cultural factors

Chronic medical illnesses[106,a]

Anxiety disorder and depression

Chronic diseases, such as anemia, respiratory failure, cardiac disease, or malignancy

Central nervous system disorders, including posttraumatic brain injury (concussion), meningitis, encephalitis, exposure to toxic inhalation, such as carbon monoxide poisoning, and increased intracranial pressure due to hydrocephalus or mass lesions

Medications[107]

Opioids

Sedation medications, which include over-the-counter medication, such as antihistamines, antidepressants (especially the tricyclic compounds), benzodiazepines, antiseizure medications, and alpha-adrenergic agonists

---

[a] Chronic medical illnesses may lead to daytime sleepiness directly or through sleep loss, but they often also lead to other symptoms that may be mistaken for sleepiness, such as fatigue and generalized weakness.

THE IMPORTANCE OF THE FAMILY PHYSICIAN, PEDIATRICIAN, AND PUBLIC HEALTH INTERVENTIONS
The Role of the Pediatrician and Family Physician

According to the Sleep in America Poll from the National Sleep Foundation in 2004, only 48% of physicians ask about the child's sleep habits, whereas 69% of parents claim that their children have sleep problems.[23] Pediatricians and family physicians have a particularly important role in the identification and assessment of sleep problems among adolescents. The minimum requirement for the clinician assessing an adolescent is to ask about the amount and quality of sleep that he or she is receiving, and whether sleep-related symptoms are present.[110] This should be part of the routine clinical evaluation of adolescents.[110] The presence of excessive daytime sleepiness can trigger further evaluation and a more detailed assessment, or referral to a specialist, when a condition such as OSA, narcolepsy, or another sleep disorder is suspected. In addition, suspicion of an anxiety disorder or depression can lead to the referral to a psychiatrist. If none of these clinical diagnoses are suspected but there is a history indicating insufficient sleep due to poor sleep habits, the assessing family physician or pediatrician can, at a minimum, educate the patient about the sleep needs of adolescents and young adults, and the serious potential consequences of sleep loss and sleepiness on well-being.[110]

There is an opportunity to decrease the rates of sleepy adolescents by attempting to influence the important modifiable risk factors of insufficient sleep.[12] There risk factors include the use of electronics at or before bed time, caffeine use, setting suitable bed times on school nights, and creating sleep-promoting environments in the home.[102,103] Physicians involved in managing sleepy older adolescents who drive can also provide relevant education about the risk of driving while sleepy and implement strong recommendations about drowsy driving.[43]

In some countries, the role of the pediatrician may be delivered by a primary care doctor, such as a family physician, or by a specialized doctor in the emergency room or during clinic visits to specialized care. In these situations, the physician expecting to play the role of the pediatrician may adopt the screening and educational tasks.

Public Health Interventions

School-based educational and behavioral interventions

School-based interventions aiming to increase hours of sleep have been assessed.[108,111,112] In general, improvement in knowledge level is observed but is seldom accompanied by behavioral change. More recent studies have reported positive findings. Tamura and Tanaka[113] performed a cluster randomized trial to assess the effect of a sleep education program with a supplementary self-help sleep promotion behavior checklist on sleep promotion behaviors, sleeping patterns, and daytime sleepiness among Japanese adolescents. Significant improvements were found for all outcomes in the intervention groups compared with baseline, and no differences were observed for the nonintervention groups.[113] Similarly, a recent pilot study in India randomized 58 adolescents (mean age of 14 years) to receive either a sleep promotion program or no program. The outcomes of interest included sleep quality, duration, onset, daytime sleepiness, and sleep hygiene. Improvements were observed in all of these outcomes but sleep hygiene.[114]

Delaying school start times

It is well documented that adolescents worldwide sleep longer on weekends in comparison to school nights, with reports of up to 91.6 minutes of extra sleep time.[21,32] Therefore, researchers and sleep experts have advocated to delay school start times for adolescents to achieve more restful sleep on a regular basis.[115]

In 2002, in one of the first studies to investigate the effect of delaying school start times on adolescents' sleep, a longitudinal study was conducted by Wahlstrom[116] to examine the impact of a shift in school start times in 7 US high schools on adolescent sleep, school enrollment, and daytime sleepiness. Compared with students who were attending schools that did not use a shift in schedule, students in later-starting schools went to bed earlier and slept an hour longer. Daytime sleepiness was also significantly reduced in students attending the late-starting schools.

Recently, a study assessed the impact of school start time by comparing American and Australian adolescents. Australian students, who start school later than American students in this particular study (at 8:30 AM and 7:45 AM, respectively), slept longer by an average of 47 minutes per school night.[100] Similarly, Wolfson and colleagues[101] found that students in late-starting schools obtained 50 more minutes of sleep per night and were less sleepy the next day, compared with their early-starting counterparts.

Owens and colleagues[14] assessed a cohort of 201 American students pre-delaying and post-delaying school start time. A 30-minute delay (from 8 to 8:30 AM) increased sleep duration by 45 minutes, advanced bed time by 18 minutes, and increased the percentage of students who obtained at least 8 hours of sleep from 16.4% to 54.7%. Moreover, the sleepiness scale scores decreased from 28.5 to 22.9, reflecting a 19.8% decrease in the mean score.

A more recent study found that the impact of delaying school start times on the total hours of sleep acquired may not be sustained.[117] Such emerging findings support the need for assessments that take place in a variety of settings to determine consistency across cultures and subgroups of adolescents.

REFERENCES

1. Harvard Medical School. Healthy sleep; the characteristics of sleep. HMS; 2008. Available at: http://www.healthysleep.med.harvard.edu/healthy/credits. Accessed December 6, 2013.
2. McGill University. The brain. Sleep and dreams. McGillu; 2013. Available at: http://www.thebrain.mcgill.ca. Accessed December 6, 2013.
3. Harris CD. Neurophysiology of sleep and wakefulness. Respir Care Clin N Am 2005;11:567–86.
4. Tarokh L, Raffray T, Van Reen E, et al. Physiology of normal sleep in adolescents. Adolesc Med State Art Rev 2010;21:401–17, vii.
5. Carskadon MA, Acebo C, Richardson GS, et al. An approach to studying circadian rhythms of adolescent humans. J Biol Rhythms 1997;12:278–89.
6. Roenneberg T, Kuehnle T, Juda M, et al. Epidemiology of the human circadian clock. Sleep Med Rev 2007;11:429–38.
7. National Sleep Foundation. How much sleep do we really need. Available at: http://www.sleepfoundation.org/article/how-sleep-works. Accessed December 6, 2013.
8. Paruthi S, Brooks LJ, D'Ambrosio C, et al. Consensus statement of the American Academy of Sleep Medicine on the recommended amount of sleep for healthy children: methodology and discussion. J Clin Sleep Med 2016;12:1549–61.
9. Paruthi S, Brooks LJ, D'Ambrosio C, et al. Recommended amount of sleep for pediatric populations:

a consensus statement of the American Academy of Sleep Medicine. J Clin Sleep Med 2016;12:785–6.

10. The American Academy of Pediatrics. Recommended amount of sleep for pediatric populations. Pediatrics 2016;138(2). pii: e20161601.

11. Hirshkowitz M, Whiton K, Albert SM, et al. National Sleep Foundation's updated sleep duration recommendations: final report. Sleep Health 2015;1:233–43.

12. Owens J, Adolescent Sleep Working Group, Committee on Adolescence. Insufficient sleep in adolescents and young adults: an update on causes and consequences. Pediatrics 2014;134:e921–32.

13. Chung KF, Cheung MM. Sleep-wake patterns and sleep disturbance among Hong Kong Chinese adolescents. Sleep 2008;31:185–94.

14. Owens JA, Belon K, Moss P. Impact of delaying school start time on adolescent sleep, mood, and behavior. Arch Pediatr Adolesc Med 2010;164: 608–14.

15. Hysing M, Pallesen S, Stormark KM, et al. Sleep patterns and insomnia among adolescents: a population-based study. J Sleep Res 2013;22: 549–56.

16. Danner F, Phillips B. Adolescent sleep, school start times, and teen motor vehicle crashes. J Clin Sleep Med 2008;4:533–5.

17. Johns MW. A new method for measuring daytime sleepiness: the Epworth Sleepiness Scale. Sleep 1991;14:540–5.

18. Carskadon MA, Dement WC. Cumulative effects of sleep restriction on daytime sleepiness. Psychophysiology 1981;18:107–13.

19. Fallone G, Acebo C, Arnedt JT, et al. Effects of acute sleep restriction on behavior, sustained attention, and response inhibition in children. Percept Mot Skills 2001;93:213–29.

20. Lo JC, Ong JL, Leong RL, et al. Cognitive performance, sleepiness, and mood in partially sleep deprived adolescents: the need for sleep study. Sleep 2016;39:687–98.

21. Gradisar M, Gardner G, Dohnt H. Recent worldwide sleep patterns and problems during adolescence: a review and meta-analysis of age, region, and sleep. Sleep Med 2011;12:110–8.

22. Ghanizadeh A, Kianpoor M, Rezaei M, et al. Sleep patterns and habits in high school students in Iran. Ann Gen Psychiatry 2008;7:5.

23. Reid A, Maldonado CC, Baker FC. Sleep behavior of South African adolescents. Sleep 2002;25:423–7.

24. Lazaratou H, Dikeos DG, Anagnostopoulos DC, et al. Sleep problems in adolescence. A study of senior high school students in Greece. Eur Child Adolesc Psychiatry 2005;14:237–43.

25. Kilani H, Al-Hazzaa H, Waly MI, et al. Lifestyle habits: diet, physical activity and sleep duration among Omani adolescents. Sultan Qaboos Univ Med J 2013;13:510–9.

26. Al-Hazzaa HM, Musaiger AO, Abahussain NA, et al. Prevalence of short sleep duration and its association with obesity among adolescents 15- to 19-year olds: a cross-sectional study from three major cities in Saudi Arabia. Ann Thorac Med 2012;7:133–9.

27. Sweileh WM, Ali IA, Sawalha AF, et al. Sleep habits and sleep problems among Palestinian students. Child Adolesc Psychiatry Ment Health 2011;5:25.

28. Shochat T, Flint-Bretler O, Tzischinsky O. Sleep patterns, electronic media exposure and daytime sleep-related behaviours among Israeli adolescents. Acta Paediatr 2010;99:1396–400.

29. Abdel-Khalek AM. Epidemiologic study of sleep disorders in Kuwaiti adolescents. Percept Mot Skills 2001;93:901–10.

30. Johansson AE, Petrisko MA, Chasens ER. Adolescent sleep and the impact of technology use before sleep on daytime function. J Pediatr Nurs 2016;31:498–504.

31. Merdad RA, Merdad LA, Nassif RA, et al. Sleep habits in adolescents of Saudi Arabia; distinct patterns and extreme sleep schedules. Sleep Med 2014;15:1370–8.

32. Olds T, Blunden S, Petkov J, et al. The relationships between sex, age, geography and time in bed in adolescents: a meta-analysis of data from 23 countries. Sleep Med Rev 2010;14:371–8.

33. Matricciani L, Olds T, Petkov J. In search of lost sleep: secular trends in the sleep time of school-aged children and adolescents. Sleep Med Rev 2012;16:203–11.

34. Marco CA, Wolfson AR, Sparling M, et al. Family socioeconomic status and sleep patterns of young adolescents. Behav Sleep Med 2011;10: 70–80.

35. Moore M, Kirchner HL, Drotar D, et al. Correlates of adolescent sleep time and variability in sleep time: the role of individual and health related characteristics. Sleep Med 2011;12:239–45.

36. Park S. Association between short sleep duration and obesity among South Korean adolescents. West J Nurs Res 2011;33:207–23.

37. Narang I, Manlhiot C, Davies-Shaw J, et al. Sleep disturbance and cardiovascular risk in adolescents. CMAJ 2012;184:E913–20.

38. Luntamo T, Sourander A, Rihko M, et al. Psychosocial determinants of headache, abdominal pain, and sleep problems in a community sample of Finnish adolescents. Eur Child Adolesc Psychiatry 2012;21:301–13.

39. Lee YJ, Cho SJ, Cho IH, et al. Insufficient sleep and suicidality in adolescents. Sleep 2012;35:455–60.

40. Pasch KE, Latimer LA, Cance JD, et al. Longitudinal bi-directional relationships between sleep and youth substance use. J Youth Adolesc 2012;41: 1184–96.

41. Arnedt JT, Owens J, Crouch M, et al. Neurobehavioral performance of residents after heavy night call vs after alcohol ingestion. JAMA 2005;294:1025–33.

42. Pack AI, Pack AM, Rodgman E, et al. Characteristics of crashes attributed to the driver having fallen asleep. Accid Anal Prev 1995;27:769–75.

43. Martiniuk ALC, Senserrick T, Lo S, et al. Sleep-deprived young drivers and the risk for crash: the DRIVE prospective cohort study. JAMA Pediatr 2013;167:647–55.

44. Kopasz M, Loessl B, Hornyak M, et al. Sleep and memory in healthy children and adolescents - a critical review. Sleep Med Rev 2010;14:167–77.

45. Dewald JF, Meijer AM, Oort FJ, et al. The influence of sleep quality, sleep duration and sleepiness on school performance in children and adolescents: a meta-analytic review. Sleep Med Rev 2010;14:179–89.

46. Shochat T, Cohen-Zion M, Tzischinsky O. Functional consequences of inadequate sleep in adolescents: a systematic review. Sleep Med Rev 2014;18:75–87.

47. Wolfson AR, Carskadon MA. Sleep schedules and daytime functioning in adolescents. Child Dev 1998;69:875–87.

48. Xu Z, Su H, Zou Y, et al. Sleep quality of Chinese adolescents: distribution and its associated factors. J Paediatr Child Health 2012;48:138–45.

49. Schmidt RE, Van der Linden M. The relations between sleep, personality, behavioral problems, and school performance in adolescents. Sleep Med Clin 2015;10:117–23.

50. American Academy of Sleep Medicine. International classification of sleep disorders. 3rd edition. Darien (IL): American Academy of Sleep Medicine; 2014.

51. Markowitz AJ, Rabow MW. Palliative management of fatigue at the close of life: "it feels like my body is just worn out". JAMA 2007;298(2):217.

52. Ji X, Liu J. Subjective sleep measures for adolescents: a systematic review. Child Care Health Dev 2016 Nov;42:825–39.

53. Spilsbury JC, Drotar D, Rosen CL, et al. The Cleveland adolescent sleepiness questionnaire: a new measure to assess excessive daytime sleepiness in adolescents. J Clin Sleep Med 2007;3:603–12.

54. Moore M, Kirchner HL, Drotar D, et al. Relationships among sleepiness, sleep time, and psychological functioning in adolescents. J Pediatr Psychol 2009;34:1175–83.

55. Drake C, Nickel C, Burduvali E, et al. The pediatric daytime sleepiness scale (PDSS): sleep habits and school outcomes in middle-school children. Sleep 2003;26:455–8.

56. Littner MR, Kushida C, Wise M, et al. Practice parameters for clinical use of the multiple sleep latency test and the maintenance of wakefulness test. Sleep 2005;28:113–21.

57. Ancoli-Israel S, Martin JL, Blackwell T, et al. The SBSM guide to actigraphy monitoring: clinical and research applications. Behav Sleep Med 2015;13(Suppl 1):S4–38.

58. Gibson ES, Powles AP, Thabane L, et al. "Sleepiness" is serious in adolescence: two surveys of 3235 Canadian students. BMC Public Health 2006;6:116–25.

59. Yang CM, Huang YS, Song YC. Clinical utility of the Chinese version of the pediatric daytime sleepiness scale in children with obstructive sleep apnea syndrome and narcolepsy. Psychiatry Clin Neurosci 2010;64:134–40.

60. Mindell JA, Owens JA. A clinical guide to pediatric sleep: diagnosis and management of sleep problems. Philadelphia: Wolters Kluwer/Lippincott Williams & Wilkins; 2015.

61. Hazama GI, Inoue Y, Kojima K, et al. The prevalence of probable delayed-sleep-phase syndrome in students from junior high school to university in Tottori, Japan. Tohoku J Exp Med 2008;216:95–8.

62. Hoban TF, Chervin RD. Assessment of sleepiness in children. Semin Pediatr Neurol 2001;8:216–28.

63. Saxvig IW, Pallesen S, Wilhelmsen-Langeland A, et al. Prevalence and correlates of delayed sleep phase in high school students. Sleep Med 2012;13:193–9.

64. Sivertsen B, Pallesen S, Stormark KM, et al. Delayed sleep phase syndrome in adolescents: prevalence and correlates in a large population based study. BMC Public Health 2013;13:1163.

65. Ohayon MM, Roberts RE, Zulley J, et al. Prevalence and patterns of problematic sleep among older adolescents. J Am Acad Child Adolesc Psychiatry 2000;39:1549–56.

66. Shirayama M, Shirayama Y, Iida H, et al. The psychological aspects of patients with delayed sleep phase syndrome (DSPS). Sleep Med 2003;4:427–33.

67. Abbott SM, Reid KJ, Zee PC. Circadian rhythm sleep-wake disorders. Psychiatr Clin North Am 2015;38:805–23.

68. Morgenthaler T, Alessi C, Friedman L, et al. Practice parameters for the use of actigraphy in the assessment of sleep and sleep disorders: an update for 2007. Sleep 2007;30:519–29.

69. Sack RL, Auckley D, Auger RR, et al. Circadian rhythm sleep disorders: part I, basic principles, shift work and jet lag disorders. An American Academy of Sleep Medicine Review. Sleep 2007;30:1460–83.

70. Wise MS. Childhood narcolepsy. Neurology 1998;50:S37–42.

71. Guilleminault C, Pelayo R. Narcolepsy in prepubertal children. Ann Neurol 1998;43:135–42.

72. Kotagal S. Narcolepsy in children. Semin Pediatr Neurol 1996;3:36–43.

73. Narcolepsy KS. In: Sheldon SH, Ferber R, Kryger MH, et al, editors. Principles and practice of pediatric sleep medicine. 2nd edition. New York: Elsevier Saunders; 2014. p. 143. Available at: https://www.elsevier.com/books/principles-and-practice-of-pediatric-sleep-medicine/sheldon/978-1-4557-0318-0.

74. Carroll JL, Loughlin GM. Obstructive sleep apnea syndrome in infants and children: clinical features and pathophysiology. In: Ferber R, Kryger M, editors. Principles and practice of sleep medicine in the child. Philadelphia: WB Saunders; 1995. p. 163.

75. Billiard M, Merle C, Carlander B, et al. Idiopathic hypersomnia. Psychiatry Clin Neurosci 1998;52:125–9.

76. Young TJ, Silber MH. Hypersomnias of central origin. Chest 2006;130:913–20.

77. Arnulf I, Zeitzer JM, File J, et al. Kleine-Levin syndrome: a systematic review of 186 cases in the literature. Brain 2005;128:2763–76.

78. Marcus CL, Brooks LJ, Draper KA, et al. Diagnosis and management of childhood obstructive sleep apnea syndrome. Pediatrics 2012;130:576–84.

79. Picchietti MA, Picchietti DL. Restless legs syndrome and periodic limb movement disorder in children and adolescents. Semin Pediatr Neurol 2008;15:91–9.

80. Picchietti DL, Stevens HE. Early manifestations of restless legs syndrome in childhood and adolescence. Sleep Med 2008;9:770–81.

81. Picchietti DL, Rajendran RR, Wilson MP, et al. Pediatric restless legs syndrome and periodic limb movement disorder: parent-child pairs. Sleep Med 2009;10:925–31.

82. Picchietti D, Allen RP, Walters AS, et al. Restless legs syndrome: prevalence and impact in children and adolescents–the Peds REST study. Pediatrics 2007;120:253–66.

83. Yilmaz K, Kilincaslan A, Aydin N, et al. Prevalence and correlates of restless legs syndrome in adolescents. Dev Med Child Neurol 2011;53:40–7.

84. Turkdogan D, Bekiroglu N, Zaimoglu S. A prevalence study of restless legs syndrome in Turkish children and adolescents. Sleep Med 2011;12:315–21.

85. Zhang J, Lam SP, Li SX, et al. Restless legs symptoms in adolescents: epidemiology, heritability, and pubertal effects. J Psychosom Res 2014;76:158–64.

86. Xue R, Liu G, Ma S, et al. An epidemiologic study of restless legs syndrome among Chinese children and adolescents. Neurol Sci 2015;36:971–6.

87. Walters AS, Hickey K, Maltzman J, et al. A questionnaire study of 138 patients with restless legs syndrome: the 'night-walkers' survey. Neurology 1996;46:92–5.

88. Whittom S, Dauvilliers Y, Pennestri MH, et al. Age-at-onset in restless legs syndrome: a clinical and polysomnographic study. Sleep Med 2007;9:54–9.

89. Montplaisir J, Boucher S, Poirier G, et al. Clinical, polysomnographic, and genetic characteristics of restless legs syndrome: a study of 133 patients diagnosed with new standard criteria. Mov Disord 1997;12:61–5.

90. Ohayon MM, O'Hara R, Vitiello MV. Epidemiology of restless legs syndrome: a synthesis of the literature. Sleep Med Rev 2012;16:283–95.

91. Picchietti DL, Walters AS. Moderate to severe periodic limb movement disorder in childhood and adolescence. Sleep 1999;22:297–300.

92. Calamaro CJ, Mason TB, Ratcliffe SJ. Adolescents living the 24/7 lifestyle: effects of caffeine and technology on sleep duration and daytime functioning. Pediatrics 2009;123:e1005–10.

93. Cain N, Gradisar M. Electronic media use and sleep in school-aged children and adolescents: a review. Sleep Med 2010;11:735–42.

94. Fossum IN, Nordnes LT, Storemark SS, et al. The association between use of electronic media in bed before going to sleep and insomnia symptoms, daytime sleepiness, morningness, and chronotype. Behav Sleep Med 2014;12:343–57.

95. Grønli J, Byrkjedal IK, Bjorvatn B, et al. Reading from an iPad or from a book in bed: the impact on human sleep. A randomized controlled cross-over trial. Sleep Med 2016;21:86–92.

96. Turton P, Piché L, Battram DS. Adolescent attitudes and beliefs regarding caffeine and the consumption of caffeinated beverages. J Nutr Educ Behav 2016;48:181–9.e1.

97. Chou KH, Bell LN. Caffeine content of prepackaged national-brand and private-label carbonated beverages. J Food Sci 2007;72:C337–42.

98. Ahluwalia N, Herrick K. Caffeine intake from food and beverage sources and trends among children and adolescents in the United States: review of national quantitative studies from 1999 to 2011. Adv Nutr 2015;6:102–11.

99. Hansen M, Janssen I, Schiff A, et al. The impact of school daily schedule on adolescent sleep. Pediatrics 2005;115:1555–61.

100. Short MA, Gradisar M, Lack LC, et al. A cross-cultural comparison of sleep duration between US and Australian adolescents: the effect of school start time, parent-set bedtimes, and extracurricular load. Health Educ Behav 2013; 40:323–30.

101. Wolfson AR, Spaulding NL, Dandrow C, et al. Middle school start times: the importance of a good night's sleep for young adolescents. Behav Sleep Med 2007;5:194–209.

102. Meijer AM, Reitz E, Dekovi· M. Parenting matters: a longitudinal study into parenting and adolescent sleep. J Sleep Res 2016;25:556–64.

103. Short MA, Gradisar M, Wright H, et al. Time for bed: parent-set bedtimes associated with improved sleep and daytime functioning in adolescents. Sleep 2011;34:797–800.

104. Radosevic-Vidacek B, Koscec A. Shiftworking families: parents' working schedule and sleep patterns of adolescents attending school in two shifts. Rev Saude Publica 2004;38(Suppl):38–46.

105. Jiang Y, Chen W, Spruyt K, et al. Bed-sharing and related factors in early adolescents. Sleep Med 2016;17:75–80.

106. Sheldon SH, Spire JP, Levy HB. Disorders of excessive somnolence. In: Sheldon SH, Spire JP, Levy HB, editors. Pediatric sleep medicine. Philadelphia: WB Saunders; 1992. p. 91.

107. Owens JA. Pharmacology of sleep. In: Sheldon SH, Ferber R, Kryger MH, et al, editors. Principles and practice of pediatric sleep medicine. 2nd edition. New York: Elsevier Saunders; 2014. p. 53.

108. Cain N, Gradisar M, Moseley L. A motivational school-based intervention for adolescent sleep problems. Sleep Med 2011;12:246–51.

109. Dagan Y, Stein D, Steinbock M, et al. Frequency of delayed sleep phase syndrome among hospitalized adolescent psychiatric patients. J Psychosom Res 1998;45:15–20.

110. Millman RP, Working Group on Sleepiness in Adolescents/Young Adults, AAP Committee on Adolescence. Excessive sleepiness in adolescents and young adults: causes, consequences, and treatment strategies. Pediatrics 2005;115:1774–86.

111. Moseley L, Gradisar M. Evaluation of a school-based intervention for adolescent sleep problems. Sleep 2009;32:334–41.

112. Cortesi F, Giannotti F, Sebastiani T, et al. Knowledge of sleep in Italian high school students: pilot-test of a school-based sleep educational program. J Adolesc Health 2004; 34:344–51.

113. Tamura N, Tanaka H. Effects of a sleep education program with self-help treatment on sleeping patterns and daytime sleepiness in Japanese adolescents: a cluster randomized trial. Chronobiol Int 2016;33:1073–85.

114. John B, Bellipady SS, Bhat SU. Sleep promotion program for improving sleep behaviors in adolescents: a randomized controlled pilot study. Scientifica (Cairo) 2016;2016:8013431.

115. Millman RP, Boergers J, Owens J. Healthy school start times: can we do a better job in reaching our goals? Sleep 2016;39:267–8.

116. Wahlstrom K. Changing times: findings from the first longitudinal study of later high school start times. Sleep 2002;86:3–21.

117. Thacher PV, Onyper SV. Longitudinal outcomes of start time delay on sleep, behavior, and achievement in high school. Sleep 2016;39(2): 271–81.

Sleepiness in the Elderly

Dora Zalai, MD[a], Arina Bingeliene, MD[b],
Colin Shapiro, MBBCh, MRC Psych, FRCP (C), PhD[b],*

KEYWORDS

• Excessive daytime sleepiness • Older adults • Elderly

KEY POINTS

- Excessive daytime sleepiness is a pathologic condition in the elderly.
- Excessive daytime sleepiness is associated with sleep and mood disorders, soporific medications, various medical conditions, and cognitive decline.
- Older adults tend to underreport excessive daytime sleepiness.
- Assessment of sleepiness in older adults may require collateral information and multiple methods.
- Management of underlying causes is pertinent; direct interventions to address sleepiness may be necessary.

INTRODUCTION

There was a time when sleep disorders were simply classified as "those that sleep too little" (insomnia); "those that sleep too much" (hypersomnia); "those that have body clock problems" (circadian sleep issues); and "the things that go bump in the night" (parasomnias). Ironically, any of the 4 above described groups can be associated with excessive daytime sleepiness (EDS). The pertinence is that patients do not present saying, for example, that "I think I have sleep apnea or narcolepsy." It is therefore up to the clinician to try to discern what the most "culpable" reason is and to treat it. There is often clear evidence of a major sleep disorder such as narcolepsy, or of a well-recognizable behavioral pattern such as a restricted time spent in bed. However, hypersomnolence/excessive sleepiness can be multifactorial, and this is particularly the case in the elderly, making both the diagnosis and the management of EDS in the elderly a "chess challenge" at a higher level. The challenge being that there are often more moving parts in the causality (eg, polypharmacy or cooccurring medical conditions and specific sleep disorders, including some that may be triggered by medications). The potential of finding a single or clear solution is less likely and may require investigation beyond the usual range of the armamentarium used in a standard sleep clinic assessment. The additional tests may include the evaluation of melatonin secretion, multiple sleep latency test (MSLT), maintenance of wakefulness test, as well as assessment of mood and cognition.

Finally, one has to appeal for modesty when it comes to treatment of excessive sleepiness in the elderly. As clinicians, we like to provide solutions. There is a narrow gap between being dismissive of problems in the elderly ("it is normal at this age") and proceeding too vigorously with a series of repeatedly failing interventions. The balance is in recognizing that there are many things we possibly still do not know and that should humble us making interventions for which we have a reason, but not to perseverate with many trials of treatment that have no substantial basis. This article describes the still limited understanding of EDS in the elderly and discusses considerations for assessment and management.

Conflict-of-Interest Statement: The authors do not have any conflict of interest with respect to the subject matter or the material discussed.
[a] Department of Psychology, Ryerson University, 790 Bay Street, Toronto, Ontario M5B 2K8, Canada;
[b] Department of Neurology, University Health Network, 399 Bathurst Street, Toronto, Ontario M5T 2S8, Canada
* Corresponding author.
E-mail address: colinshapiro@rogers.com

NORMAL SLEEP IN OLDER ADULTS

Total sleep time, sleep continuity, and sleep architecture change with healthy aging. Total sleep time declines by an average 10 minutes per decade, more in women and less in men,representing a large effect size of aging on sleep duration.[1] Sleep continuity also decreases with aging, because of the increase of both wake after sleep onset (WASO) and sleep onset latency (SOL). Time spent awake during the night lengthens by 10 minutes in every 10 years of life and becomes noticeable from the third decade of age. Increase of SOL is more subtle and becomes noticeable only in older adulthood (greater than 80), when it is 10 minutes longer compared with the SOL of people in their 20s. The above changes in SOL and WASO contribute the decline of sleep efficiency, most prominently from the 40s by 3% per decade. With respect to the composition of sleep, proportions of stage 1 and stage 2 of sleep slowly and gradually increase between the ages of 20 and 70, whereas the percentage of slow wave sleep (SWS) and rapid eye movement (REM) sleep decreases with aging. Although the effect sizes are small for stage 1, stage 2, and moderate for REM sleep, there is a robust decline of SWS with aging.

Because SWS is a marker of the sleep homeostat, the question arises whether diminishing SWS is a sign of declining efficiency of the sleep homeostat to dispense sleep drive during the night or is it simply the result of less accumulation of sleep drive and decreased biological need for deep sleep in older age. If sleep pressure remains high but older adults are unable to produce enough deep sleep at night, they should feel sleepier during the day and/or nap more than younger and middle-aged adults do even if the circadian wake-promoting mechanisms are active. Conversely, if sleep need declines with age, the less efficient and more "shallow" sleep of older adults should be sufficient to maintain normal level of sleepiness, alertness, and cognitive functioning during the day.

Experiments applying extended wakefulness and total sleep deprivation paradigms have shown that older adults are more alert; less sleepy; able to stay awake better; and able to maintain attention and cognitive performance more effectively than younger adults can after sleep deprivation.[2–5] In addition, older adults have normal increase of daytime sleep propensity and normal SWS rebound and increase in slow-wave sleep activity in response to nighttime experimental SWS disruption, suggesting that the sleep homeostasis is intact in old age.[2,6] The circadian distribution of sleep propensity during the daytime hours is similar in older to that in younger adults, providing further support to the observation that healthy older adults are not sleepier during the day than adults of younger age.[7,8]

Collectively, the above findings indicate that sleep in healthy older adults adequately maintains normal daytime sleep propensity and alertness despite the normal, age-related changes in sleep duration, continuity, and architecture. Indeed, epidemiologic studies have shown that the prevalence of EDS and hypersomnolence is similar or even lower in older than in younger and middle-aged adults, confirming that excessive sleepiness and hypersomnia are not normal states in healthy old adulthood.[9–11] Thus, when excessive daytime sleepiness and hypersomnolence are detected in older adults, these conditions should be viewed as warning signals for the presence of pathologic conditions; nonadaptive sleep-specific or daytime behavioral habits; or environmental factors that interfere with normal sleep and wake regulation, sleep quality, and maintenance of wakefulness during the day.

SLEEP, MOOD, AND COGNITIVE CHANGES ASSOCIATED WITH EXCESSIVE DAYTIME SLEEPINESS IN OLDER ADULTS

Chronic medical conditions, including sleep, psychiatric, and neurologic conditions, as well as certain prescribed medications are associated with EDS in older adults (**Fig. 1, Table 1**).[11–13] EDS, increased frequency of napping, or unintentional dozing may be the first or most readily noticeable signal of the presence of an undiagnosed sleep disorder, depression, latent neurodegenerative disorder, or cognitive decline. It is important to note that EDS is not simply a benign risk factor, symptom, or consequence of other condition. EDS independently impairs functioning; interferes with activities of daily living; decreases exercise frequency; increases the risk for falls and cognitive decline; and increases mortality in the elderly.[14–19] Hence, it is crucial to recognize EDS, identify and eliminate the conditions that may contribute to it, or to address EDS directly, if the causes cannot be eliminated.

SLEEP-RELATED FACTORS ASSOCIATED WITH EXCESSIVE DAYTIME SLEEPINESS IN OLDER ADULTS
Sleep-Related Breathing Disorders

The most common sleep disorders associated with EDS in older adults are sleep-related breathing disorders (SRBD). The prevalence of SRBD increases with age and reaches an exceptionally

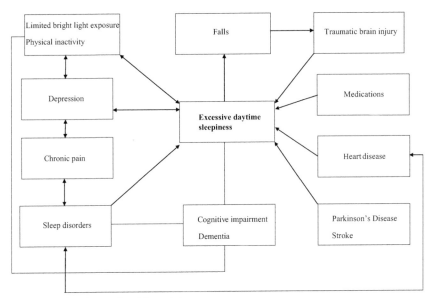

Fig. 1. Factors associated with EDS in older adults.

high (20%–80%) rate in old adulthood.[20–23] There is a weaker association between SRBD and EDS in older than in younger adults, but when EDS is present in the elderly, it should be an alerting sign for a possibly undiagnosed SRBD.[24,25] Moderate and severe sleep apnea (apnea hypopnea index, AHI ≥20) associated with subjective EDS has been found to double the likelihood for all-cause mortality within 14 years in old adults (independently of their sex), whereas sleep apnea or EDS alone was not associated with increased mortality.[26] This finding speaks to idea that the combination of EDS and moderate to severe obstructive sleep apnea (OSA) represents a "deadly phenotype" that, if effectively treated, may increase longevity even when the patients are in their late 70s.[27] The mechanisms that explain the interaction between sleep apnea and EDS with respect to mortality in this age group are not clearly elucidated and may be explained with elevated level of inflammatory factors associated with fatigue, metabolic syndrome, and cardiovascular disorders. It has been shown that the combination of self-reported habitual snoring and subjective EDS (but not snoring or EDS alone) increased the odds of incident cardiovascular events in a cohort of 70- to 79-year-old adults who were followed for an average of 9.9 years.[28] There was a high rate of diabetes mellitus, low high-density lipoprotein cholesterol, and metabolic syndrome in the group of individuals who reported snoring and sleepiness, but the role of these factors in mediating increased risk for cardiovascular events (and possible for mortality) should be further explored.

Advanced Sleep Phase

Under controlled conditions, older adults go to bed on average 1 hour earlier and wake up 1.3 hours earlier than younger adults, showing that there is inherent phase advance of the sleep-wake cycle in older age.[29] This notion has been supported in experiments demonstrating that older adults wake up closer to the nadir of their core body temperature and melatonin crest; have shorter REM latencies close to the falling limb and the initial part of the rising limb of the body temperature rhythm; and have more REM sleep in the nighttime hours of the circadian phase than younger adults do.[7,29] Because older adults wake up early in their circadian phase, the morning light exposure in the early phase of the circadian cycle may cause further phase advance. These changes do not significantly affect the circadian variation of sleep propensity in healthy older people but may be attenuated by a dearth of bright light exposure and diminished melatonin secretion in individuals with dementia and in older adults living in nursing homes.[30–38] The combined effects of intrinsic biological changes in the sleep-wake phase relative to the circadian cycle, minimal exposure to natural light, and lack of regular sleep-wake schedule may lead to the disruption of the circadian rhythm of sleep and wakefulness and manifest as disrupted nighttime sleep and daytime napping in these groups of older adults.

When older adults maintain the bed time and rise time they were accustomed to when they

Table 1
Sedative medications commonly used in the elderly

	Medication	Indication	Common Side Effects
Benzodiazepines	Temazepam Clonazepam Lorazepam Diazepam Alprazolam	Sleep disturbances Anxiety and agitation	Muscle hypotonia Behavioral disturbances Retrograde amnesia, cognitive deficit, drowsiness, clumsiness, slurred speech, and dizziness
Hypnotic agents	Zopiclone Zolpidem	Sleep disturbances	More than double risks of falls and hip fractures due to drowsiness, dizziness Headache Activities such as driving, cooking, or eating while asleep (parasomnia)
Opioid analgesics	Codeine Fentanyl Hydrocodone Hydrocodone/ acetaminophen Hydromorphone Meperidine Methadone	Acute and chronic pain management	Sedation, dizziness Nausea, vomiting, constipation Respiratory depression
Muscle relaxants (centrally acting)	Carisoprodol Cyclobenzaprine Metaxalone	Low back pain, neck pain Fibromyalgia Tension headaches Myofascial pain syndrome	Confusion, drowsiness, dizziness and weakness, fatigue, blurred vision Dry mouth Constipation
Anticholinergics (centrally acting)	Atropine Benzatropine Biperiden Chlorpheniramine Dicyclomine Dimenhydrinate Diphenhydramine	Gastrointestinal disorders Genitourinary disorders Respiratory disorders Insomnia (although usually only on a short-term basis) Dizziness (including vertigo and motion sickness–related symptoms)	Confusion, disorientation, agitation Euphoria or dysphoria Respiratory depression Memory problems, inability to concentrate Wandering thoughts Incoherent speech Irritability Mental confusion (brain fog) Unusual sensitivity to sudden sounds Visual disturbances
Antihistamines	Brompheniramine Cetirizine Chlorpheniramine Clemastine Diphenhydramine Fexofenadine Loratadine	Hay fever Hives, itching, and insect bites and stings May be used to help reduce nausea and vomiting	Dry mouth Drowsiness, dizziness Nausea and vomiting Restlessness or moodiness (in some children) Dysuria Blurred vision Confusion
Antiemetics	Cyclizine Diphenhydramine Dimenhydrinate Ondansetron Domperidone Metoclopramide	Nausea and vomiting	Drowsiness Dizziness Constipation or diarrhea Dry mouth Fatigue

(continued on next page)

Table 1
(continued)

	Medication	Indication	Common Side Effects
Antipsychotics	Quetiapine Olanzapine Clozapine Risperidone Haloperidol Aripiprazole	Psychosis Bipolar mood disorder	Blurred vision Dry mouth Drowsiness, sedation Muscle spasms or tremors (extrapyramidal symptoms) Weight gain Metabolic syndrome Hypotension Anticholinergic effects Sexual dysfunction Cardiac arrhythmias
	Gabapentin	Chronic pain, mood stabilizer	Sleepiness, dizziness, fatigue Clumsiness while walking Visual changes, including double vision Tremor Weight gain
	Pregabalin	Chronic pain Fibromyalgia Mood stabilizer	Ataxia, blurred vision Dizziness, drowsiness, fatigue, headache Peripheral edema Tremor Weight gain Visual field loss
Anticonvulsants	Carbamazepine	Antiseizure medication Trigeminal neuralgia	Dizziness, drowsiness Nausea, vomiting Dry mouth, swollen tongue
	Valproate	Antiepileptic drug Mood stabilizer Migraines	Somnolence Elevated liver enzymes Mild drowsiness or weakness Diarrhea, constipation, upset stomach

Antidepressants	Amitriptyline	Sleep disturbances
		Depression
		Chronic pain
			Drowsiness
			Constipation, diarrhea,
			  nausea, vomiting, upset
			  stomach; unusual taste,
			  appetite, or weight changes
			Dysuria
			Decreased libido/impotence

	Trazodone	Mood disorder	Headache
			Nausea, vomiting, loss of
			  appetite
			Constipation or diarrhea
			Decreased libido, erectile
			  dysfunction
			Dizziness
			Dry mouth or dry eyes
			Numbness, burning, or
			  tingling sensations

	Mirtazapine	Mood disorder	Drowsiness, dizziness Vision changes Dry mouth Constipation Increased appetite/weight gain

(continued on next page)

Table 1
(continued)

	Medication	Indication	Common Side Effects
Antihypertensive medications	Alpha-blockers	Hypertension Benign prostatic hyperplasia Nightmares	Hypotension Dizziness Heart fibrillation, chest pain
	Beta-blockers	Hypertension Cardiac arrhythmias	Fatigue Dizziness Headache Constipation, diarrhea Shortness of breath
Drugs for Parkinson disease	Sinemet	Parkinson disease Parkinsonism	Involuntary body movements, confusion, nausea, hallucinations
	Selegiline		Dizziness, abdominal pain, dry mouth, nausea, stomach upset, trouble sleeping, and headache
	Levodopa/ Carbidopa		Mild nausea, dry mouth, loss of appetite, heartburn, diarrhea, constipation Headache Dizziness, drowsiness, blurred vision Cold symptoms Insomnia Muscle pain, numbness, or tingly feeling
	Pramipexole		Dry mouth, stomach pain, vomiting, constipation, appetite or weight changes Headache, dizziness, spinning sensation, mild drowsiness, blurred vision Insomnia, unusual dreams Amnesia, forgetfulness, thinking problems
	Bromocriptine		Dizziness, mild drowsiness, fatigue Mild headache Depressed mood Insomnia Dry mouth Upset stomach, nausea, vomiting, stomach pain, loss of appetite, diarrhea, constipation

were younger, they may experience insomnia due to extended time in bed in the morning after their final awakening, sleep deprivation due to the relatively late bed time, and consequently, daytime sleepiness. It is important to note that older adults with insomnia tend to misperceive short daytime naps as wakefulness, which may result in the underestimation of subjective daytime sleepiness in this group.[39]

Depression and Excessive Daytime Sleepiness in the Elderly

EDS and hypersomnolence have been found to be associated with depressive symptoms in older adults in both cross-sectional and longitudinal studies. In the largest prospective study ($N = 3824$) measuring the association between EDS and depression in older adults, EDS was more strongly associated with incidence depression symptoms than insomnia was.[40] Furthermore, EDS was significantly associated with depression symptoms at both shorter- (2 years) and longer-term (4 years) follow-up, whereas insomnia was significantly associated with self-reported depression symptoms only at the final follow-up assessment. It is important to note that subjective measures (eg, the Epworth Sleepiness Scale, ESS) capture sleepiness better than objective measures of sleep propensity (ie, MSLT) in adults with mood disorders, and only subjective sleepiness (as opposed to sleep propensity measured by the MSLT) is associated longitudinally with depression.[41,42]

Late-onset depression is underdiagnosed, in part because the clinical presentation is more subtle; depressed mood, guilt, and suicidal ideation are less prevalent, whereas somatic symptoms are more likely endorsed in late-onset than in early-onset depression. Thus, when older adults report subjective EDS, the assessment of depression symptoms, using tools validated for this age group, is warranted.

Excessive Daytime Sleepiness and Cognitive Decline

According to cross-sectional, population-based studies, EDS is associated with cognitive impairment in older adults.[43,44] Longitudinal studies have also demonstrated that older adults with EDS are more likely to develop dementia than those without EDS. For example, in a cohort of 2346 older Japanese men without dementia (Honolulu Asian Aging Study), EDS at baseline indicated a 2-fold risk for development of dementia within 3 years.[18] Consistent findings emerged from the French, "Three City Study" (N = 4894), that involved older adults of both sexes and had a longer (8-year) follow-up period.[19] This study revealed a 30% increased risk for global cognitive decline in older adults with EDS who developed dementia during follow-up. Similarly to the findings of the Honolulu Asian Aging Study, EDS emerged as a risk factor independently of depression and other potential confounding factors.

The mechanism linking EDS to dementia is unknown. One can speculate that SRBD could contribute to the observed relationship between EDS and cognitive decline. It is well established that OSA is associated with cognitive changes, including poor attention/working memory, executive functions, and verbal memory (in particular, immediate and delayed recall) compared with healthy controls.[45–53]

Recent, large-scale longitudinal studies also revealed that SRBD predicts cognitive decline.

The first prospective study on SDBS and cognitive impairment followed close to 300 older women (mean age = 82.3 years) for 5 years. The women with SRBD (AHI >15) at baseline were more likely to develop mild cognitive impairment and dementia (odds ratio, OR = 2.36) after adjustment of relevant demographic, medical, and lifestyle factors as well as of baseline cognitive performance.[54] In a more recent Taiwanese nationwide study using the health insurance data of more than 1400 individuals (both sexes, older than 40, newly diagnosed OSA), an increased risk for dementia (hazard ratio = 1.44) was shown over a 5-year period compared with controls, after adjustment for relevant comorbidities. Only Alzheimer disease and vascular dementia diagnoses were made; the risk was increased only for vascular dementia.[55] In keeping with these findings, sleep apnea was associated with a 2-fold likelihood of developing vascular (but not Alzheimer) dementia in a cohort of Welsh elderly in a decade following the baseline sleep assessment. Importantly, this study also collected information about subjective EDS and found a strong relationship (OR = 4.4) between EDS and vascular dementia.

Because none of the longitudinal studies concerning the relationship between EDS and dementia has examined the role of SRBD, the possible effect of SRBD on the relationship between EDS and cognitive decline remains to be elucidated.

In addition to SRBD, neuropathologic processes affecting the brain areas responsible for sleep-wake regulation could also explain the relationship between EDS and cognitive decline in individuals who subsequently develop dementia. Indeed, EDS is common among adults with neurodegenerative disorders and is associated with poor cognitive performance. For example, 16% to 74% of patients with Parkinson disease suffer from subjective EDS, whereas approximately 50% of patients have objective EDS based on MSLT.[56,57] In Parkinson disease, EDS has been associated with dementia in both prospective and cross-sectional observational studies, and the prevalence of EDS in Parkinson disease increases over time in tandem with the cognitive decline.[58–61]

EDS is more common among individuals with Parkinson disease and Lewy body disease than in people with Alzheimer disease, suggesting that EDS may be partly related to the disease process than to dementia per se.[58] The neuropathologic changes in Parkinson disease involve the neuronal networks and transmitter systems involved in sleep homeostasis (locus coeruleus, pedunculopontine nucleus, dorsal raphe nucleus, and the lateral hypothalamus) from the prodromal stages of the disease. Because the cell abnormality in these brain regions precedes the critical the cell loss in the substantia nigra, EDS often predates the onset of motor symptoms of Parkinson disease.[43]

EDS is also a common daytime symptom of parasomnias, for example, REM behavioral disorder (RBD). RBD traditionally has been regarded as a rare, usually benign, idiopathic sleep disorder in middle-aged men, or as a side effect of antidepressant medications. There has been a major shift in the perception of the clinical significance of RBD recently, because longitudinal studies have shown that 70% to 80% of those with RBD develop a Lewy body disease (Parkinson's disease [PD], dementia with Lewy bodies, or multiple system atrophy) within 10 to 20 years.[62–65] As RBD is rare in the general population, and the conversion rate to the above neurodegenerative disorders is high, RBD in combination with other prodromal PD symptoms is considered to be the most specific potential biomarker of prodromal Parkinson disease.[66]

Because the motor symptoms are salient and quintessential for diagnosis, it is less appreciated that approximately 20% to 40% of individuals with Parkinson disease also have mild cognitive impairment by the time they receive the diagnosis. Given the association between EDS and cognitive decline in Parkinson disease, EDS may be an important warning sign for a presence of subtle cognitive changes in the prodromal stage of the disease. Given that there is a quest for interventions that could slow the cognitive decline or ease the burden of cognitive impairment in Parkinson disease, the potential relationship between EDS and cognition in the context of Parkinson disease is a pertinent topic to explore.

ASSESSMENT OF EXCESSIVE DAYTIME SLEEPINESS IN OLDER ADULTS

In an ideal situation, assessment of EDS in older adults involves multiple methods and sources of information about sleepiness and sleep propensity. A clinical interview should include questions about the nighttime sleep as well as frequency, duration, and diurnal pattern of subjective sleepiness, intended naps, and unintended "sleep attacks." Napping in older adults occurs both during the day and in the evening.[67] It is important to keep in mind that evening naps (within 2 hours before bed time) are characteristic of old age and specifically should be enquired about.[68] Self-report tools, for example, the ESS have been widely used in both clinical practice and research to assess EDS in the elderly. The ESS has yielded high response rates in large research studies, implying the older adults are able to complete this assessment tool. Nevertheless, there has been a concern about difficulties that independently living older adults and their caregivers may face when completing the ESS, especially in cultures where certain items (eg, the ones related to commuting with a car) are less applicable to this age group.[69]

Importantly, older adults tend to underreport sleepiness and napping compared with information obtained from collateral reports and objective assessment.[39,67,69] For example, when sleep propensity was assessed using self-report and information obtained from caregivers, older adults consistently had lower scores (on average by 2.8 points) on the ESS than what their caregivers assigned to them.[69] Twenty percent of older adults whose self-report score was below the cut-off for EDS were identified as excessively sleepy by the caregivers. Older age and poorer cognition accounted for the difference between these discrepancies. Older adults also tend to underreport naps, particularly evening naps, on sleep diaries compared with actigraphy and polysomnography (PSG) recordings. Furthermore, older adults with mild insomnia misperceive daytime sleep (measured by MSLT) as wakefulness, especially when the naps are short and have short N2 and N3 periods.[39] These individuals also have lower ESS scores than those who are aware of dozing off during the MSLT, suggesting that they generally underestimate their level of sleepiness and sleep propensity. Those with lower global cognitive performance and less severe insomnia more likely underperceive their naps.

In the light of the above, it is advisable to collect collateral information about sleep propensity and evening naps as part of the EDS assessment in older adults. Objective assessment tools are invaluable when collateral information is not available and when subjective reports have limited validity due to impaired cognition. Actigraphy can be used to record sleep and circadian rhythm patterns in community-dwelling healthy older adults and is recommended for the diagnosis when advanced sleep phase syndrome contributes to evening naps and early morning awakenings.[70] It also provides useful information about sleep patterns of older people living in nursing homes. In addition, actigraphy can be used to establish if the patient has adequate sleep pattern and duration before an MSLT is conducted.

PSG is recommended for older adults with EDS to obtain information about SRBD and other sleep disorders that can be detected primarily with PSG. If the patient reports symptoms of narcolepsy, the PSG should be followed by an MSLT. Given the association between EDS and depression in older adults, it is recommended that the sleep assessment is complemented with an assessment of depression symptoms, using assessment tools validated in this age group. It is also pertinent to obtain information about cognitive functioning and arrange formal cognitive assessment, especially if the EDS does not respond to treatment. When evaluating the risk for depression or cognitive decline, one has to remember that subjective sleepiness is more informative than sleep propensity measured with the MSLT.

TREATMENT CONSIDERATIONS OF EXCESSIVE DAYTIME SLEEPINESS IN OLDER ADULTS

The general principles of management of EDS in the elderly is "the same but different" to that of managing the EDS in young adults. It is the same in the sense that one needs to identify the cause irrespective of age, but it is different in the sense that in older adults EDS is much more likely to be multifaceted, because of associated medical conditions and the pharmacologic treatment of those conditions in part contributing to the sleepiness. It is therefore often necessary to undertake a review of all aspects of the older patients' health and of the treatments they receive. It is common that there are other physicians involved in the patients' care, and they may need to be consulted. As was alluded to in the introduction, one may need to test 3 or 4 interventions before one has a resolution of the complaint of EDS in the elderly.

The interventions often will be behavioral as well as pharmacologic. Daily, regular exposure to external cues (bright light, regular meals, social activities) that entrain the circadian system is imperative to maintain normal circadian phase, decrease EDS, and improve sleep in older adults with and without dementia.[71–73]

Older adults with EDS often attribute their sleepiness to getting an inadequate amount of sleep during the night. They explain their sleepiness with reduced amount of sleep, rather than with low sleep quality because they are more cognizant of a relatively small decrease in sleep duration than to the much more dramatic decline in proposition of deep sleep. Many older adults who complain of "not getting enough sleep" will quickly change their tune when asked if "more" or "better-quality" sleep is what they seek. Simple, nonpharmacologic interventions, for example, regular, light exercise, have been shown to increase the proportion of slow-wave sleep and improve cognition in this age group.[74,75]

Evening light exposure has been shown to be an efficacious, optional therapy for older adults with advanced sleep phase syndrome.[76] When EDS is associated with insomnia, the first treatment choice is cognitive behavioral therapy.[77] This treatment is as effective in older as in younger adults and not only alleviates insomnia but also improves the mood and the quality of life of the elderly.[78–80]

With respect to pharmacologic interventions, a first step can be to taper off soporific medications and substitute these with ones that do not cause sleepiness or to change to medications that increase alertness. A simple example may be switching from a beta-blocker for hypertension that is highly lipophilic to one that is not (and therefore less likely to cause central effects of sleepiness while having the same antihypertensive effects). There are specific agents that include a stimulant component that may be substituted for an agent that does not have a stimulant component. For example, the underutilized benefit of selegiline hydrochloride (morning and midday) rather than a more sedating dopaminergic agonist for restless legs syndrome or periodic leg movement disorder can help with alleviating sleepiness in these conditions.

When sleepiness presents in the context of depression, it may be caused by the mood disorder per se; it may be the side effect of sedentary antidepressants; or it may be that the antidepressant medication disrupts sleep quality (ie, it suppresses REM sleep, increases arousal rate, or suppresses SWS), resulting in nonrestorative sleep and EDS. This effect can have a delayed onset, because the metabolite of the antidepressant could be more sleep disruptive than the parent compound. In a sleepy individual, fluoxetine in the morning may be a specifically useful treatment approach for depression. Conversely, mirtazapine taken 2 to 3 hours before bed time may be the best treatment choice in a person with multiple brief arousals across the night, because this medication been shown to consolidate sleep and decrease daytime sleepiness based on MSLT measures.[81]

The treatment of sleep disorders, discontinuing soporific medications, changing class of dopaminergic medications, prescribing psychostimulants or melatonin, has been suggested for the management of EDS in Parkinson disease.[82] It has been less emphasized that the pharmacologic management of EDS can be complemented with nonpharmacologic interventions, in particular, maintaining a regular activity routine, introducing regular physical activity, restricting daytime napping, and scheduling bright light exposure. An advantage of the behavioral strategies is that these interventions also effectively lift depression, which also might benefit both sleep and cognition.[83–86]

Although it is generally presumed that treatment of sleep apnea with continuous positive airway pressure therapy will invariably lead to a resolution of the sleepiness in patients with OSA, evidence from large studies suggests that a significant proportion (10%–65%) of patients suffer from ongoing sleepiness.[87] The use of an alertness-enhancing agent such as modafinil in this population is probably grossly underutilized. However, caution should be taken when prescribing modafinil to adults older than 65, because of limited evidence concerning its efficacy and side effects and because the elimination of the drug and its metabolites may be slow in this age group. It is recommended starting at a low (ie, 100 mg) single dose in the morning, while closely monitoring side effects.

SUMMARY

EDS has pathologic causes and numerous adverse consequences, and therefore, it requires medical attention in older adults. Excessive sleepiness in older adults is often multifactorial and may signal an underlying sleep disorder, chronic medical condition, undiagnosed mood disorder, or side effects of medications. Furthermore, it is associated with increased risk for cognitive decline and dementia in the elderly. Excessive sleepiness often requires a multi-method assessment in this age group. It is pertinent to take a systematic, step-by-step treatment approach geared toward the underlying cause and to treat sleepiness directly, when the cause cannot be eliminated in order to prevent adverse outcomes.

REFERENCES

1. Ohayon MM, Carskadon MA, Guilleminault C, et al. Meta-analysis of quantitative sleep parameters from childhood to old age in healthy individuals: developing normative sleep values across the human lifespan. Sleep 2004;27(7):1255–73.
2. Dijk DJ, Groeger JA, Stanley N, et al. Age-related reduction in daytime sleep propensity and nocturnal slow wave sleep. Sleep 2010;33(2):211–23.
3. Duffy JF, Willson HJ, Wang W, et al. Healthy older adults better tolerate sleep deprivation than young adults. J Am Geriatr Soc 2009;57(7):1245–51.
4. Buysse DJ, Monk TH, Reynolds CF 3rd, et al. Patterns of sleep episodes in young and elderly adults during a 36-hour constant routine. Sleep 1993;16(7): 632–7.
5. Reynolds CF 3rd, Jennings JR, Hoch CC, et al. Daytime sleepiness in the healthy "old old": a comparison with young adults. J Am Geriatr Soc 1991; 39(10):957–62.
6. Bonnet MH. Effect of 64 hours of sleep deprivation upon sleep in geriatric normals and insomniacs. Neurobiol Aging 1986;7(2):89–96.
7. Dijk DJ, Duffy JF, Riel E, et al. Ageing and the circadian and homeostatic regulation of human sleep during forced desynchrony of rest, melatonin and temperature rhythms. J Physiol 1999;516(Pt 2): 611–27.
8. Haimov I, Lavie P. Circadian characteristics of sleep propensity function in healthy elderly: a comparison with young adults. Sleep 1997;20(4):294–300.
9. Hara C, Lopes Rocha F, Lima-Costa MF. Prevalence of excessive daytime sleepiness and associated factors in a Brazilian community: the Bambui study. Sleep Med 2004;5(1):31–6.
10. Bixler EO, Vgontzas AN, Lin HM, et al. Excessive daytime sleepiness in a general population sample: the role of sleep apnea, age, obesity, diabetes, and depression. J Clin Endocrinol Metab 2005;90(8):4510–5.
11. Ohayon MM. Determining the level of sleepiness in the American population and its correlates. J Psychiatr Res 2012;46(4):422–7.
12. Pack AI, Dinges DF, Gehrman PR, et al. Risk factors for excessive sleepiness in older adults. Ann Neurol 2006;59(6):893–904.
13. Whitney CW, Enright PL, Newman AB, et al. Correlates of daytime sleepiness in 4578 elderly persons: the Cardiovascular Health Study. Sleep 1998;21(1): 27–36.
14. Hayley AC, Williams LJ, Kennedy GA, et al. Excessive daytime sleepiness and falls among older men and women: cross-sectional examination of a population-based sample. BMC Geriatr 2015;15:74.
15. Gooneratne NS, Weaver TE, Cater JR, et al. Functional outcomes of excessive daytime sleepiness in older adults. J Am Geriatr Soc 2003;51(5):642–9.
16. Chasens ER, Sereika SM, Weaver TE, et al. Daytime sleepiness, exercise, and physical function in older adults. J Sleep Res 2007;16(1):60–5.
17. Wu S, Wang R, Ma X, et al. Excessive daytime sleepiness assessed by the Epworth Sleepiness Scale and its association with health related quality of life: a population-based study in China. BMC Public Health 2012;12:849.
18. Foley D, Monjan A, Masaki K, et al. Daytime sleepiness is associated with 3-year incident dementia and cognitive decline in older Japanese-American men. J Am Geriatr Soc 2001;49(12):1628–32.
19. Jaussent I, Bouyer J, Ancelin ML, et al. Excessive sleepiness is predictive of cognitive decline in the elderly. Sleep 2012;35(9):1201–7.
20. Ancoli-Israel S, Kripke DF, Klauber MR, et al. Sleep-disordered breathing in community-dwelling elderly. Sleep 1991;14(6):486–95.
21. Young T, Shahar E, Nieto FJ, et al. Predictors of sleep-disordered breathing in community-dwelling adults: the Sleep Heart Health Study. Arch Intern Med 2002;162(8):893–900.
22. Hoch CC, Reynolds CF 3rd, Monk TH, et al. Comparison of sleep-disordered breathing among healthy

elderly in the seventh, eighth, and ninth decades of life. Sleep 1990;13(6):502–11.

23. Bixler EO, Vgontzas AN, Ten Have T, et al. Effects of age on sleep apnea in men: I. Prevalence and severity. Am J Respir Crit Care Med 1998;157(1):144–8.

24. Morrell MJ, Finn L, McMillan A, et al. Aging reduces the association between sleepiness and sleep disordered breathing. Eur Respir J 2012;40(2):386–93.

25. Sforza E, Pichot V, Martin MS, et al. Prevalence and determinants of subjective sleepiness in healthy elderly with unrecognized obstructive sleep apnea. Sleep Med 2015;16(8):981–6.

26. Gooneratne NS, Richards KC, Joffe M, et al. Sleep disordered breathing with excessive daytime sleepiness is a risk factor for mortality in older adults. Sleep 2011;34(4):435–42.

27. Mokhlesi B, Pamidi S, Yaggi HK. Sleep disordered breathing and subjective sleepiness in the elderly: a deadly combination? Sleep 2011;34(4):413–5.

28. Endeshaw Y, Rice TB, Schwartz AV, et al. Snoring, daytime sleepiness, and incident cardiovascular disease in the health, aging, and body composition study. Sleep 2013;36(11):1737–45.

29. Duffy JF, Dijk DJ, Klerman EB, et al. Later endogenous circadian temperature nadir relative to an earlier wake time in older people. Am J Physiol 1998;275(5 Pt 2):R1478–87.

30. Jacobs D, Ancoli-Israel S, Parker L, et al. Twenty-four-hour sleep-wake patterns in a nursing home population. Psychol Aging 1989;4(3):352–6.

31. Pat-Horenczyk R, Klauber MR, Shochat T, et al. Hourly profiles of sleep and wakefulness in severely versus mild-moderately demented nursing home patients. Aging (Milano) 1998;10(4):308–15.

32. Ancoli-Israel S, Klauber MR, Jones DW, et al. Variations in circadian rhythms of activity, sleep, and light exposure related to dementia in nursing-home patients. Sleep 1997;20(1):18–23.

33. Campbell SS, Kripke DF, Gillin JC, et al. Exposure to light in healthy elderly subjects and Alzheimer's patients. Physiol Behav 1988;42(2):141–4.

34. Shochat T, Martin J, Marler M, et al. Illumination levels in nursing home patients: effects on sleep and activity rhythms. J Sleep Res 2000;9(4):373–9.

35. Bordet R, Devos D, Brique S, et al. Study of circadian melatonin secretion pattern at different stages of Parkinson's disease. Clin Neuropharmacol 2003; 26(2):65–72.

36. Skene DJ, Swaab DF. Melatonin rhythmicity: effect of age and Alzheimer's disease. Exp Gerontol 2003; 38(1–2):199–206.

37. Harper DG, Volicer L, Stopa EG, et al. Disturbance of endogenous circadian rhythm in aging and Alzheimer disease. Am J Geriatr Psychiatry 2005; 13(5):359–68.

38. Harper DG, Stopa EG, McKee AC, et al. Differential circadian rhythm disturbances in men with

Alzheimer disease and frontotemporal degeneration. Arch Gen Psychiatry 2001;58(4):353–60.

39. Nguyen-Michel VH, Levy PP, Pallanca O, et al. Underperception of naps in older adults referred for a sleep assessment: an insomnia trait and a cognitive problem? J Am Geriatr Soc 2015;63(10): 2001–7.

40. Jaussent I, Bouyer J, Ancelin ML, et al. Insomnia and daytime sleepiness are risk factors for depressive symptoms in the elderly. Sleep 2011;34(8): 1103–10.

41. Plante DT, Finn LA, Hagen EW, et al. Longitudinal associations of hypersomnolence and depression in the Wisconsin Sleep Cohort Study. J Affect Disord 2017;207:197–202.

42. Plante DT, Finn LA, Hagen EW, et al. Subjective and objective measures of hypersomnolence demonstrate divergent associations with depression among participants in the Wisconsin Sleep Cohort Study. J Clin Sleep Med 2016;12(4):571–8.

43. Merlino G, Piani A, Gigli GL, et al. Daytime sleepiness is associated with dementia and cognitive decline in older Italian adults: a population-based study. Sleep Med 2010;11(4):372–7.

44. Ohayon MM, Vecchierini MF. Daytime sleepiness and cognitive impairment in the elderly population. Arch Intern Med 2002;162(2):201–8.

45. Daurat A, Ricarrere M, Tiberge M. Decision making is affected in obstructive sleep apnoea syndrome. J Neuropsychol 2013;7(1):139–44.

46. Lis S, Krieger S, Hennig D, et al. Executive functions and cognitive subprocesses in patients with obstructive sleep apnoea. J Sleep Res 2008;17(3): 271–80.

47. Salorio CF, White DA, Piccirillo J, et al. Learning, memory, and executive control in individuals with obstructive sleep apnea syndrome. J Clin Exp Neuropsychol 2002;24(1):93–100.

48. Saunamaki T, Jehkonen M. A review of executive functions in obstructive sleep apnea syndrome. Acta Neurol Scand 2007;115(1):1–11.

49. Wallace A, Bucks RS. Memory and obstructive sleep apnea: a meta-analysis. Sleep 2013;36(2):203–20.

50. Sagaspe P, Philip P, Schwartz S. Inhibitory motor control in apneic and insomniac patients: a stop task study. J Sleep Res 2007;16(4):381–7.

51. Greneche J, Krieger J, Bertrand F, et al. Short-term memory performances during sustained wakefulness in patients with obstructive sleep apnea-hypopnea syndrome. Brain Cogn 2011;75(1):39–50.

52. Daurat A, Foret J, Bret-Dibat JL, et al. Spatial and temporal memories are affected by sleep fragmentation in obstructive sleep apnea syndrome. J Clin Exp Neuropsychol 2008;30(1):91–101.

53. Bawden FC, Oliveira CA, Caramelli P. Impact of obstructive sleep apnea on cognitive performance. Arq Neuropsiquiatr 2011;69(4):585–9.

54. Yaffe K, Laffan AM, Harrison SL, et al. Sleep-disordered breathing, hypoxia, and risk of mild cognitive impairment and dementia in older women. JAMA 2011;306(6):613–9.

55. Chang WP, Liu ME, Chang WC, et al. Sleep apnea and the risk of dementia: a population-based 5-year follow-up study in Taiwan. PLoS One 2013; 8(10):e78655.

56. Tan EK, Lum SY, Fook-Chong SM, et al. Evaluation of somnolence in Parkinson's disease: comparison with age- and sex-matched controls. Neurology 2002; 58(3):465–8.

57. Ghorayeb I, Loundou A, Auquier P, et al. A nationwide survey of excessive daytime sleepiness in Parkinson's disease in France. Movement Disord 2007;22(11):1567–72.

58. Boddy F, Rowan EN, Lett D, et al. Subjectively reported sleep quality and excessive daytime somnolence in Parkinson's disease with and without dementia, dementia with Lewy bodies and Alzheimer's disease. Int J Geriatr Psychiatry 2007;22(6):529–35.

59. Compta Y, Santamaria J, Ratti L, et al. Cerebrospinal hypocretin, daytime sleepiness and sleep architecture in Parkinson's disease dementia. Brain 2009; 132(Pt 12):3308–17.

60. Gjerstad MD, Aarsland D, Larsen JP. Development of daytime somnolence over time in Parkinson's disease. Neurology 2002;58(10):1544–6.

61. Hely MA, Reid WG, Adena MA, et al. The Sydney Multicenter Study of Parkinson's Disease: the inevitability of dementia at 20 years. Movement Disord 2008;23(6):837–44.

62. Schenck CH, Boeve BF, Mahowald MW. Delayed emergence of a parkinsonian disorder or dementia in 81% of older men initially diagnosed with idiopathic rapid eye movement sleep behavior disorder: a 16-year update on a previously reported series. Sleep Med 2013;14(8):744–8.

63. Iranzo A, Tolosa E, Gelpi E, et al. Neurodegenerative disease status and post-mortem pathology in idiopathic rapid-eye-movement sleep behaviour disorder: an observational cohort study. Lancet Neurol 2013;12(5):443–53.

64. Postuma RB, Gagnon JF, Vendette M, et al. Quantifying the risk of neurodegenerative disease in idiopathic REM sleep behavior disorder. Neurology 2009;72(15):1296–300.

65. Wing YK, Li SX, Mok V, et al. Prospective outcome of rapid eye movement sleep behaviour disorder: psychiatric disorders as a potential early marker of Parkinson's disease. J Neurol Neurosurg Psychiatry 2012;83(4):470–2.

66. Postuma RB. Predicting neurodegenerative disease in idiopathic rapid eye movement (REM) sleep behavior disorder: conference proceedings, REM Sleep Behavior Symposium 2011. Sleep Biol Rhythms 2013;11(Suppl 1):75–81.

67. Dautovich ND, McCrae CS, Rowe M. Subjective and objective napping and sleep in older adults: are evening naps "bad" for nighttime sleep? J Am Geriatr Soc 2008;56(9):1681–6.

68. Yoon IY, Kripke DF, Youngstedt SD, et al. Actigraphy suggests age-related differences in napping and nocturnal sleep. J Sleep Res 2003;12(2):87–93.

69. Onen F, Moreau T, Gooneratne NS, et al. Limits of the Epworth Sleepiness Scale in older adults. Sleep Breath 2013;17(1):343–50.

70. Morgenthaler T, Alessi C, Friedman L, et al. Practice parameters for the use of actigraphy in the assessment of sleep and sleep disorders: an update for 2007. Sleep 2007;30(4):519–29.

71. Zisberg A, Gur-Yaish N, Shochat T. Contribution of routine to sleep quality in community elderly. Sleep 2010;33(4):509–14.

72. Brown CA, Berry R, Tan MC, et al. A critique of the evidence base for non-pharmacological sleep interventions for persons with dementia. Dementia (London) 2013;12(2):210–37.

73. Mishima K, Okawa M, Hishikawa Y, et al. Morning bright light therapy for sleep and behavior disorders in elderly patients with dementia. Acta Psychiatr Scand 1994;89(1):1–7.

74. Naylor E, Penev PD, Orbeta L, et al. Daily social and physical activity increases slow-wave sleep and daytime neuropsychological performance in the elderly. Sleep 2000;23(1):87–95.

75. Vitiello MV, Prinz PN, Schwartz RS. Slow wave sleep but not overall sleep quality of healthy older men and women is improved by increased aerobic fitness. Sleep Research 1994;23:149.

76. Auger RR, Burgess HJ, Emens JS, et al. Clinical practice guideline for the treatment of intrinsic circadian rhythm sleep-wake disorders: advanced sleep-wake phase disorder (ASWPD), delayed sleep-wake phase disorder (DSWPD), non-24-hour sleep-wake rhythm disorder (N24SWD), and irregular sleep-wake rhythm disorder (ISWRD). An update for 2015: an American Academy of Sleep Medicine Clinical Practice Guideline. J Clin Sleep Med 2015; 11(10):1199–236.

77. Morgenthaler T, Kramer M, Alessi C, et al. Practice parameters for the psychological and behavioral treatment of insomnia: an update. An American Academy of Sleep Medicine report. Sleep 2006; 29(11):1415–9.

78. Karlin BE, Trockel M, Spira AP, et al. National evaluation of the effectiveness of cognitive behavioral therapy for insomnia among older versus younger veterans. Int J Geriatr Psychiatry 2015;30(3): 308–15.

79. Morin CM, Bootzin RR, Buysse DJ, et al. Psychological and behavioral treatment of insomnia: update of the recent evidence (1998-2004). Sleep 2006; 29(11):1398–414.

80. Irwin MR, Cole JC, Nicassio PM. Comparative meta-analysis of behavioral interventions for insomnia and their efficacy in middle-aged adults and in older adults 55+ years of age. Health Psychol 2006;25(1):3–14.

81. Shen J, Hossain N, Streiner DL, et al. Excessive daytime sleepiness and fatigue in depressed patients and therapeutic response of a sedating antidepressant. J Affect Disord 2011;134(1–3):421–6.

82. Videnovic A, Golombek D. Circadian and sleep disorders in Parkinson's disease. Exp Neurol 2013;243: 45–56.

83. Dobson KS, Hollon SD, Dimidjian S, et al. Randomized trial of behavioral activation, cognitive therapy, and antidepressant medication in the prevention of relapse and recurrence in major depression. J Consult Clin Psychol 2008;76(3):468–77.

84. Manber R, Edinger JD, Gress JL, et al. Cognitive behavioral therapy for insomnia enhances depression outcome in patients with comorbid major depressive disorder and insomnia. Sleep 2008; 31(4):489–95.

85. Berman MG, Kross E, Krpan KM, et al. Interacting with nature improves cognition and affect for individuals with depression. J Affect Disord 2012;140(3): 300–5.

86. Koenig AM, Butters MA. Cognition in late life depression: treatment considerations. Curr Treat Options Psychiatry 2014;1(1):1–14.

87. Gasa M, Tamisier R, Launois SH, et al. Residual sleepiness in sleep apnea patients treated by continuous positive airway pressure. J Sleep Res 2013;22(4):389–97.

Hypersomnia in Neurodegenerative Diseases

Sushanth Bhat, MD*, Sudhansu Chokroverty, MD, FRCP

KEYWORDS

- Hypersomnia • Hypersomnolence • Excessive daytime sleepiness • Neurodegenerative diseases
- Alzheimer disease • Parkinson disease • Multiple system atrophy • Progressive supranuclear palsy

KEY POINTS

- Hypersomnia is a common complaint in many patients with neurodegenerative diseases and is usually multifactorial in cause.
- Circadian rhythm disorder, or non-24-hour syndrome, is a common cause of hypersomnia in patients with Alzheimer disease.
- Dopaminergic therapy is an important factor associated with hypersomnia in Parkinson disease.
- Although sleep-disordered breathing has not been demonstrated to be more prevalent in patients with neurodegenerative disorders, it contributes to hypersomnia when present.
- Other primary sleep disorders (eg, restless legs syndrome, periodic limb movements in sleep, rapid eye movement [REM]–sleep behavior disorder), disrupted sleep architecture, and depletion of orexin neurons are common in many neurodegenerative diseases, but the extent of their contribution to hypersomnia remains unclear.

INTRODUCTION

The term, "neurodegenerative diseases" refers to a broad, highly heterogeneous group of disorders affecting both the central nervous system (CNS) and the peripheral nervous system, characterized by insidious, irreversible, relentlessly progressive loss of previously intact neurologic function, worsening with age. In most cases, they are sporadic and the exact cause remains unknown (although a genetic basis had been identified in a few disorders and in small subsets of others). The degenerative process usually begins before clinical symptoms develop and involves abnormal intracellular processing and deposition of proteinaceous material; in many cases, a characteristic histopathological pattern is found. **Box 1** lists some common neurodegenerative conditions seen in clinical practice. A detailed discussion of the pathophysiology, clinical findings, diagnosis, and treatment of neurodegenerative diseases is beyond the scope of this article but readers are referred to several excellent resources on the subject.[1,2]

Sleep disorders are very common in patients with neurodegenerative diseases.[3] Patients complain of both daytime hypersomnia and disturbed nocturnal sleep, the latter of which may be related to associated sleep-disordered breathing (both obstructive sleep apnea [OSA] and central sleep apnea [CSA]), sleep fragmentation caused by parasomnias, restless legs syndrome (RLS), periodic limb movements of sleep (PLMS), circadian rhythm disorders, side-effects of agents used in the treatment of the underlying condition, and factors intrinsic to the disease itself causing degeneration of putative

Disclosure Statement: The authors have nothing to disclose with regard to conflicts of interest relevant to this article.
Division of Sleep Medicine, Department of Neuroscience, JFK Neuroscience Institute, Seton Hall University, 65 James Street, Edison, NJ 08818, USA
* Corresponding author.
E-mail address: sbhat2012@yahoo.com

Sleep Med Clin 12 (2017) 443–460
http://dx.doi.org/10.1016/j.jsmc.2017.03.017
1556-407X/17/© 2017 Elsevier Inc. All rights reserved.

sleep-wake centers. Associated complaints may also include daytime fatigue, lack of concentration, impaired motor skills, morning headaches, and absence of symptom relief from additional sleep. Management of such complaints can be challenging, and unfortunately these complaints frequently get overlooked in general practice and neurology clinics. Nevertheless, they often have profound impact on quality of life of both patients and caregivers, and successful management can be very rewarding for all concerned. This article discusses the mechanisms underlying hypersomnia in patients with the more common neurodegenerative diseases, as well as currently available treatment options and recommendations.

DETERMINANTS OF WAKEFULNESS AND SLEEP

The mechanisms underlying cycling between wakefulness, nonrapid eye movement (NREM) sleep and rapid eye movement (REM) sleep are quite complex with multiple theories proposed. Although the following brief discussion is intended to serve the purpose of describing sleep dysfunction in neurodegenerative diseases, interested readers are referred to several other resources that discuss the role of various centers and neurotransmitters in sleep neurobiology in much greater detail.[4,5]

There are multiple CNS centers that control wakefulness and sleep, with several neurotransmitters involved in these pathways.[6] Variation in firing rates in the neurons in these centers results in the cycling between wakefulness, NREM sleep, and REM sleep. These centers are all discrete but highly interrelated through widespread projections that are both facilitatory and inhibitory, thereby modulating wake or sleep activity in the CNS as a whole.

Multiple independent centers are responsible for promoting the wakeful state. The ascending reticular activating system (ARAS), consisting of several groups of neurons with a diffuse, widespread presence in large sections of the brainstem (but particularly the mesencephalon) and extending into the posterior hypothalamus, mediates wakefulness through a variety of neurotransmitters, such as acetylcholine, glutamate, and monoamines like histamine, dopamine, norepinephrine, and serotonin, through projections to the thalamus and, from there, to the cortex. Wake-promoting aminergic neurons are also present in the noradrenergic locus coeruleus (LC) and serotonergic dorsal raphe nucleus (DR) of the pons (which also serve as REM-off cells; see later discussion). The tuberomammillary nucleus (TMN) of the posterior hypothalamus is the main source of brain histamine, and increases its firing rate during wakefulness, with lower firing rates during NREM sleep and the lowest during REM sleep. Orexin-A and B (also known as hypocretin-1 and 2), are secreted by the lateral and posterior hypothalamus, which have widespread, heavy projection to multiple other centers, causing excitation of TMN, LC, and DR (thereby promoting wakefulness and suppressing REM sleep), and inhibition of the ventrolateral preoptic (VLPO) and median preoptic (MnPO) nuclei of the anterior hypothalamus (thereby suppressing NREM sleep). The cholinergic basal forebrain increases its firing rate during wakefulness and REM sleep, and decreases its firing rate in NREM sleep.

NREM sleep, in turn, is promoted by centers such as the VLPO and MnPO nuclei, which secrete the inhibitory neurotransmitters, γ-aminobutyric acid (GABA), and galanin. These in turn have reciprocal projections to multiple other centers, including inhibitory pathways to the wake-promoting neurons of the TMN, LC, DR, orexin-producing cells, and the basal forebrain. Adenosine is a neuro-transmitter that inhibits most wake-promoting centers, decreasing cholinergic firing of the basal forebrain while disinhibiting VLPO and MnPO, thereby promoting NREM sleep.

The seat of generation and inhibition of REM sleep lies in the pons, and lesions that affect the pons cause REM dysfunction. REM sleep is promoted by cholinergic neurons in the laterodorsal tegmental (LDT) and pedunculopontine tegmental (PPT) nuclei at the pontomesencephalic junction, as well as sublaterodorsal nucleus in the pons, which are designated as REM-on cells. Conversely, increased firing of LC, DR, ventrolateral periaqueductal gray, and lateral pontine tegmentum, called REM off-cells, inhibits REM sleep and promotes wakefulness. Descending pathways from the pons and ventrolateral medulla are responsible for inhibition of the cranial and spinal motor neurons in REM sleep, producing REM atonia, through glycinergic and GABA-ergic pathways; disruption of these pathways leads to REM without atonia (RWA), seen in REM sleep behavior disorder (RBD).

Many neurodegenerative diseases are a result of neuronal death, usually as a result of excessive protein misfolding and intracellular protein aggregation, leading to the deposition of abnormal inclusion bodies, such as neurofibrillary plaques and tangles or Lewy bodies. Therefore, it is not surprising that the neurodegenerative process may also involve centers for wakefulness and sleep, leading to insomnia, hypersomnia, and REM dysfunction, as well as the respiratory neurons in the brainstem, resulting in sleep-disordered breathing. Additionally, medications used to treat or manage the symptoms of neurodegenerative diseases act through inhibition or augmentation of the effect of many of the aforementioned neurotransmitters, often leading to imbalance in their actions and consequent sleep dysfunction.

DIAGNOSTIC APPROACH TO HYPERSOMNIA IN PATIENTS WITH NEURODEGENERATIVE DISEASES

As with the diagnosis of any condition, the first step in managing patients with neurodegenerative diseases and sleep complaints is a thorough history and physical examination. A detailed family history and medication history is crucial as well. Sleep complaints may often be the prodromal manifestation of an undiagnosed neurodegenerative disease. For example, RBD may precede the overt symptoms of Parkinson disease (PD) by several decades. However, patients presenting with disrupted sleep and dream enactment may exhibit subtle early extrapyramidal signs, such as subtle cogwheel rigidity, positive glabellar tap, orthostatic dysfunction due to dysautonomia, or decreased sense of smell. Similarly, a circadian rhythm disorder causing daytime hypersomnolence may prompt more detailed neuropsychiatric evaluation that reveals early cognitive dysfunction in patients with Alzheimer disease (AD).

In patients with previously diagnosed neurodegenerative diseases, a thorough sleep history is essential. Review of sleep schedule, hours of sleep, and daytime napping may suggest a circadian rhythm disorder such as non-24 hour rhythm, which frequently occurs in AD (see later discussion). Particular attention should be paid to the occurrence of parasomnias, such as dream-enacting behavior seen in RBD, which tends to occur in the early hours of the morning and can be reported by the bedpartner. Questions regarding RLS (recently renamed Willis-Ekbom disease) should be incorporated in the routine evaluation of these patients because severe RLS symptoms frequently occur in patients with many neurodegenerative diseases and may contribute to sleep initiation, maintenance insomnia, and, subsequently, daytime hypersomnia. All patients with neurodegenerative diseases and complaints of daytime sleepiness should be screened for sleep-disordered breathing by eliciting information about snoring, choking, or gasping in sleep, and about witnessed apneas.

Patients with suspected sleep-disordered breathing should undergo polysomnography (PSG). When parasomnias (particularly RBD) are suspected, it is crucial that the evaluation be performed in the sleep laboratory, rather than in an ambulatory setting, so that visual analysis can be performed. Also, it is helpful to use additional electromyography channels to evaluate for RWA. Patients with suspected circadian rhythm disorders should be asked to fill out sleep logs; actigraphy may provide additional objective evidence of sleep schedules. In the evaluation of patients with hypersomnia and suspected narcoleptic phenotype, a multiple sleep latency test (MSLT) is indicated to evaluate for short sleep latencies and the presence of sleep-onset REM periods (SOREMPs).

The diagnostic approach to hypersomnia in patients with neurodegenerative diseases is summarized in **Box 2**.

HYPERSOMNIA IN TAUOPATHIES

Tau proteins belong to the family of microtubule-associated proteins involved in maintaining cell shape and serve as tracks for axonal transport.

Box 2
Diagnostic approach to hypersomnia in patients with neurodegenerative diseases

History
- Screening for sleep-disordered breathing (snoring, choking or gasping for air, witnessed apneas)
- Parasomnias (NREM parasomnias, such as sleepwalking and dream-enacting behavior; REM parasomnias, such as RBD)
- RLS symptoms
- Family history
- Medication history (dopaminergic agents, opioids, benzodiazepines, benzodiazepine agonists)

Physical examination
- Neurologic examination for extrapyramidal signs (bradykinesia, cogwheel rigidity, gait instability, resting tremor, glabellar tap response, orthostatic hypotension, extraocular movement abnormalities, axial rigidity) and frontal release signs
- Mental status examination (mini-mental status testing, MoCA scale) for early cognitive changes
- Risk factors for sleep-disordered breathing (overweight, large neck circumference, narrow oropharynx, nasal obstruction)

Laboratory testing
- Sleep logs and/or actigraphy for suspected circadian rhythm disorders
- PSG or ambulatory sleep study (if sleep-disordered breathing is suspected)
- PSG with multiple muscle montage for parasomnias such as RBD
- MSLT for suspected narcolepsy or narcoleptic phenotype
- CSF orexin levels for suspected narcolepsy or idiopathic hypersomnia

Abbreviations: CSF, cerebrospinal fluid; MoCA, Montreal cognitive assessment.

The main tauopathies include AD, progressive supranuclear palsy (PSP), corticobasal degeneration (CBD), and frontotemporal dementia (FTD).

ALZHEIMER DISEASE

AD accounts for over half of all cases of chronic dementia; its prevalence increases with age.[7] The characteristic clinical picture is that of progressive memory and intellectual deterioration, usually beginning in middle to late adult life, with motor dysfunction occurring only late in the disease. AD is associated with diffuse cerebral atrophy, especially in the parietal and posterior temporal lobes. There is often associated neuronal loss in the nucleus basalis of Meynert, resulting in alteration of forebrain cholinergic and, to a lesser degree, noradrenergic systems, which has profound implications for cognition and daytime alertness. Histopathologically, the defining lesions in AD are abundant neurofibrillary tangles consisting of tau protein and beta-amyloid neuritic plaque deposits with amyloid angiopathy. AD remains a predominantly sporadic acquired disorder of unclear cause. Fewer than 25% of cases are familial, with autosomal dominant mutations in genes coding for presenilin 1 and 2, and amyloid precursor protein being implicated. Inheritance of the E4 allele of apolipoprotein E (Apoe4) is believed to be an important genetic risk factor.

Sleep disturbances occur early in the course of AD and progressively worsen in tandem with cognitive deterioration. There are demonstrable PSG changes in patients with AD, although the results vary somewhat from study to study. These include reduced sleep efficiency, decreased REM and slow-wave sleep, loss of phasic components (spindles and K complexes) of NREM sleep, and sleep-wake rhythm disturbances.[3] The interactions between sleep and cognitive performance in AD seem to be complex and bidirectional. There is a growing body of literature that suggests that sleep disturbances themselves are among the earliest clinical manifestations of AD[8] and may not even be noticed by patients in the initial stages. A recent study showed that objective sleep disturbances, as detected by PSG and actigraphy, even in the absence of subjective complaints, were more common in cognitively intact patients with the ApoE4 allele than controls, although it remains to be seen whether this is necessarily predictive of the development of AD.[9] Many reports also suggest that in AD, sleep complaints may be predictive of the degree of cognitive impairment; depression may explain this association.[10] Sleep quality also predicts pathologic changes in patients with diagnosed AD.[11] Recent data suggest that amyloid deposition (as determined by cerebrospinal fluid [CSF] A beta-42 levels) in the preclinical stage of AD seems to be associated with worse sleep quality (but not sleep quantity)[12] and, even in normal adults, poor sleep efficiency mediates the relationship between amyloid deposition and poor cognitive performance.[13] A recent meta-analysis suggested that individuals with sleep problems had a 1.68 times higher risk for the combined outcome of cognitive impairment or AD.[14] Sleep disturbances, particularly sleep deprivation, are thus increasingly being investigated as potential modifiable factors in the development and progression of cognitive deficits in patients with AD.[15]

Hypersomnia is a major complaint in patients with AD. It is reportedly less frequent than in those with other neurodegenerative diseases, such as PD disease or diffuse Lewy body disease with dementia (DLBD).[16] However, when present, hypersomnia in AD patients has been found to be associated with greater functional impairment.[17] Chronic daytime somnolence is associated with a distinctive decline in verbal memory, even in cognitively normal ApoE4 homozygotes, a group at particularly high risk of developing AD.[18] The mechanisms underlying hypersomnia in patients with AD remain to be elucidated but, in most cases, are likely to be multifactorial. One major contributory factor is potential sleep-disordered breathing. Between 33% to 70% of patients with AD have coexistent OSA, greater than in the general population, and there is a demonstrated association between the presence of the ApoE4 gene and OSA,[19] with OSA predicting poorer performance on cognitive tests that require both memory and executive function engagement in these patients.[20] Treatment with continuous positive airway pressure (CPAP) has been demonstrated to improve the degree of hypersomnia.[21] Although it is less certain whether untreated OSA is a risk factor for the development of AD, and whether treatment of OSA with CPAP improves cognitive outcomes in patients with AD, animal models suggest that recurrent hypoxemic episodes, as occur in OSA, lead to increasing amyloid deposition.[22] Several small studies have demonstrated some slowing of cognitive decline with therapeutic CPAP use in patients with AD and OSA, which seems to be sustained.[23–25] Daytime hypersomnia in patients with AD is also commonly caused by circadian rhythm abnormalities, particularly the non-24-hour rhythm, thought to be due to degeneration of the suprachiasmatic nucleus of the hypothalamus and the circadian pacemaker, as well as the nucleus basalis of Meynert, the main cholinergic pathway promoting both wakefulness and REM sleep. Sundowning, or cyclic nocturnal agitation syndrome, is an extreme form of this phenomenon, with inversion of sleep schedule (wakefulness and agitation at night and somnolence in the daytime). This is particularly disruptive to caregivers and families and a frequent cause of institutionalization, which, paradoxically, may worsen the problem. Sundowning has been shown to be a predictor of faster cognitive decline. Factors such as early bedtimes, increased use of sedatives, advanced cognitive impairment, and associated medical conditions may all contribute to sundowning.[26] In addition to intrinsic sleep-wake disturbances, many institutionalized patients with AD are particularly underexposed to sufficient levels of light.[27] In several reports, an improvement in nighttime sleep and a decrease in daytime sleepiness after bright light exposure in the evening in patients with AD and related dementias has been reported.[28–31] A combination of nighttime melatonin (5 mg) and bright light (2500 lux) exposure for 1 hour the next morning improved daytime activity levels and wake time in a group of institutionalized patients with AD but not those receiving placebo and bright light only.[32] Structured exercise schedules daily in the morning and evening have been shown to improve the circadian rhythmicity in elderly controls and demented subects. In sundowning syndrome, aerobic exercise and cognitive behavioral therapy (CBT) has been shown to improve agitation and reduce serum cortisol levels.[33] There has recently been increasing interest in the role of the orexins in sleep disturbances in patients with AD, with early results somewhat discordant. Small preliminary autopsy studies in patients with AD suggest that both the number of orexin-producing cells and ventricular CSF orexin-A levels are decreased compared with controls.[34] Notably, however, other investigators have found increased levels of CSF orexin in patients with AD, which correlated to tau levels, sleep disturbances, and cognitive decline.[35] Another group found no difference in the circadian rhythm of CSF orexin production between patients with AD and controls, although there was a correlation between mean A beta-42 levels and mean orexin-A levels.[36] Clearly, the orexin system plays a role in both sleep disturbances in, and pathogenesis of, AD; however, its exact nature is unclear and more research needs to be done in this field. Unfortunately, there have been no high-quality studies regarding the use of pharmacologic agents such as benzodiazepines or benzodiazepine receptor agonists for insomnia, nor of wakefulness-promoting agents such as modafinil or of stimulants such as methylphenidate or dextroamphetamines for hypersomnia in patients with AD and circadian abnormalities, although these are often prescribed in clinical practice with mixed results.

FRONTOTEMPORAL DEMENTIA

FTD is distinct from AD in cause, clinical presentation, and histopathological findings. The clinical features of FTD include younger age of onset than AD (usually sixth decade), early loss of insight and disinhibition, social decline, personal conduct defects, emotional blunting, relative preservation of perception and memory (in contrast to AD), reduced speech output and hyperorality, perseverance, and echolalia.[1] There are many variants, including behavioral variant FTD or frontal variant FTD, and the primary progressive aphasias (further subdivided into progressive nonfluent aphasia, semantic dementia, and logopenic progressive aphasia). In recent years, there has been a lot of progress in characterizing its genetic basis, including the identification of multiple mutations in the microtubule-associated protein tau (MAPT) gene, located on chromosome 17, associated with FTD syndromes and insoluble tau deposits.[37] Some cases exhibit ubiquitin immunoreactive inclusions in the cytoplasm or nucleus or ubiquitin immunoreactive neuritis, linked to the progranulin gene on chromosome 17.[38] Neuroimaging shows greater frontal and anterior temporal atrophy compared with the insular and posterior temporoparietal atrophy seen in AD.[39]

Sleep disturbances are common in FTD. However, most studies are limited by having been conducted in small numbers of subjects. It has been reported that, compared with subjects with AD, subjects with FTD exhibit sleep disturbances earlier in the course of the disease, and the deterioration of sleep quality is more rapid. Subjects with AD had better preservation of sleep parameters and macrostructure than those with FTD over the course of 1 study.[40] Subjects with FTD have decreased sleep time and sleep efficiency compared with controls and with subjects with AD. They show increased nocturnal and decreased morning activity, worsening with disease progression, suggesting a possible phase delay type of circadian rhythm disruption.[41,42] Insomnia or disturbed nocturnal sleep and hypersomnia occur frequently. RLS, OSA, and circadian rhythm abnormalities have all been described.[43] There are conflicting reports about how commonly RBD co-occurs[43–45] and it is unclear how much RBD contributes to daytime sleepiness in this condition. It is also uncertain whether patients with FTD have low CSF orexin levels. One study that measured plasma (not CSF) orexin levels found that subjects with FTD had lower levels than subjects with AD and PD.[46] Two patients in the study had low short sleep latency on MSLT but no SOREMPs; it is unclear whether those 2 subjects also had low plasma orexin levels. Another study found that subjects with FTD were more likely than controls to complain of hypersomnia if they had low CSF orexin levels (although orexin levels and hypersomnia did not differ significantly from controls).[47]

PROGRESSIVE SUPRANUCLEAR PALSY

PSP, also known as Steele-Richardson-Olszewski syndrome, is a degenerative condition characterized by akinetic rigidity, dystonia, early gait disturbances, pseudobulbar palsy, and characteristic supranuclear extraocular movement abnormality that is manifested initially by impaired voluntary vertical eye movements, particularly downward gaze, but which later involves movements in all directions. Mean age of onset is in the seventh decade. The pathologic hallmark of PSP is the presence of gliosis and abnormal tau deposition resulting in neuronal loss with globose neurofibrillary tangles in multiple subcortical nuclei, including the LC, with relative preservation of the cortex and hippocampus. Abnormalities near or in the gene coding for tau protein are implicated in the pathogenesis of PSP. However, as with most neurodegenerative diseases, most cases are sporadic, acquired, and idiopathic.

Most studies suggest that sleep disturbances in PSP are more severe than in other neurodegenerative diseases. As with AD, sleep disturbances are common and occur early in PSP and, as with PD, the sleep disturbances worsen with greater motor involvement. Sleep architectural changes in PSP are prominent and include suppression of REM sleep, decreased slow-wave sleep, and abnormal NREM sleep with blunting of sleep spindles.[48,49] Total sleep time and sleep efficiency worsen with disease progression[50] and the degree of impairment is greater than that seen in PD.[51] There is more significant brainstem pathologic abnormality in patients with PSP than in those with AD or PD, especially in the pontine tegmentum (that generates REM sleep) and the connections between the ARAS and the thalamus (which generates sleep spindles), explaining the greater degree of sleep architectural changes and subjective sleep disturbances. Insomnia is more common than with AD, likely due both to the underlying degenerative changes, as well as discomfort due to immobility and difficulty turning in bed. Other factors for sleep deprivation and fragmentation include depression, dysphasia, and frequent nocturia. All these factors play a role in the daytime hypersomnia in these patients. RLS occurs in more than half the patients with PSP[52] and is another cause of sleep fragmentation, insomnia, and hypersomnia. Although patients with PSP and hypersomnia should be screened for OSA and treated appropriately, there are no definitive data to suggest that PSP confers a greater risk for sleep-disordered breathing.[53] As a tauopathy, it is generally assumed that RBD is less common in PSP than in PD,[54,55] although this has been disputed.[56]

There have been reports of a narcoleptic phenotype (DR2/DQB1 positivity, abnormal MSLT, and low CSF orexin levels) in patients with PSP.[57] Degeneration of orexin-producing cells has been speculated to be a cause of hypersomnia in these patients.[58] Low CSF levels of orexin correlate with disease severity. In fact, the finding of low CSF hypocretin sets PSP and CBD (see later discussion) apart from other neurodegenerative conditions, but this remains to be validated with larger studies. Treatment of underlying motor abnormalities and RLS in patients with PSP may help sleep fragmentation and insomnia, thereby relieving hypersomnia, but there are only a few large-scale studies to guide treatment at this time.

CORTICOBASAL DEGENERATION

CBD is a rare tauopathy, characterized by unilateral or asymmetric signs of rigidity, action or stimulus-sensitive myoclonus, and apraxia often associated with circumscribed higher cortical deficits. The other characteristic features include cortical sensory loss consisting of agraphesthesia, astereognosis, and sensory extinction in presence of intact primary sensory modalities, as well as alien limb phenomenon in which the patient cannot recognize his own affected limb, which may be performing purposeful movements not intended by the patient. The pathologic hallmarks of CBD are gliosis and large achromatic balloon neurons distributed asymmetrically in discrete frontal or parietal cortical areas and in subcortical regions.[59]

Given the relative rarity of the disease, sleep abnormalities in CBD have yet to be definitely characterized. Sleep disturbances were reported to be less common in patients with CBD compared with those with atypical parkinsonian syndromes such as DLBD, PSP, and multiple system atrophy (MSA).[60] This may be because intracellular tau aggregates occur more commonly in the cortex than the brainstem in this disease.[61] It is unclear whether patients with CBD suffer from excessive hypersomnia to the same degree as those with other neurodegenerative diseases. Insomnia, PLMS, OSA,[62,63] and RBD[54,64] have all been described in small case series, in addition to low CSF orexin levels.[58] These factors could all potentially contribute to hypersomnia; however, all studies have been conducted in small numbers of patients, so further studies in an adequate number of subjects are needed.

HYPERSOMNIA IN SYNUCLEINOPATHIES

Alpha-synuclein is a protein that helps transportation of dopamine-laden vesicles from the cell body to the synapses. Synucleinopathies are a group of disorders with abnormal deposition of alpha-synuclein in the cytoplasm of neurons or glial cells, as well as extracellular deposits of amyloid. The main synucleinopathies include PD, DLBD, and MSA. These 3 conditions are also classified as atypical parkinsonian syndromes.

PARKINSON DISEASE

PD is the most common neurodegenerative movement disorder. It is characterized by a combination of rest tremor, bradykinesia or akinesia, rigidity, gait instability, impaired postural reflexes, and prominent dysautonomia. The mean age of onset is the sixth decade. Histologically, degenerative changes occur in the zona compacta of substantia nigra and cytoplasmic inclusion bodies composed of alpha-synuclein (Lewy bodies) in surviving neurons. Similar abnormalities may be present in the LC, dorsal motor nucleus of vagus nerve, other pigmented brainstem nuclei, substantia innominata, and intermediolateral cell column of the spinal cord. Depletion of dopaminergic neurons of substantia nigra is believed to be the main biochemical abnormality in PD. Almost all cases are idiopathic; however, a small number of cases of early-onset PD have been found to have a genetic basis. Mutations in SNCA (PARK1- 4) and LRRK2 (PARK8) are responsible for autosomal dominant forms, and mutations in Parkin (PARK2), PINK1 (PARK6), DJ-1 (PARK7), and ATP13A2 (PARK9) are accountable for an autosomal recessive mode of inheritance. The subject of the genetics of PD is complex and beyond the scope of this article; however, interested readers are referred to several excellent resources for further discussion.[65]

Sleep disturbance is near-universal in patients with PD and is a major nonmotor manifestation with a significant impact on quality of life.[66] With the exception of RBD, most sleep complaints do not seem to precede the diagnosis of PD, in contrast to AD.[67] Sleep fragmentation leading to poor nocturnal sleep and insomnia is a major complaint that in turn results in hypersomnia. Most patients complain of insomnia and PSG analysis shows that sleep architecture is markedly disturbed in patients with idiopathic PD, with reductions in the total sleep time and slow-wave and REM sleep.[68] Motor disturbances (bradykinesia and stiffness in bed causing difficulty with postural changes), pain, and discomfort, as well as rest tremor and temperature dysregulation due to dysautonomia, contribute to sleep onset and maintenance problems. Additionally, patients with PD frequently suffer from RLS, leading to sleep onset and maintenance insomnia.[69] The relationship between RLS and PD, however, is poorly understood. There are some data to suggest an association between RLS and PD with Parkin mutations.[70,71] Most studies report that RLS symptoms develop after treating the PD patients with dopaminergic medications,[72] suggesting that RLS may be provoked through a process of augmentation even in those who do not have RLS.[73,74] It is also unclear what impact RLS has on daytime sleepiness in patients with PD. Agents used in its treatment, such as dopaminergic therapy, opioids, gabapentin, and pregabalin, may in turn cause hypersomnia, further confounding the issue. Notably, a recent study suggested that dopaminergic therapy and RLS were the 2 strongest predictors of hypersomnia in patients with PD.[75]

Subjective hypersomnia occurs in 30% to 55% of subjects with PD,[76,77] more commonly than in controls,[78] even before initiation of treatment.[79] However, many of these subjects do not exhibit short sleep latency on MSLT.[80] As in most neurodegenerative diseases, hypersomnia in PD is multifactorial in cause. It is worse with older age of onset,[81] is associated with severe depression and poorer quality of life, and is predictive of impaired cognitive performance[82,83] and falls.[84] It has been suggested that OSA is more common in subjects with PD than age-matched controls,[85] although that finding is disputed.[86,87] When present, OSA undoubtedly contributes to the hypersomnia that these subjects experience,[88] although some investigators suggest that its overall role in this regard may be limited.[89] Inability to turn in bed may worsen the degree of sleep-disordered breathing in subjects with positional OSA.[90] Of note, a recent report suggested that use of dopamine agonists promoted central apneic events in subjects with PD; however, in general, subjects with PD do not exhibit greater central apnea indices than controls with sleep-disordered breathing.[85] Additionally, although 1 study found that OSA in subjects with PD is worse in NREM sleep than REM sleep, possibly due to reduced REM atonia,[85] another study found that OSA is more frequent and more severe in subjects with RBD than in subjects without, and that RBD increases the risk of hypoxemia during sleep.[91] CPAP treatment is effective in improving subjective and objective hypersomnia in subjects with PD and OSA.[92]

Dopamine therapy has consistently been shown to be 1 of the most reliable predictors of hypersomnia in subjects with PD.[75,79,93–95] A recent longitudinal study using Scales for Outcomes in Parkinson's disease (SCOPA)-SLEEP-daytime sleepiness scores[94] reported that longer duration of disease is associated with increased daytime somnolence in subjects with PD. The following factors were noted to be associated with hypersomnia: male gender, poorer nighttime sleep, cognitive and autonomic dysfunction, hallucinations, less severe dyskinesias, higher dose of dopamine agonists, and use of antihypertensive medications; whereas use of benzodiazepines was associated with less daytime sleepiness. Subjects with PD are also prone to irresistible sleep attacks,[95] which are sudden episodes of sleep that appear without warning in a patient who does not otherwise feel sleepy. This is relatively rare and some investigators think that it is related to high doses of dopaminergic therapy. Subjects with PD, both with and without irresistible sleep attacks, may exhibit a narcoleptic phenotype, including cataplexy[96] and SOREMPs on MSLT.[97] However, CSF orexin levels in patients with PD are normal.[58] A recent study showed that, although PD subjects with dementia complain of greater hypersomnia than those without dementia, CSF orexin levels in both groups, as well as in normal controls, do not differ significantly.[98] Nevertheless, postmortem studies demonstrate that, compared with controls, subjects with PD have a significantly reduced number of orexin neurons, markedly lower orexin-A concentration in ventricular CSF, and decreased orexin-A concentrations in prefrontal cortex,[99] which worsens with disease progression.[100] This pattern of normal CSF orexin levels in living patients with findings of orexin cell loss on autopsy is also noted with MSA and DLBD (see later discussion). Thus, the exact role that orexin deficiency plays in the hypersomnia of PD remains to be elucidated. Although patients with PD, as with all synucleinopathies, often exhibit motor dyscontrol in REM sleep that leads to RWA and RBD, there is no clear evidence to suggest that it is a cause of hypersomnia[101] or that its treatment improves daytime alertness. However, a recent study suggested that daytime sleepiness in patients with idiopathic RBD predicts more rapid conversion to parkinsonism and dementia, suggesting that daytime sleepiness may be an early marker of neuronal loss in brainstem arousal systems.[101] Finally, although preliminary data from studies involving 24-hour melatonin monitoring in subjects with PD demonstrate possible circadian rhythm abnormalities that conceivably contribute to hypersomnia; more analysis needs to be done in this field.[102]

MULTIPLE SYSTEM ATROPHY

MSA is a sporadic, adult-onset neurodegenerative disorder characterized by parkinsonism, autonomic failure, and dysfunction of cerebellar and corticospinal systems.[103,104] Two motor phenotypes have been clinically identified: parkinsonian, which is characterized by substantia nigra pallor; and cerebellar, characterized by cerebellar atrophy. Alternatively, the condition is often referred to as Shy-Drager syndrome (SDS) when autonomic failure predominates, as striatonigral degeneration when parkinsonism predominates, and as sporadic olivopontocerebellar atrophy (OPCA) when cerebellar dysfunction predominates (see later discussion). The pathologic features of MSA consist of degeneration and gliosis in basal ganglia, brainstem, cerebellum, and spinal cord with characteristic oligodendroglial cytoplasmic inclusions consisting of an accumulation of protein alpha-synuclein.

Sleep architectural changes are not pronounced in MSA, except for decreased total sleep time.[105] However, sleep complaints lead to poor quality of life in patients with all subtypes of MSA[106] and are more common than in patients with PD.[107] Daytime sleepiness, in particular, occurs in nearly a quarter of patients with MSA[108] and, unlike in patients with PD, seems to occur independently of dopaminergic therapy.[75] Poor sleep efficiency and sleep-disordered breathing seem to be stronger predictors of hypersomnolence in MSA. There have, however, been reports of irresistible sleep attacks occurring in the context of a levodopa challenge in subjects with MSA.[109,110] Although sleep-disordered breathing is often seen in patients with MSA, there are no data to suggest that MSA itself confers a greater risk for OSA. Rarely, patients with MSA may present with pure CSA,[111] Cheyne-Stokes respiration,[112] or treatment-emergent CSA.[113] It is thought that degeneration of respiratory centers in the brainstem is the cause. Patients with MSA are at particular risk for the development of nocturnal laryngeal stridor, hypothesized to be due to degeneration of the laryngeal adductor muscles.[114] Laryngeal stridor may also be the presenting feature of MSA. Sudden nocturnal death is the most serious consequence of this untreated respiratory dysrhythmia. Although CPAP is usually first-line treatment (due to patients' resistance to tracheostomy for social reasons), tracheostomy is often required as definitive treatment, especially when stridor occurs in the daytime.[115] It remains uncertain, however, whether nocturnal stridor is a contributory factor in the development of hypersomnia in MSA patients. There have been reports of advanced sleep phase syndrome, a circadian rhythm disorder with daytime hypersomnia and nocturnal insomnia, in patients with MSA.[116] RLS occurs with greater frequency in patients with MSA than in the general population and may contribute to sleep fragmentation resulting in hypersomnia.[117] The data are less clear for PLMS, with some studies suggesting that PLMS is less frequent in MSA than in PD, although more than that noted in general population.[118] RBD is seen in virtually all patients with MSA, and RWA, the physiologic marker of RBD, occurs in the PSG of almost all patients with MSA, even in those that do not report dream-enacting behavior.[119] However, as with other neurodegenerative diseases, it is unclear whether RBD or PLMS contribute to daytime sleepiness in patients with MSA. Although autopsy studies of some subjects with MSA have demonstrated decreased orexin neurons in the lateral hypothalamus,[120] decreased CSF orexin levels have not been found.[121,122] Thus, the role of orexin in hypersomnia in patients with MSA remains unclear. However, a proposed theory is loss of mesopontine cholinergic neurons in LDT and PPT nuclei, which mediate both alertness and REM sleep; this theory would also explain REM dysfunction that occurs in these patients.[123]

DIFFUSE LEWY BODY DISEASE WITH DEMENTIA

DLBD is a neurodegenerative synucleinopathy characterized by the onset of dementia (impaired executive function) within 12 months of onset of motor symptoms of parkinsonism, such as akinesia or bradykinesia, postural instability, and rigidity without the characteristic parkinsonian tremor. Early visual hallucinations are prominent and often a defining feature. There is also visuospatial dysfunction, fluctuating cognitive function, and hypersensitivity to neuroleptics. The pathologic criteria include the presence of Lewy bodies in limbic, paralimbic, and neocortical regions, in addition to midbrain substantia nigra, LC, and raphe nuclei. Senile plaques are present in most individuals with DLBD, although neurofibrillary tangles are typically sparse.

As with most synucleinopathies, RBD occurs very frequently in DLBD, and is so common as to be considered a core feature of the disease.[124] There is also a high prevalence of PLMS in DLBD.[125] RLS also occurs[126] but seems to be less frequent in DLBD than in PD, MSA, or PSP.[127] Similar to other neurodegenerative diseases, the contribution of RBD, RLS, or PLMS to hypersomnia in these patients is unclear. Hypersomnia occurs more commonly in DLBD than in PD, AD, or the general population.[128,129] DLBD patients have several sleep problems (eg, insomnia, RLS, and RBD) co-occurring at the same time, requiring screening and accurate assessment of sleep disturbance.[130] A recent study found that subjects with DLBD had shorter mean sleep latency on MSLT than in those with AD. However, unlike in subjects with AD, the mean MSLT latency was unrelated to the degree of cognitive impairment, the degree of motor impairment, sleep efficiency the night before, visual hallucinations, or RBD,[131] suggesting that excessive daytime sleepiness is a unique feature in DLBD unrelated to sleep fragmentation or other cardinal features of the disease. Hypersomnia and poor nocturnal sleep are associated with depression in DLBD.[132] Studies have not found significantly low CSF orexin levels in patients with DLBD[133] despite reduced neocortical orexin immunoreactivity in DLBD subjects correlating with hypersomnolence and alpha-synuclein levels.[134] This discrepancy, similar to what is observed in patients with PD and MSA, may reflect that a significant neuronal loss in orexin-producing cells is needed for CSF orexin levels to become abnormal. In a recent study,[135] subjects with a postmortem diagnosis of DLBD manifested greater disturbances of circadian rhythm of locomotor activity than subjects with AD, possibly suggesting greater sleep disturbances in this population.

HYPERSOMNIA IN OTHER NEURODEGENERATIVE DISEASES
Cerebellar and Spinocerebellar Degeneration

OPCA defines chronic progressive hereditary, usually dominant (occasionally recessive, rarely sporadic) cerebellar degeneration, often accompanied by parkinsonism and associated with atrophy of the pontine nuclei, cerebellar cortex, and olivopontocerebellar regions. Cerebellar influence on the sleep-wakefulness mechanism has been demonstrated in animal experiments.[136] However, there has been very little research into sleep dysfunction, including hypersomnia, in subjects with OPCA or spinocerebellar ataxias (SCA). Most studies have focused on the prevalence of primary sleep disorders. Brainstem neurons, which undergo degeneration in OPCA, lie close to the hypnogenic and respiratory neurons. Thus, hypersomnia and other sleep dysfunction may be expected in OPCA. Central, obstructive, and mixed apneas have been described in sleep in many subjects with OPCA,[137,138] but respiratory disturbances are less frequent and intense than in SDS. RBD, PLMS, and RLS have also been described in several cases of OPCA,[139] SCA-1, SCA-2, Machado-Joseph disease (SCA3), and SCA-13.[140–144] Whether this results in hypersomnia is unknown. Both NREM parasomnias and

RBD have been described in SCA3.[145] One recent study in a family with SCA-2 suggested that depression was the main determinant of both insomnia and hypersomnia.[146] Recent studies in subjects with SCA-3 suggested that poor sleep efficiency and REM sleep aberrations are the characteristics of sleep structure disruption in SCA3 as the disease progresses, but the incidence of respiratory disturbance during sleep or hypersomnia was not significantly higher in SCA3 subjects than controls.[147,148] Compared with matched controls, subjects with SCA-6 have greater frequency of PLMS and RLS,[149] a reduction in slow-wave sleep, and a higher frequency of snoring and respiratory disorders during sleep.[150] They also have impaired subjective sleep quality and tend to have greater daytime sleepiness,[151] but the mechanisms underlying this have yet to be elucidated.

Huntington Disease

Huntington disease (HD) is an inherited, autosomal dominant neurodegenerative disease caused by the expansion of a cysteine-adenosine-guanine repeat encoding a polyglutamine tract in the N-terminus of the protein product called huntingtin, whose gene is located on the short arm of chromosome 4. It is characterized by relentlessly progressive dementia and chorea, which begins at a relatively young age (mean age of onset is the fourth decade). The most striking neuropathology in HD occurs within the neostriatum, in which gross atrophy of the caudate nucleus and putamen is accompanied by selective neuronal loss and astrogliosis. Marked neuronal loss also is seen in deep layers of the cerebral cortex. Other regions, including the globus pallidus, thalamus, subthalamic nucleus, substantia nigra, and cerebellum, show varying degrees of atrophy, depending on the pathologic grade. N-terminal fragments of mutant huntingtin accumulate and form inclusions in the cell nucleus in these regions.

Although sleep has been found to be variably impaired in HD, sleep disturbances are not well-characterized. Sleep dysfunction is worse in those patients with more advanced disease and includes increased sleep onset latency, reduced sleep efficiency, frequent nocturnal awakenings, increased wake-after-sleep onset, and decreased slow-wave and REM sleep.[152,153] Although not all patients show architectural abnormalities,[154] they may occur very early in the disease course and may precede subjective sleep complaints.[155] A characteristic PSG finding in HD is increased sleep spindle density in contrast to decreased number of spindles in most other neurodegenerative diseases.[156] The significance, however, of this finding remains undetermined. In presymptomatic patients, sleep disturbances predict poorer neuropsychiatric outcomes and, in those patients already symptomatic, are additionally associated with accelerated thalamic degeneration.[157] Subjectively, both complaints of disturbed nocturnal sleep and hypersomnia are common.[158] Nocturnal sleep disturbances and circadian rhythm abnormalities, particularly delayed sleep phase syndrome,[159] have been described in HD. In addition to conceivably contributing to hypersomnia, they are correlated to depression and poor cognitive performance in these patients. Sleep-disordered breathing does not seem to be a major concern in patients with HD,[160] nor does RBD.[161] Both RLS and PLMS have been described in HD, but their impact on hypersomnia is unclear.[161,162] CSF orexin levels in patients with HD are normal.[163,164]

Potential causes of hypersomnia in patients with neurodegenerative diseases are summarized in **Box 3**.

MANAGEMENT OF HYPERSOMNIA IN NEURODEGENERATIVE DISEASES

The management of hypersomnia in patients with neurodegenerative diseases should be tailored to the underlying cause, if identifiable. If sleep fragmentation occurs due to motor discomfort associated with the underlying neurodegenerative disease, optimization of therapy may alleviate insomnia and thereby improve daytime hypersomnia. Sedating medications should be avoided as best possible, or appropriately timed to cause the least daytime drowsiness. Treatment of hypersomnia in reference to PD merits a special mention. Levodopa has a dual effect on sleep; low doses of levodopa have a sedating effect, whereas high doses have a stimulating effect. Thus, a small dose of levodopa with a second dose later on awakening at night may help with both sleep onset and sleep maintenance insomnia. Alternatively, longer acting preparations taken near bedtime may also help. However, it is increasingly realized that excessive daytime sleepiness and sleep attacks may be related to dopaminergic therapy. Levodopa monotherapy carries the lowest risk for sleep attacks, followed by dopamine agonist monotherapy. Use of multiple dopaminergic agents likely increases the risk for hypersomnia. Thus, as a general guideline, minimal effective doses of dopaminergic therapy should be used in an individual patient, and patients should be cautioned against driving when a dopaminergic agent is initiated.[3] Patients with sleep-disordered breathing, whether OSA, CSA, complex sleep

---

Box 3
Potential causes of hypersomnia in patients with neurodegenerative diseases

Disrupted nocturnal sleep

- Abnormal sleep architecture (reduced sleep efficiency and total sleep time, increased sleep latency, decreased slow-wave sleep, decreased REM sleep)
- Motor dysfunction causing sleep fragmentation
- Insomnia
- Depression

Circadian rhythm abnormalities

- Non-24-hr circadian rhythm (described most commonly in AD)
- Delayed sleep-phase syndrome (has been described in FTD)

Coexistent primary sleep disorders

- Sleep-disordered breathing (OSA, CSA)
- RLS (most commonly seen in tauopathies)
- PLMS (most commonly seen in tauopathies)
- Parasomnias (REM parasomnias such as RBD, most commonly seen in synucleinopathies; NREM parasomnias such as sleepwalking)
- Coexistent narcolepsy or narcoleptic phenotype (most frequently described in PD)

Medications

- Dopaminergic therapy (particularly in PD)
- Benzodiazepines (such as clonazepam used to treat RBD or alprazolam used to treat anxiety and insomnia), benzodiazepine agonists, opioids, certain antidepressants (SSRI, MAO-I)

Due to underlying degenerative process

- Low CSF orexin levels (described in PSP and CBD) or degeneration of orexin cells (seen in AD, MSA, PSP, PD)
- Degeneration of wake-promoting neurons, such as in basal forebrain, ARAS, posterior hypothalamus (includes circadian rhythm abnormalities previously listed, due to degeneration of circadian pacemaker in the suprachiasmatic nucleus)

Note: Many of the above mechanisms are proposed, with limited data regarding contribution to hypersomnia in patients with neurodegenerative diseases (see article for details).
Abbreviations: MAO-I, monoamine oxidase inhibitor; SSRI, selective serotonin reuptake inhibitor.

apnea, or laryngeal stridor, should be treated with upper airway pressurization (CPAP, bilevel positive airway pressure with back-up rate as needed for central apneas, adaptive servoventilation for patients with Cheyne-Stokes respirations), with tracheostomy as a last resort. Patients with circadian rhythm abnormalities should undergo actigraphy to properly delineate their sleep habits and then bright-light or melatonin therapy in an attempt to stabilize their sleep-wake cycle. In patients with advanced neurodegenerative disease, especially AD, who have non-24-hour circadian rhythm abnormality, this may not always be successful. Patients with sleep disruption due to RBD are often treated with clonazepam; however, this may worsen daytime sleepiness. Melatonin remains an alternative option. Unfortunately, many patients with neurodegenerative diseases have a multifactorial cause for hypersomnia and treatment of underlying conditions and comorbid sleep disorders may not completely alleviate daytime sleepiness. Although stimulants such as methylphenidate and dextroamphetamines, and wakefulness-promoting agents such as modafinil and armodafinil have been used clinically, there have been few high-quality random controlled studies regarding their role in treating hypersomnia in patients with neurodegenerative diseases and their use remains off-label.[165]

Treatment strategies for hypersomnia in patients with neurodegenerative diseases are summarized in **Box 4**.

Box 4
Management of hypersomnia in patients with neurodegenerative diseases

- Minimize sedating medications (eg, dopaminergic therapy, benzodiazepines, benzodiazepine agonists, opioids)
- Identify and treat coexistent primary sleep disorders (upper airway pressurization for sleep-disordered breathing, optimization of medication regimen for RLS, treatment of underlying parasomnias with benzodiazepines)
- Identify and treat primary insomnia and mood disorders (CBT, medications)
- Identify and treat circadian rhythm disorders (bright light or melatonin therapy)
- Identify and treat narcolepsy or narcoleptic phenotype
- Limited data exit for use of wakefulness-promoting agents such as modafinil and armodafinil, or stimulants such as methylphenidate or dextroamphetamines

---

SUMMARY

Hypersomnia is a common complaint in patients with neurodegenerative diseases, and a major factor causing decreased quality of life. In most patients, its cause is multifactorial. Sleep architecture is affected in almost all the neurodegenerative conditions, leading to decreased total sleep time, decreased sleep efficiency, and sleep architectural changes, including frequent arousals, decreased REM and slow-wave sleep, and decreased sleep spindles, all of which may result in unrefreshing sleep. Additionally, nocturnal sleep is also disrupted by commonly occurring comorbid conditions such as RLS, as well as by motor discomfort and pain from the underlying neurodegenerative condition itself (both very common in PD and the atypical parkinsonian syndromes), further worsening hypersomnia. Insomnia is also a common complaint in neurodegenerative conditions. Treatment of these complaints is usually by agents (dopaminergic therapy, benzodiazepines, and benzodiazepine-receptor agonists) that may worsen daytime hypersomnia. Dopaminergic therapy, in particular, is a leading cause of hypersomnia in patients with PD. Many patients have coincidental sleep-disordered breathing, causing hypersomnia, although there are little data suggesting that patients with neurodegenerative conditions are at increased risk. Circadian rhythm disorders are common causes of nocturnal insomnia and daytime hypersomnia, especially in the tauopathies (AD and FTD). Although RBD has been reported in most of the synucleinopathies, it is unclear that it is a major cause of daytime hypersomnia. Similarly, it is unclear whether PLMS, also seen in patients with neurodegenerative diseases, causes daytime sleepiness. There has been a lot of interest in the role of orexin deficiency in causing hypersomnia in neurodegenerative diseases; however, although autopsy studies show orexin cell loss, low CSF orexin levels have been demonstrated in only a few neurodegenerative conditions. Treatment of hypersomnia has to be individualized and directed at the underlying causes if found. There are no clear guidelines on the use of stimulants or wakefulness-promoting agents in the treatment of hypersomnia in patients with neurodegenerative diseases at this time.

REFERENCES

1. Galimberti D, Scarpini E. Neurodegenerative diseases: clinical aspects, molecular genetics and biomarkers. London: Springer-Verlag; 2014.
2. Litvan I. Atypical Parkinsonian disorders: clinical and research aspects. Totowa (NJ): Humana Press; 2005.

3. Chokroverty S. Sleep and neurodegenerative diseases. Semin Neurol 2009;29:446–68.

4. Monti JM, Pandi-Perumal SR, Sinton CM, editors. Neurochemistry of sleep and wakefulness. Cambridge (United Kingdom): Cambridge University Press; 2008.

5. Chokroverty S, Provini F. Sleep, breathing and neurologic disorders. In: Chokroverty S, editors. Sleep disorders medicine: basic science, technical considerations and clinical aspects. 4th edition. Springer; in press.

6. España RA, Scammell TE. Sleep neurobiology from a clinical perspective. Sleep 2011;34(7):845–58.

7. Dos Santos Picanço LC, Ozela PF, de Fátima de Brito Brito M, et al. Alzheimer's disease: a review from the pathophysiology to diagnosis, new perspectives for pharmacological treatment. Curr Med Chem 2016. [Epub ahead of print].

8. Kabeshita Y, Adachi H, Matsushita M, et al. Sleep disturbances are key symptoms of very early stage Alzheimer disease with behavioral and psychological symptoms: a Japan multi-center cross-sectional study (J-BIRD). Int J Geriatr Psychiatry 2017;32(2):222–30.

9. Drogos LL, Gill SJ, Tyndall AV, et al. Evidence of association between sleep quality and APOE ε4 in healthy older adults: a pilot study. Neurology 2016;87(17):1836–42.

10. Hahn EA, Wang HX, Andel R, et al. A change in sleep pattern may predict Alzheimer disease. Am J Geriatr Psychiatry 2014;11:1262–71.

11. Branger P, Arenaza-Urquijo EM, Tomadesso C, et al. Relationships between sleep quality and brain volume, metabolism, and amyloid deposition in late adulthood. Neurobiol Aging 2016;41: 107–14.

12. Ju YE, McLeland JS, Toedebusch CD, et al. Sleep quality and preclinical Alzheimer disease. JAMA Neurol 2013;70(5):587–93.

13. Molano JR, Roe CM, Ju YS. The interaction of sleep and amyloid deposition on cognitive performance. J Sleep Res 2016. http://dx.doi.org/10.1111/jsr.12474.

14. Bubu OM, Brannick M, Mortimer J, et al. Sleep, Cognitive impairment and Alzheimer's disease: a systematic review and meta-analysis. Sleep 2016. pii: sp-00173–16. [Epub ahead of print].

15. Busche MA, Kekuš M, Förstl H. Connections between sleep and Alzheimer's disease: insomnia, amnesia and amyloid. Nervenarzt 2017;88(3): 215–21 [in German].

16. Boddy F, Rowan EN, Lett D, et al. Subjectively reported sleep quality and excessive daytime somnolence in Parkinson's disease with and without dementia, dementia with Lewy bodies and Alzheimer's disease. Int J Geriatr Psychiatry 2007; 22(6):529–35.

17. Lee JH, Bliwise DL, Ansari FP, et al. Daytime sleepiness and functional impairment in Alzheimer disease. Am J Geriatr Psychiatry 2007;15(7):620–6.

18. Caselli RJ, Reiman EM, Hentz JG, et al. A distinctive interaction between memory and chronic daytime somnolence in asymptomatic APOE e4 homozygotes. Sleep 2002;25(4):447–53.

19. Bliwise DL. Sleep apnea, APOE4 and Alzheimer's disease 20 years and counting? J Psychosom Res 2002;53(1):539–46.

20. Nikodemova M, Finn L, Mignot E, et al. Association of sleep disordered breathing and cognitive deficit in APOE ε4 carriers. Sleep 2013;36(6):873–80.

21. Chong MS, Ayalon L, Marler M, et al. Continuous positive airway pressure reduces subjective daytime sleepiness in patients with mild to moderate Alzheimer's disease with sleep disordered breathing. J Am Geriatr Soc 2006;54(5):777–81.

22. Shiota S, Takekawa H, Matsumoto SE, et al. Chronic intermittent hypoxia/reoxygenation facilitate amyloid-β generation in mice. J Alzheimers Dis 2013;37(2):325–33.

23. Troussière AC, Charley CM, Salleron J, et al. Treatment of sleep apnoea syndrome decreases cognitive decline in patients with Alzheimer's disease. J Neurol Neurosurg Psychiatry 2014;85(12): 1405–8.

24. Ancoli-Israel S, Palmer BW, Cooke JR, et al. Cognitive effects of treating obstructive sleep apnea in Alzheimer's disease: a randomized controlled study. J Am Geriatr Soc 2008;56(11):2076–81.

25. Cooke JR, Ayalon L, Palmer BW, et al. Sustained use of CPAP slows deterioration of cognition, sleep, and mood in patients with Alzheimer's disease and obstructive sleep apnea: a preliminary study. J Clin Sleep Med 2009;5(4):305–9.

26. Gnanasekaran G. "Sundowning" as a biological phenomenon: current understandings and future directions: an update. Aging Clin Exp Res 2016; 28(3):383–92.

27. Campbell SS, Kripke DF, Gillin JC, et al. Exposure to light in healthy elderly subjects and Alzheimer's patients. Physiol Behav 1988;42(2):141–4.

28. Fetveit A, Bjorvatn B. Bright-light treatment reduces actigraphic-measured daytime sleep in nursing home patients with dementia: a pilot study. Am J Geriatr Psychiatry 2005;13(5):420–3.

29. Ancoli-Israel S, Gehrman P, Martin JL, et al. Increased light exposure consolidates sleep and strengthens circadian rhythms in severe Alzheimer's disease patients. Behav Sleep Med 2003;1(1):22–36.

30. Skjerve A, Holsten F, Aarsland D, et al. Improvement in behavioral symptoms and advance of activity acrophase after short-term bright light treatment in severe dementia. Psychiatry Clin Neurosci 2004;58(4):343–7.

31. Wu YH, Swaab DF. Disturbance and strategies for reactivation of the circadian rhythm system in aging and Alzheimer's disease. Sleep Med 2007; 8(6):623–36.

32. Dowling GA, Burr RL, Van Someren EJ, et al. Melatonin and bright-light treatment for rest-activity disruption in institutionalized patients with Alzheimer's disease. J Am Geriatr Soc 2008;56(2): 239–46.

33. Venturelli M, Sollima A, Cè E, et al. Effectiveness of exercise- and cognitive-based treatments on salivary cortisol levels and sundowning syndrome symptoms in patients with Alzheimer's disease. J Alzheimers Dis 2016;53(4):1631–40.

34. Fronczek R, van Geest S, Frölich M, et al. Hypocretin (orexin) loss in Alzheimer's disease. Neurobiol Aging 2012;33(8):1642–50.

35. Liguori C, Romigi A, Nuccetelli M, et al. Orexinergic system dysregulation, sleep impairment, and cognitive decline in Alzheimer disease. JAMA Neurol 2014;71(12):1498–505.

36. Slats D, Claassen JA, Lammers GJ, et al. Association between hypocretin-1 and amyloid-β42 cerebrospinal fluid levels in Alzheimer's disease and healthy controls. Curr Alzheimer Res 2012;9(10): 1119–25.

37. Hutton M, Lendon CL, Rizzu P, et al. Association of missense and 5'-splice-site mutations in tau with the inherited dementia FTDP-17. Nature 1998; 393(6686):702–5.

38. Cruts M, Gijselinck I, van der Zee J, et al. Null mutations in progranulin cause ubiquitin-positive frontotemporal dementia linked to chromosome 17q21. Nature 2006;442(7105):920–4.

39. Rabinovici GD, Seeley WW, Kim EJ, et al. Distinct MRI atrophy patterns in autopsy-proven Alzheimer's disease and frontotemporal lobar degeneration. Am J Alzheimers Dis Other Demen 2007; 22(6):474–88.

40. Bonakis A, Economou NT, Paparrigopoulos T, et al. Sleep in frontotemporal dementia is equally or possibly more disrupted, and at an earlier stage, when compared to sleep in Alzheimer's disease. J Alzheimers Dis 2014;38(1):85–91.

41. Anderson KN, Hatfield C, Kipps C, et al. Disrupted sleep and circadian patterns in frontotemporal dementia. Eur J Neurol 2009;16(3):317–23.

42. Merrilees J, Hubbard E, Mastick J, et al. Disruption in a patient with frontotemporal dementia. Neurocase 2009;15(6):515–26.

43. McCarter SJ, St Louis EK, Boeve BF. Sleep disturbances in frontotemporal dementia. Curr Neurol Neurosci Rep 2016;16(9):85.

44. Pistacchi M, Gioulis M, Contin F, et al. Sleep disturbance and cognitive disorder: epidemiological analysis in a cohort of 263 patients. Neurol Sci 2014;35(12):1955–62.

45. Lo Coco D, Cupidi C, Mattaliano A, et al. REM sleep behavior disorder in a patient with frontotemporal dementia. Neurol Sci 2012;33(2):371–3.

46. Çoban A, Bilgiç B, Lohmann E, et al. Reduced orexin-A levels in frontotemporal dementia: possible association with sleep disturbance. Am J Alzheimers Dis Other Demen 2013;28(6):606–11.

47. Liguori C, Romigi A, Mercuri NB, et al. Cerebrospinal-fluid orexin levels and daytime somnolence in frontotemporal dementia. J Neurol 2014;261(9): 1832–6.

48. Gross RA, Spehlmann R, Daniels JC. Sleep disturbances in progressive supranuclear palsy. Electroencephalogr Clin Neurophysiol 1978;45:16–25.

49. Aldrich MS, Foster NL, White RF, et al. Sleep abnormalities in progressive supranuclear palsy. Ann Neurol 1989;25(6):577–81.

50. Lee S. The neuropsychiatric evolution of a case of progressive supranuclear palsy. Br J Psychiatry 1991;158:273–5.

51. Sixel-Döring F, Schweitzer M, Mollenhauer B, et al. Polysomnographic findings, video-based sleep analysis and sleep perception in progressive supranuclear palsy. Sleep Med 2009;10(4):407–15.

52. Gama RL, Távora DG, Bomfim RC, et al. Sleep disturbances and brain MRI morphometry in Parkinson's disease, multiple system atrophy and progressive supranuclear palsy - a comparative study. Parkinsonism Relat Disord 2010;16(4): 275–9.

53. De Bruin VS, Machado C, Howard RS, et al. Nocturnal and respiratory disturbances in Steele-Richardson-Olszewski syndrome (progressive supranuclear palsy). Postgrad Med J 1996; 72(847):293–6.

54. Cooper AD, Josephs KA. Photophobia, visual hallucinations, and REM sleep behavior disorder in progressive supranuclear palsy and corticobasal degeneration: a prospective study. Parkinsonism Relat Disord 2009;15(1):59–61.

55. Nomura T, Inoue Y, Takigawa H, et al. Comparison of REM sleep behaviour disorder variables between patients with progressive supranuclear palsy and those with Parkinson's disease. Parkinsonism Relat Disord 2012;18(4):394–6.

56. Arnulf I, Merino-Andreu M, Bloch F, et al. REM sleep behavior disorder and REM sleep without atonia in patients with progressive supranuclear palsy. Sleep 2005;28(3):349–54.

57. Hattori Y, Hattori T, Mukai E, et al. Excessive daytime sleepiness and low CSF orexin-A/hypocretin-I levels in a patient with probable progressive supranuclear palsy. No To Shinkei 2003;55(12): 1053–6 [in Japanese].

58. Yasui K, Inoue Y, Kanbayashi T, et al. CSF orexin levels of Parkinson's disease, dementia with Lewy bodies, progressive supranuclear palsy and

corticobasal degeneration. J Neurol Sci 2006; 250(1–2):120–3.

59. Wakabayashi K, Takahashi H. Pathological heterogeneity in progressive supranuclear palsy and corticobasal degeneration. Neuropathology 2004; 24(1):79–86.

60. Colosimo C, Morgante L, Antonini A, et al. Non-motor symptoms in atypical and secondary parkinsonism: the PRIAMO study. J Neurol 2010;257:5.

61. Arai T, Ikeda K, Akiyama H, et al. Intracellular processing of aggregated tau differs between corticobasal degeneration and progressive supranuclear palsy. Neuroreport 2001;12(5):935–8.

62. Wetter TC, Brunner H, Collado-Seidel V, et al. Sleep and periodic limb movements in corticobasal degeneration. Sleep Med 2002;3(1):33–6.

63. Roche S, Jacquesson JM, Destee A, et al. Sleep and vigilance in corticobasal degeneration: a descriptive study. Neurophysiol Clin 2007;37(4): 261–4.

64. Kimura K, Tachibana N, Aso T, et al. Subclinical REM sleep behavior disorder in a patient with corticobasal degeneration. Sleep 1997;20(10):891–4.

65. Klein C, Westenberger A. Genetics of Parkinson's disease. Cold Spring Harb Perspect Med 2012; 2(1):a008888.

66. Gulyani S, Salas R, Mari Z, et al. Evaluating and managing sleep disorders in the Parkinson's disease clinic. Basal Ganglia 2016;6(3):165–72.

67. Prudon B, Duncan GW, Khoo TK, et al. Primary sleep disorder prevalence in patients with newly diagnosed Parkinson's disease. Mov Disord 2014; 29(2):259–62.

68. Selvaraj VK, Keshavamurthy B. Sleep dysfunction in Parkinson's disease. J Clin Diagn Res 2016; 10(2):OC09–12.

69. Bro D, O'Hara R, Primeau M, et al. Association of restless legs syndrome with incident Parkinson disease sleep. J Clin Diagn Res 2016. pii: sp-00400–16. [Epub ahead of print].

70. Adel S, Djarmati A, Kabakci K, et al. Co-occurrence of restless legs syndrome and Parkin mutations in two families. Mov Disord 2006;21(2):258–63.

71. Limousin N, Konofal E, Karroum E, et al. Restless legs syndrome, rapid eye movement sleep behavior disorder, and hypersomnia in patients with two parkin mutations. Mov Disord 2009; 24(13):1970–6.

72. Poewe W, Högl B. Akathisia, restless legs and periodic limb movements in sleep in Parkinson's disease. Neurology 2004;63(8 Suppl 3):S12–6.

73. Marchesi E, Negrotti A, Angelini M, et al. A prospective study of the cumulative incidence and course of restless legs syndrome in de novo patients with Parkinson's disease during chronic dopaminergic therapy. J Neurol 2016; 263(3):441–7.

74. Allen RP, Earley CJ. Augmentation of the restless legs syndrome with carbidopa/levodopa. Sleep 1996;19(3):205–13.

75. Moreno-López C, Santamaría J, Salamero M, et al. Excessive daytime sleepiness in multiple system atrophy (SLEEMSA study). Arch Neurol 2011; 68(2):223–30.

76. Setthawatcharawanich S, Limapichat K, Sathirapanya P, et al. Excessive daytime sleepiness and nighttime sleep quality in Thai patients with Parkinson's disease. J Med Assoc Thai 2014; 97(10):1022–7.

77. Babkina OV, Poluektov MG, Levin OS. Heterogeneity of excessive daytime sleepiness in Parkinson's disease. Zh Nevrol Psikhiatr Im S S Korsakova 2016;116(6 Vyp 2. Neurology and psychiatry of elderly):60–70 [in Russian].

78. Tandberg E, Larsen JP, Karlsen K. Excessive daytime sleepiness and sleep benefit in Parkinson's disease: a community-based study. Mov Disord 1999;14(6):922–7.

79. Tholfsen LK, Larsen JP, Schulz J, et al. Development of excessive daytime sleepiness in early Parkinson disease. Neurology 2015;85(2):162–8.

80. Cochen De Cock V, Bayard S, Jaussent I, et al. Daytime sleepiness in Parkinson's disease: a reappraisal. PLoS One 2014;9(9):e107278.

81. Mahale R, Yadav R, Pal PK. Quality of sleep in young onset Parkinson's disease: any difference from older onset Parkinson's disease. Parkinsonism Relat Disord 2015;21(5):461–4.

82. Goldman JG, Ghode RA, Ouyang B, et al. Dissociations among daytime sleepiness, nighttime sleep, and cognitive status in Parkinson's disease. Parkinsonism Relat Disord 2013;19(9):806–11.

83. Gong Y, Liu CF. An analysis of clinical characteristics and factors in Parkinson's disease patients with excessive daytime sleepiness. Zhonghua Nei Ke Za Zhi 2016;55(7):515–9 [in Chinese].

84. Spindler M, Gooneratne NS, Siderowf A, et al. Daytime sleepiness is associated with falls in Parkinson's disease. J Parkinsons Dis 2013;3(3):387–91.

85. Valko PO, Hauser S, Sommerauer M, et al. Observations on sleep-disordered breathing in idiopathic Parkinson's disease. PLoS One 2014;9(6):e100828.

86. Nomura T, Inoue Y, Kobayashi M, et al. Characteristics of obstructive sleep apnea in patients with Parkinson's disease. J Neurol Sci 2013;327(1–2):22–4.

87. da Silva-Júnior FP Jr, do Prado GF, Barbosa ER, et al. Sleep disordered breathing in Parkinson's disease: a critical appraisal. Sleep Med Rev 2014;18(2):173–8.

88. Yeh NC, Tien K, Yang CM, et al. Increased risk of Parkinson's disease in patients with obstructive sleep apnea: a population-based, propensity score-matched, longitudinal follow-up study. Medicine (Baltimore) 2016;95(2):e2293.

89. Cochen De Cock V, Abouda M, Leu S, et al. Is obstructive sleep apnea a problem in Parkinson's disease? Sleep Med 2010;11(3):247–52.

90. Cochen De Cock V, Benard-Serre N, Driss V, et al. Supine sleep and obstructive sleep apnea syndrome in Parkinson's disease. Sleep Med 2015; 16(12):1497–501.

91. Zhang LY, Liu WY, Kang WY, et al. Association of rapid eye movement sleep behavior disorder with sleep-disordered breathing in Parkinson's disease. Sleep Med 2016;20:110–5.

92. Neikrug AB, Liu L, Avanzino JA, et al. Continuous positive airway pressure improves sleep and daytime sleepiness in patients with Parkinson disease and sleep apnea. Sleep 2014;37(1):177–85.

93. Ataide M, Franco CM, Lins OG. Daytime sleepiness in Parkinson's disease: perception, influence of drugs, and mood disorder. Sleep Disord 2014; 2014:939713.

94. Zhu K, van Hilten JJ, Marinus J. Course and risk factors for excessive daytime sleepiness in Parkinson's disease. Parkinsonism Relat Disord 2016;24:34–40.

95. Pal S, Bhattacharya KF, Agapito C, et al. A study of excessive daytime sleepiness and its clinical significance in three groups of Parkinson's disease patients taking pramipexole, cabergoline and levodopa mono and combination therapy. J Neural Transm 2001;108(1):71–7.

96. Ylikoski A, Martikainen K, Sarkanen T, et al. Parkinson's disease and narcolepsy-like symptoms. Sleep Med 2015;16(4):540–4.

97. Bliwise DL, Trotti LM, Juncos JJ, et al. Daytime REM sleep in Parkinson's disease. Parkinsonism Relat Disord 2013;19(1):101–3.

98. Compta Y, Santamaria J, Ratti L, et al. Cerebrospinal hypocretin, daytime sleepiness and sleep architecture in Parkinson's disease dementia. Brain 2009;132(Pt 12):3308–17.

99. Fronczek R, Overeem S, Lee SY, et al. Hypocretin (orexin) loss in Parkinson's disease. Brain 2007; 130(Pt 6):1577–85.

100. Thannickal TC, Lai YY, Siegel JM. Hypocretin (orexin) cell loss in Parkinson's disease. Brain 2007;130(Pt 6):1586–95.

101. Arnulf I, Neutel D, Herlin B, et al. Sleepiness in idiopathic REM sleep behavior disorder and Parkinson disease. Sleep 2015;38(10):1529–35.

102. Videnovic A, Noble C, Reid KJ, et al. Circadian melatonin rhythm and excessive daytime sleepiness in Parkinson disease. JAMA Neurol 2014; 71(4):463–9.

103. Gilman S, Low P, Quinn N, et al. Consensus on the diagnosis of multi-system atrophy. Neurologia 1999;14(9):425–8 [in Spanish].

104. Gilman S, Wenning GK, Low PA, et al. Second consensus statement on the diagnosis of multiple system atrophy. Neurology 2008;71(9):670–6.

105. Nam H, Hong YH, Kwon HM, et al. Does multiple system atrophy itself affect sleep structure? Neurologist 2009;15(5):274–6.

106. Zhang L, Cao B, Ou R, et al. Non-motor symptoms and the quality of life in multiple system atrophy with different subtypes. Parkinsonism Relat Disord 2017;35:63–8.

107. Ghorayeb I, Yekhlef F, Chrysostome V, et al. Sleep disorders and their determinants in multiple system atrophy. J Neurol Neurosurg Psychiatry 2002;72(6): 798–800.

108. Shimohata T, Nakayama H, Tomita M, et al. Daytime sleepiness in Japanese patients with multiple system atrophy: prevalence and determinants. BMC Neurol 2012;12:130.

109. Hogl B, Seppi K, Brandauer E, et al. Irresistible onset of sleep during acute levodopa challenge in a patient with multiple system atrophy (MSA): placebo-controlled, polysomnographic case report. Mov Disord 2001;16(6):1177–9.

110. Seppi K, Hogl B, Diem A, et al. Levodopa-induced sleepiness in the Parkinson variant of multiple system atrophy. Mov Disord 2006;21(8):1281–3.

111. Garcia-Sanchez A, Fernandez-Navarro I, Garcia-Rio F. Central apneas and REM sleep behavior disorder as an initial presentation of multiple system atrophy. J Clin Sleep Med 2016;12(2):267–70.

112. Shimohata T, Shinoda H, Nakayama H, et al. Daytime hypoxemia, sleep-disordered breathing, and laryngopharyngeal findings in multiple system atrophy. Arch Neurol 2007;64(6):856–61.

113. Suzuki M, Saigusa H, Shibasaki K, et al. Multiple system atrophy manifesting as complex sleep-disordered breathing. Auris Nasus Larynx 2010; 37(1):110–3.

114. Ozawa T, Sekiya K, Aizawa N, et al. Laryngeal stridor in multiple system atrophy: clinicopathological features and causal hypotheses. J Neurol Sci 2016;361:243–9.

115. Ferini-Strambi L, Marelli S. Sleep dysfunction in multiple system atrophy. Curr Treat Options Neurol 2012;14(5):464–73.

116. Shukla G, Kaul B, Gupta A, et al. Parkinsonian syndromes presenting with circadian rhythm sleep disorder- advanced sleep-phase type. Natl Med J India 2015;28(5):233–5.

117. Ghorayeb I, Dupouy S, Tison F, et al. Restless legs syndrome in multiple system atrophy. J Neural Transm (Vienna) 2014;121(12):1523–7.

118. Wetter TC, Collado-Seidel V, Pollmacher T, et al. Sleep and periodic leg movement patterns in drug-free patients with Parkinson's disease and multiple system atrophy. Sleep 2000;23(3):361–7.

119. Palma JA, Fernandez-Cordon C, Coon EA, et al. Prevalence of REM sleep behavior disorder in multiple system atrophy: a multicenter study and meta-analysis. Clin Auton Res 2015;25(1):69–75.

120. Benarroch EE, Schmeichel AM, Low PA, et al. Depletion of putative chemosensitive respiratory neurons in the ventral medullary surface in multiple system atrophy. Brain 2007;130(Pt 2):469–75.

121. Martinez-Rodriguez JE, Seppi K, Cardozo A, et al. Cerebrospinal fluid hypocretin-1 levels in multiple system atrophy. Mov Disord 2007;22(12):1822–4.

122. Abdo WF, Bloem BR, Kremer HP, et al. CSF hypocretin-1 levels are normal in multiple-system atrophy. Parkinsonism Relat Disord 2008;14(4): 342–4.

123. Schmeichel AM, Buchhalter LC, Low PA, et al. Mesopontine cholinergic neuron involvement in Lewy body dementia and multiple system atrophy. Neurology 2008;70(5):368–73.

124. Ferman TJ, Boeve BF, Smith GE, et al. Inclusion of RBD improves the diagnostic classification of dementia with Lewy bodies. Neurology 2011;77(9): 875–82.

125. Hibi S, Yamaguchi Y, Umeda-Kameyama Y, et al. The high frequency of periodic limb movements in patients with Lewy body dementia. J Psychiatr Res 2012;46(12):1590–4.

126. Fujishiro H. Effects of gabapentin enacarbil on restless legs syndrome and leg pain in dementia with Lewy bodies. Psychogeriatrics 2014;14(2):132–4.

127. Bhalsing K, Suresh K, Muthane UB, et al. Prevalence and profile of restless legs syndrome in Parkinson's disease and other neurodegenerative disorders: a case-control study. Parkinsonism Relat Disord 2013;19(4):426–30.

128. Scharre DW, Chang SI, Nagaraja HN, et al. Paired studies comparing clinical profiles of Lewy Body Dementia with Alzheimer's and Parkinson's Diseases. J Alzheimers Dis 2016;54(3):995–1004.

129. Cagnin A, Fragiacomo F, Camporese G, et al. Sleep-Wake profile in dementia with Lewy Bodies, Alzheimer's Disease, and normal aging. J Alzheimers Dis 2017;55(4):1529–36.

130. Chwiszczuk L, Breitve M, Hynninen M, et al. Higher frequency and complexity of sleep disturbances in dementia with Lewy Bodies as compared to Alzheimer's Disease. Neurodegener Dis 2016;16(3–4): 152–60.

131. Ferman TJ, Smith GE, Dickson DW, et al. Abnormal daytime sleepiness in dementia with Lewy bodies compared to Alzheimer's disease using the multiple sleep latency test. Alzheimers Res Ther 2014; 6(9):76.

132. Elder GJ, Colloby SJ, Lett DJ, et al. Depressive symptoms are associated with daytime sleepiness and subjective sleep quality in dementia with Lewy bodies. Int J Geriatr Psychiatry 2016;31(7):765–70.

133. Baumann CR, Dauvilliers Y, Mignot E, et al. Normal CSF hypocretin-1 (orexin A) levels in dementia with Lewy bodies associated with excessive daytime sleepiness. Eur Neurol 2004;52(2):73–6.

134. Lessig S, Ubhi K, Galasko D, et al. Reduced hypocretin (orexin) levels in dementia with Lewy bodies. Neuroreport 2010;21(11):756–60.

135. Harper DG, Stopa EG, McKee AC, et al. Dementia severity and Lewy bodies affect circadian rhythms in Alzheimer disease. Neurobiol Aging 2004;25(6): 771–81.

136. Cunchillos JD, De Andrés I. Participation of the cerebellum in the regulation of the sleep-wakefulness cycle. Results in cerebellectomized cats. Electroencephalogr Clin Neurophysiol 1982;53(5):549–58.

137. Kitamura J, Kubuki Y, Tsuruta K, et al. A new family with Joseph disease in Japan. Homovanillic acid, magnetic resonance, and sleep apnea studies. Arch Neurol 1989;46(4):425–8.

138. Chokroverty S, Sachdeo R, Masdeu J. Autonomic dysfunction and sleep apnea in olivopontocerebellar degeneration. Arch Neurol 1984;41(9):926–31.

139. Salva MA, Guilleminault C. Olivopontocerebellar degeneration, abnormal sleep, and REM sleep without atonia. Neurology 1986;36(4):576–7.

140. Pedroso JL, Braga-Neto P, Escorcio-Bezerra ML, et al. Non-motor and extracerebellar features in spinocerebellar Ataxia Type 2. Cerebellum 2017; 16(1):34–9.

141. Abele M, Bürk K, Laccone F, et al. Restless legs syndrome in spinocerebellar ataxia types 1, 2, and 3. J Neurol 2001;248(4):311–4.

142. Friedman JH. Presumed rapid eye movement behavior disorder in Machado-Joseph disease (spinocerebellar ataxia type 3). Mov Disord 2002; 17(6):1350–3.

143. Iranzo A, Muñoz E, Santamaria J, et al. REM sleep behavior disorder and vocal cord paralysis in Machado-Joseph disease. Mov Disord 2003; 18(10):1179–83.

144. Kapoor M, Greenough G. Spectrum of sleep disorders in a patient with spinocerebellar ataxia 13. J Clin Sleep Med 2015;11(2):177–9.

145. Silva GM, Pedroso JL, Dos Santos DF, et al. NREM-related parasomnias in Machado-Joseph disease: clinical and polysomnographic evaluation. J Sleep Res 2016;25(1):11–5.

146. Hsu CH, Chen YL, Pei D, et al. Depression as the primary cause of insomnia and excessive daytime sleepiness in a family with multiple cases of spinocerebellar ataxia. J Clin Sleep Med 2016;12(7): 1059–61.

147. Chi NF, Shiao GM, Ku HL, et al. Sleep disruption in spinocerebellar ataxia type 3: a genetic and polysomnographic study. J Chin Med Assoc 2013; 76(1):25–30.

148. Pedroso JL, Braga-Neto P, Felício AC, et al. Sleep disorders in machado-joseph disease: frequency, discriminative thresholds, predictive values, and correlation with ataxia-related motor and non-motor features. Cerebellum 2011;10(2):291–5.

149. Boesch SM, Frauscher B, Brandauer E, et al. Restless legs syndrome and motor activity during sleep in spinocerebellar ataxia type 6. Sleep Med 2006; 7(6):529–32.

150. Rueda AD, Pedroso JL, Truksinas E, et al. Polysomnography findings in spinocerebellar ataxia type 6. J Sleep Res 2016;25(6):720–3.

151. Howell MJ, Mahowald MW, Gomez CM. Evaluation of sleep and daytime somnolence in spinocerebellar ataxia type 6 (SCA6). Neurology 2006;66(9): 1430–1.

152. Wiegand M, Möller AA, Lauer CJ, et al. Nocturnal sleep in Huntington's disease. J Neurol 1991; 238(4):203–8.

153. Spire JP, Bliwise DL, Noronha ABC, et al. Sleep profiles in Huntington disease. Neurology 1981; 31(2):151.

154. Emser W, Brenner M, Stober T, et al. Changes in nocturnal sleep in Huntington's and Parkinson's disease. J Neurol 1988;235(3):177–9.

155. Goodman AO, Rogers L, Pilsworth S, et al. Asymptomatic sleep abnormalities are a common early feature in patients with Huntington's disease. Curr Neurol Neurosci Rep 2011;11(2):211–7.

156. Morton AJ. Circadian and sleep disorders in Huntington's disease [review]. Exp Neurol 2013;243: 34–44.

157. Baker CR, Domínguez DJF, Stout JC, et al. Subjective sleep problems in Huntington's disease: a pilot investigation of the relationship to brain structure, neurocognitive, and neuropsychiatric function. J Neurol Sci 2016;364:148–53.

158. Videnovic A, Leurgans S, Fan W, et al. Daytime somnolence and nocturnal sleep disturbances in Huntington disease. Parkinsonism Relat Disord 2009;15(6):471–4.

159. Aziz NA, Anguelova GV, Marinus J, et al. Sleep and circadian rhythm alterations correlate with depression and cognitive impairment in Huntington's disease. Parkinsonism Relat Disord 2010;16(5): 345–50.

160. Cuturic M, Abramson RK, Vallini D, et al. Sleep patterns in patients with Huntington's disease and their unaffected first-degree relatives: a brief report. Behav Sleep Med 2009;7(4):245–54.

161. Piano C, Losurdo A, Della Marca G, et al. Polysomnographic findings and clinical correlates in Huntington disease: a cross-sectional cohort study. Sleep 2015;38(9):1489–95.

162. Savva E, Schnorf H, Burkhard PR. Restless legs syndrome: an early manifestation of Huntington's disease? Acta Neurol Scand 2009;119(4):274–6.

163. Meier A, Mollenhauer B, Cohrs S, et al. Normal hypocretin-1 (orexin-A) levels in the cerebrospinal fluid of patients with Huntington's disease. Brain Res 2005;1063(2):201–3.

164. Gaus SE, Lin L, Mignot E. CSF hypocretin levels are normal in Huntington's disease patients. Sleep 2005;28(12):1607–8.

165. Sheng P, Hou L, Wang X, et al. Efficacy of modafinil on fatigue and excessive daytime sleepiness associated with neurological disorders: a systematic review and meta-analysis. PLoS One 2013;8(12): e81802.

Pharmacologic Management of Excessive Daytime Sleepiness

Shinichi Takenoshita, MD, MPH, Seiji Nishino, MD, PhD*

KEYWORDS

- Stimulants • Excessive daytime sleepiness • Narcolepsy • Idiopathic hypersomnia

KEY POINTS

- Excessive daytime sleepiness (EDS) is related to medical and social problems, including mental disorders, physical diseases, poor quality of life, and so forth.
- Several different types of stimulants (or wake-promoting compounds) are available to treat EDS, and a variety of new drugs are under development.
- The side effects of some of the stimulants are potent, and careful selection and management is required.

INTRODUCTION

EDS is defined as "irresistible sleepiness in a situation when an individual would be expected to be awake, and alert."[1] EDS has been a big concern not only from a medical but also from a public health point of view. According to recently published articles, the prevalence of patients who suffer from EDS is approximately 20% in the world.[2–4] Patients with EDS have the possibility of falling asleep even when they should wake up and concentrate, for example, when they drive, play sports, or walk outside. Subjects who have EDS encounter a lower quality of life and have a higher odds ratio of developing a mental disorder, cognitive impairment, and motor vehicle accidents.[5–8]

Although nonpharmacologic treatments (ie, napping and work accommodations) are often helpful, a large majority of the diagnosed patients reported using pharmacologic therapies, mostly stimulant medications.[9]

Historically, EDS was also a large concern in the military. Many countries let soldiers take stimulants when they were engaged in military service in World War II. Currently, preventing sleepiness caused by sleep deprivation is still a major research project by the Defense Advanced Research Projects Agency in the United States.

In 1931, the first stimulant (ie, amphetamine) was applied to treat EDS associated with narcolepsy.[10] Since then, many new stimulants have developed to treat EDS, and many patients received benefits. Stimulants, however, are drugs with strong side effects (ie, sympathomimetic) and addiction potential and these treatments are mostly symptomatic; they improve the level of alertness by simply suppressing sleepiness.

Abuse potential of stimulants is a problem especially when diagnoses of hypersomomnias are loosely made, and this is particularly true for narcolepsy, where stimulant abuse is rare among patients with well-defined narcolepsy.[11–14] In this article, clinical characteristics of common hypersomnias and pharmacologic treatments of each hypersomnia are described. New treatment options under development for treating EDS associated with these hypersomnias are also

Disclosure Statement: S. Nishino had a sponsored research contract (SPO#50970) with Ono Pharmacutical Co. Ltd.
Sleep and Circadian Neurobiology Laboratory, Department of Psychiatry and Behavioral Sciences, Stanford University School of Medicine, Stanford University, Palo Alto, CA, USA
* Corresponding author. 3155 Porter Drive, Room 2141, Palo Alto, CA 94304.
E-mail address: nishino@stanford.edu

Sleep Med Clin 12 (2017) 461–478
http://dx.doi.org/10.1016/j.jsmc.2017.03.019

discussed. The hypersomnias focused on in this article are narcolepsy type 1, narcolepsy type 2, idiopathic hypersomnia, and hypersomnia due to a medical disorder, defined in the *International Classification of Sleep Disorders, Third Edition* (*ICSD-3*).

TYPES OF HYPERSOMNIAS

According to the *ICDS-3*, published in 2014, diseases that result from EDS are listed as narcolepsy type 1, narcolepsy type 2, idiopathic hypersomnia, Kleine-Levin syndrome, hypersomnia due to a medical disorder, hypersomnia due to a medication or substance, hypersomnia associated with a psychiatric disorder, and insufficient sleep syndrome.[15]

This review covers the pharmacologic treatments of EDS associated with narcolepsy type 1,

narcolepsy type 2, idiopathic hypersomnia, and hypersomnia due to a medical disorder, because relatively consistent guidelines for the pharmacotherapy of these diseases are available. The *ICSD-3* diagnostic criteria of these hypersomnias are summarized in **Table 1**. For the treatment of Kleine-Levin syndrome and other hypersomnias, see the article by Arnulf.[16]

NARCOLEPSY
Symptoms of Narcolepsy

Narcolepsy is a syndrome characterized by "EDS that is typically associated with cataplexy and other [rapid eye movement] REM sleep phenomena such as sleep paralysis and hypnagogic hallucinations."[17] The prevalence of narcolepsy with cataplexy has been examined in many studies and falls between 25 and 50 per 100,000 people

Table 1
Diagnostic criteria, *International Classification of Sleep Disorders, Third Edition*

Narcolepsy Type 1	Narcolepsy Type 2	Idiopathic Hypersomnia	Hypersomnia due to a Medical Disorder
Criteria A and B	All Criteria A–E	All Criteria A–F	All Criteria A–D

A. Daily periods of irrepressible need to sleep or daytime lapses into sleep, present for at least 3 mo
B. Either 1 or 2 or both
  1. Cataplexy and mean sleep latency ≤8 min and 2 or more SOREM periods on MSLT. REM within 15 min of sleep onset on the preceding nocturnal polysomnogram may replace one of SOREM periods.
  2. Low CSF hypocretin-1 concentration (<110 pg/mL or less than one-third of control values)
	A. Daily periods of irrepressible need to sleep or daytime lapses into sleep, present for at least 3 mo
	B. Mean sleep latency ≤8 min and 2 or more SOREM periods on MSLT. REM within 15 min of sleep onset on the preceding nocturnal polysomnogram may replace one of the SOREM periods.
	C. No cataplexy
	D. CSF hypocretin-1 concentration has not been measured or CSF hypocretin-1 concentration is ≥110 pg/mL or greater than one-third of control values.
	E. The hypersomnolence and/or MSLT findings are not better explained by other causes.
		A. Daily periods of irrepressible need to sleep or daytime lapses into sleep, present for at least 3 mo
		B. Fewer than 2 SOREM periods on MSLT (or fewer than one of nocturnal REM latency was ≤15 min)
		C. No cataplexy
		D. Either 1 or 2 or both
		  1. Mean sleep latency ≤8 min on MSLT
		  2. Total 24-h sleep time ≥660 min on 24-h polysomnographic monitoring or wrist actigraphy (averaged over ≥7 d)
		E. Insufficient sleep syndrome is ruled out.
		F. The hypersomnolence and/or MSLT findings are not better explained by other causes.
			A. Daily periods of irrepressible need to sleep or daytime lapses into sleep, present for at least 3 mo
			B. The daytime sleepiness occurs as a consequence of a significant underlying medical or neurologic condition.
			C. Mean sleep latency is ≤8 min, and fewer than 2 SOREM periods are observed.
			D. The symptoms are not better explained by another untreated sleep disorder, a mental disorder, or the effects of medications or drugs.

From International classification of sleep disorders: diagnostic and coding manual, 3rd edition. Westchester (IL): American Academy of Sleep Medicine; 2014; with permission.

(0.025%–0.05%).[18,19] The onset of the disease is most often seen during adolescence around puberty.[20] As with the sleepiness of other sleep disorders, sleepiness or EDS of narcolepsy presents with an increased propensity to fall asleep, nodding, or easily dozing in relaxed or sedentary situations or a need to exert extra effort to avoid sleeping in these situations.[21] Additionally, irresistible or overwhelming urges to sleep commonly occur from time to time during wakeful periods in untreated narcolepsy patients. These so-called sleep attacks are not instantaneous lapses into sleep, as is often thought by the general public, but represent episodes of profound sleepiness experienced by those with marked sleep deprivation or other severe sleep disorders. This feeling is most often relieved by short naps (15–30 minutes), but in most cases the refreshed sensation only lasts a short time after awaking. The refreshing value of short naps is of considerable diagnostic value for EDS associated with narcolepsy.

EDS can be objectively measured with the standardized multiple sleep latency test (MSLT), and the MSLT findings (mean sleep latency <8 minutes) were included in the diagnostic criteria of EDS associated with narcolepsy and other hypersomnias (see **Table 1**).[17] The maintenance of wakefulness test (MWT) was also developed to measure how alert patients are when they are set in a boring situation during the day.[22] Although the MWT is not included in the diagnostic criteria of any hypersomnias, many researchers believe that the MWT is more sensitive in evaluating effects of treatments, such as by pharmacotherapy with wake-promoting compounds. One of the reasons for this is the floor effects seen with MSLT; when the EDS is sever, it is often difficult to detect the therapeutic effects (to sleep vs to stay awake with MWT) with the MSLT protocol. Therefore, the MWT is often used to examine the therapeutic effects of wake-promoting compounds. There is not enough evidence, however, to set the cutoff value even when the MWT is used to measure the effect of the treatment of diseases.[23,24]

In addition to EDS, narcoleptic patients exhibit cataplexy and other abnormal manifestations of REM sleep, such as hypnagogic hallucinations and sleep paralysis.[25] Cataplexy, the sudden occurrence of muscle weakness in association with emotions, such as laughing, joking, or anger, has long been considered a pathognomonic symptom of the syndrome.[21,26,27] Cataplectic events usually last from a few seconds to 2 or 3 minutes but occasionally continue longer.[28] Patients are usually alert and oriented during the event despite their inability to respond. Positive emotions, such as laughter, more commonly trigger cataplexy than negative emotions; however, any strong emotion is a potential trigger.[29]

Hypnagogic or hypnopompic hallucinations may be visual, tactile, auditory, or multisensory events, usually brief but occasionally continuing for a few minutes, that occur at transitions from wakefulness to sleep (hypnagogic) or from sleep to wakefulness (hypnopompic).[21] Hallucinations may contain combined elements of dream sleep and consciousness and are often bizarre or disturbing to patients.

Sleep paralysis is the inability to move, lasting from a few seconds to a few minutes, during the transition from sleep to wakefulness or from wakefulness to sleep. Episodes of sleep paralysis may alarm patients, particularly those who experience the sensation of being unable to breathe. Although accessory respiratory muscles may not be active during these episodes, diaphragmatic activity continues, and air exchange remains adequate.

One of the most frequently associated symptoms is insomnia, best characterized as a difficulty to maintain nighttime sleep. Typically, narcoleptic patients fall asleep easily, only to wake up after a short nap and are unable to return to sleep for another hour or so. Narcoleptic patients do not usually sleep more than normal individuals over the 24-hour cycle[30–32] but frequently have disrupted nighttime sleep.[30–32] Frequently associated problems are periodic leg movements,[33,34] REM behavior disorder, other parasomnias,[35,36] and obstructive sleep apnea.[34,37,38]

Other commonly reported symptoms include automatic behavior — absent-minded behavior or speech that is often nonsensical that the patient does not remember. Hypnagogic hallucinations, sleep paralysis, and automatic behavior are nonspecific to narcolepsy and occur in other sleep disorders (as well as in healthy individuals); however, these symptoms are far more common and occur with much greater frequency in narcolepsy.[39]

Hypocretin/Orexin Deficiency in Type 1 Narcolepsy

In most patients with cataplexy, a deficiency in the hypocretin neuropeptide system is involved in the pathophysiology of human narcolepsy.[40] The observation that cerebrospinal fluid (CSF) hypocretin-1 levels are decreased in patients with narcolepsy provides a new diagnostic tool and refines the nosologic considerations for narcolepsy.

Using a large sample of patients and controls, the authors determined that 110 pg/mL (30% of mean control values) was the most specific and sensitive cutoff value for diagnosing narcolepsy.[41] Most samples had undetectable levels (<40 pg/mL), and a few had detectable but very diminished levels. None of the patients with idiopathic hypersomnia, sleep apnea, restless legs syndrome, or insomnia had abnormal hypocretin levels. Because the specificity of the CSF finding is also high, low CSF hypocretin-1 levels were included in the *International Classifications of Sleep Disorder, Second Edition*, as a positive diagnosis for narcolepsy-cataplexy.[42] In the most recent revision of the *ICSD*, *ICSD-3*, published in 2014,[15] narcolepsy-cataplexy was renamed narcolepsy type 1, or hypocretin deficiency syndrome, whereas narcolepsy without cataplexy was renamed narcolepsy type 2 (hypocretin nondeficient) to emphasize the pathophysiologic basis of the diseases.

Immune System and Narcolepsy

It has been reported that a large majority people with narcolepsy have the tissue-type HLA DR2.[21,28] High-resolution typing revealed that narcolepsy has the closest association with HLA-DQB1*0602, which is found in 95% of narcoleptic patients with cataplexy and 41% of patients with narcolepsy without cataplexy but only 18% to 35% of the general population.[21,43] The tight association between narcolepsy and an antigen-presenting class II HLA type suggests that autoimmune processes may play a critical role in type 1 narcolepsy because many autoimmune diseases exhibit tight associations with class II HLA haplotypes. Type 1 narcolepsy cases could thus involve an autoimmune alteration of hypocretin-containing cells in the central nervous system (CNS), but the antigen for this pathologic process has not yet been identified. Dauvilliers and colleagues[44] reported an HLA-DQB1*0602–positive monozygotic twin pair discordant for narcolepsy and CSF hypocretin-1 (only the affected subject had a low hypocretin-1 level), suggesting that altered CSF hypocretin levels are state dependent and not trait dependent and likely an acquired deficit. In other words, the genetic background is likely not sufficient to develop an abnormality in the hypocretin system. This finding is also complementary to the autoimmune hypothesis.

Considerations for the Pathophysiology of Type 2 Narcolepsy

There are debates about the pathophysiology of narcolepsy with normal hypocretin levels (ie, type 2 narcolepsy). More than 90% of the patients with narcolepsy without cataplexy show normal CSF hypocretin levels, yet they show apparent REM sleep abnormalities (ie, sleep-onset REMs [SOREMs]). Furthermore, even if the strict criteria for narcolepsy-cataplexy are applied, up to 10% of patients with narcolepsy-cataplexy show normal CSF hypocretin levels. Considering that occurrence of cataplexy is tightly associated with hypocretin deficiency, impaired hypocretin neurotransmission is still likely involved in narcolepsy-cataplexy with normal CSF hypocretin levels. Conceptually, there are 2 possibilities to explain these mechanisms: (1) specific impairment of hypocretin receptor and their downstream pathway and (2) partial/localized loss of hypocretin ligand (yet normal CSF levels exhibited). A good example for the former is Hcrtr 2-mutated narcoleptic dogs; they exhibit normal CSF hypocretin-1 levels[45] while having full-blown narcolepsy. Thannickal and colleagues[46] reported 1 narcolepsy without cataplexy patient (HLA typing was unknown) who had an overall loss of 33% of hypocretin cells compared with normal, with maximal cell loss in the posterior hypothalamus. This result favors the second hypothesis, but studies with more cases are needed.

Treatment of Excessive Daytime Sleepiness Associated with Narcolepsy Types 1 and 2

Nonpharmacologic treatments (ie, behavioral modification, such as regular napping and work accommodations) are often helpful. In a survey by a patient group organization,[47–49] however, 94% of all patients reported using pharmacologic therapies, mostly stimulant medications.[50]

Sleepiness is usually treated using amphetamine-like CNS stimulants (ie, methylphenidate) or modafinil (ie, 2-[(diphenylmethy)sulfinyl]acetamide) and its R-enantiomer, armodafinil, which are wake-promoting compounds unrelated to amphetamines (**Table 2**[51]). More recently, the American Academy of Sleep Medicine (AASM) recommended the use of sodium oxybate, a short-lasting sedative of unknown mechanisms, as first-line treatment of EDS and cataplexy, The most commonly used amphetamine-like compounds are methylphenidate, methamphetamine, D-amphetamine (all schedule II compounds), and mazindol (a schedule IV compound) (**Fig. 1**; see **Table 2**). The clinical use of stimulants in narcolepsy often has been the subject of standards of practice published by AASM.[52] Typically, a patient is started on a low dose, which is then increased progressively to obtain satisfactory results. Studies have shown that daytime sleepiness can be greatly improved subjectively, but sleep variables are never completely normalized by stimulant treatments.[53] Milder stimulants with low efficacy and potency, such as modafinil or armodafinil, are usually tried first (see **Fig. 1**). More effective amphetamine-like

Table 2
Current pharmacologic treatment of excessive daytime sleepiness associated with narcolepsy

Compound	Scheduled Class[a]	Usual Daily Doses	Half-Life (h)	Side Effects/Notes
Modafinil	IV	100–400 mg	9–14[b]	No peripheral sympathomimetic action, headaches, nausea
Armodafinil	IV	100–300 mg	10–15[b]	Similar to those of modafinil
Mazindol	IV	2–8 mg	10–13	Reduction of appetite or increase in blood pressure
Methylphenidate hydrochloride	II	≤80 mg	2–4	Same as amphetamines; less reduction of appetite or increase in blood pressure
Methamphetamine	II	5–80 mg	9–12	Irritability, mood changes, headache, palpitations, tremors, excessive sweating, insomnia
D-Amphetamine sulfate	II	≤60 mg	10–28	Irritability, mood changes, headache, palpitations, tremors, excessive sweating, insomnia
Sodium oxybate	III	4.5–9 g	0.5–1	Overdoses (a single dose of 60–100 mg/kg) induce dizziness, nausea, vomiting, confusion, agitation, epileptic seizures, hallucinations, coma with bradycardia, and respiratory depression; evidence of withdrawal syndrome

[a] All compounds in the list are scheduled and the class is listed.
[b] The half-life of the S-enantiomer of modafinil is short (approximately 3–4 h), so the half-life of racemic modafinil mostly reflects the R-enantiomer (armodafinil).

stimulants (methylphenidate, D-amphetamine, and methamphetamine) are then used if needed (see **Fig. 1**). Stimulant compounds are generally well tolerated in patients with narcolepsy. Minor adverse effects, such as headaches, irritability, nervousness, tremors, anorexia, palpitations, sweating, and gastric discomfort, are common. Cardiovascular impact, such as increased blood pressure, is possible, considering that sympathomimetic effects of these classes of compounds have been established in animals, although they have been remarkably difficult to document in human studies. Surprisingly, tolerance rarely occurs in this patient population and drug holidays are not recommended by the AASM.[52] Stimulant abuse is rare among patients with well-defined narcolepsy.[11–14] A compliance study has shown that approximately 50% of patients who receive stimulants reduce or withdraw stimulant medications by themselves.[54] Exceptionally, psychotic complications may be observed, most often when the medications are used at high doses and chronically disrupt nocturnal sleep.[55]

Modafinil/armodafinil

Modafinil (2-[(diphenylmethyl)sulfinyl]acetamide) is a chemically unique compound developed in France. Modafinil has been available in France since 1984 on a compassionate mode and was officially approved in France in 1992. Modafinil (and its R-enantiomer) has been approved in 1998 in the United States for the treatment of narcolepsy, shift-work disorder, and residual sleepiness in treated patients with sleep apnea syndrome.

Armodafinil, the R-enantiomer of racemic modafinil, with a longer half-life, was also recently approved by the Food and Drug Administration (FDA) for EDS associated with narcolepsy as well as for residual sleepiness in nasal continuous positive airway pressure–treated individuals and sleepiness in shift work sleep disorder. Importantly, the R-enantiomer of modafinil has a half-life of 10 hours to 15 hours, which is longer than that of the S-enantiomer of modafinil (3–4 hours).[56] The dual pharmacokinetic properties of the racemic mixture may explain why modafinil is

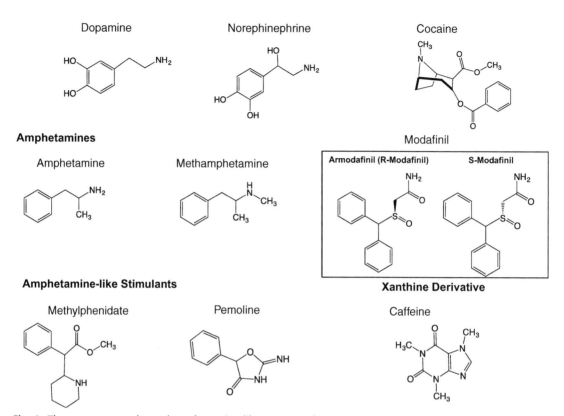

Fig. 1. The most commonly used amphetamine-like compounds.

often more potent when taken twice per day at the beginning of therapy, during the period of drug accumulation. In terms of plasma concentrations, armodafinil is higher than modafinil late in the day on a milligram-to-milligram basis.[57] That is the reason why modafinil is given twice a day at the beginning of therapy, and armodafinil is given once a day.

Several randomized trials have shown that modafinil is effective against EDS in narcolepsy compared with placebo.[58,59] Armodafinil improves the MWT compared with placebo among narcolepsy patients.[60] Both modafinil and armodafinil are classified as schedule IV (defined as drugs with low potential for abuse and low risk of dependence) (see **Table 2**).[61]

The prevalence of side effects of modafinil/armodafinil is not high, and headache, nausea, dry mouth, and anorexia are the known side effects.[62] Modafinil can cause a serious rash in children, although rarely.[63]

In clinical practice, modafinil is given once a day in the morning on an empty stomach in bed to maximize the effect of the drug. The starting dose is usually 200 mg, and the dose range can vary between 100 mg and 400 mg, as needed, depending on the effect.[64] If the maximum dose

(400 mg/d) is not sufficient to treat EDS among narcolepsy patients, then it is recommended to increase the dose up to 600 mg per day.

As discussed previously, armodafinil is usually given once a day in the early morning, and the dose range of armodafinil is 100 mg to 300 mg each morning.

The mechanism of action of modafinil/armodafinil is highly debated. There are few studies addressing the mode of action of armodafinil, and this review mostly discusses the action of racemic modafinil. Modafinil/armodafinil has not been shown to bind to or inhibit any receptors or enzymes of known neurotransmitters.[65,66] In vitro, modafinil/armodafinil binds to the dopamine transporter [DAT] and inhibits dopamine (DA) reuptake.[66,67] These binding inhibitory effects have been shown associated with increased extracellular DA levels in the striatum in rats and dog brain.[68,69]

The most striking finding was that DAT knockout mice were completely unresponsive to the wake-promoting effects of methamphetamine, GBR12909 (a selective DAT blocker), and modafinil. These results further confirm the critical role of DAT in mediating the wake-promoting effects of amphetamines and modafinil and that an intact DAT molecule is required for mediating the arousal effects of these compounds.[69] Qu and colleagues[70] further demonstrated that wake-promoting effects of modafinil were attenuated in D2 receptor knockout mice and were completely abolished in D2 receptor knockout mice with D1 antagonist, confirming the importance of dopaminergic neurotransmission for the modes of the action of modafinil.

Furthermore, a recent human PET study in 10 healthy humans with [11C] cocaine (DAT radioligand) and [11C] raclopride (D2/D3 radioligand sensitive to changes in endogenous DA) also demonstrated that modafinil (200 mg and 400 mg given orally) decreased [11C] cocaine binding potential in the caudate (53.8%), putamen (47.2%), and nucleus accumbens (39.3%).[71] In addition, modafinil also reduced binding potential of [11C] raclopride in these structures, suggesting the increases in extracellular DA were caused by DAT blockades.[71] These results are highly consistent with the results of the animal studies, discussed previously; modafinil's effects on alertness are entirely abolished in mice without the DAT protein[69] and in animals lacking D1 and D2 receptor functions.[70]

Methylphenidate and amphetamines

In 1935, amphetamine was used for the first time for the treatment of narcolepsy. Narcolepsy was possibly the first condition for which amphetamine was used clinically. It revolutionized therapy for the condition, even though it was not curative. Methylphenidate, the piperazine derivative of amphetamine, was introduced for the treatment of narcolepsy in 1959, and both compounds share similar pharmacologic properties.[72] Phenylisopropylamine (amphetamine) has a simple chemical structure resembling endogenous catecholamines.

Amphetamine-like compounds, such as methylphenidate, pemoline, and fencamfamine, are structurally similar to amphetamines; all compounds include a benzene core with an ethylamine group side chain (phenethylamine derivatives). Methylphenidate has been commonly used for the treatment of EDS in narcolepsy, and a racemic mixture of both the D-enantiomer and L-enantiomer is used, but D-methylphenidate mainly contributes to clinical effects, especially after oral administration.

Molecular targets mediating amphetamine-like stimulant effects are complex and vary depending on the specific analog/isomer and the dose administered. Amphetamine per se increases catecholamine (DA and norepinephrine [NE]) release and inhibits reuptake. These effects are mediated by specific catecholamine transporters (ie, DAT and NE transporter).[73] Amphetamine derivatives inhibit the uptake and enhance the release of DA, NE, or both by interacting with these molecules. These mechanisms, as well as the reverse transport (ie, exchange diffusion) and the blocking of reuptake of DA/NE by amphetamine, all lead to an increase in NE and DA synaptic concentrations.[73]

Methylphenidate is now recommended for use as one of the second-line options. Because there are new medicines available, like sodium oxybate and modafinil/armodafinil, methylphenidate is used when patients do not response to these new classes of drugs.

The mechanism of action of methylphenidate is similar to that of amphetamines and mainly increases the extracellular concentration of DA by blockage of the DAT and also, to a lesser degree, increases DA release.[74,75]

The side effects of methylphenidate are reduced appetite, nausea, headache, insomnia, and psychosis, which are similar to that of amphetamine.[74] It has been said that methylphenidate increases the risk of cardiovascular events in children and adults[76]; however, a large cohort, including more than 1 million children and young adults, has shown that the cardiovascular events risk is not strongly associated with attention deficit-hyperactivity disorder drugs, which is mainly methylphenidate.[77]

In clinical practice, methylphenidate is initially prescribed 10 mg per day at first. The recommended maximum dose is up to 80 mg per day.

Sodium oxybate

Sodium oxybate, the sodium salt of γ-hydroxybutyrate (GHB), taken in the evening and once again during the night, reduces daytime sleepiness, cataplectic attacks, and other manifestations of REM sleep.[78–82] GHB has been used in Canada and European countries for the treatment of narcolepsy-cataplexy. The administration of GHB was followed by a significant decrease in number of stage shifts and awakenings, wakefulness after sleep onset, and percentage of sleep stage 1. Sleep efficiency and slow-wave sleep percentage increased REM latency decreased significantly.[83] Although improvement in sleepiness occurs relatively quickly, anticataplectic effects appear 1 week to 2 weeks after the initiation of the treatment. Due to its positive effects on mood and libido, its slow-wave sleep–enhancing properties, and a subsequent increase in growth hormone release, GHB is widely abused by athletes and other populations.[84,85] In addition, because of its euphorigenic, behavioral disinhibitive, and amnestic properties, coupled with simple administration (ie, high solubility, colorlessness, and tastelessness when mixed with a drink), the abuse/misuse of GHB as a recreational substance and as a date rape drug has risen sharply in recent years, leading to an increased number of overdoses and intoxications for which no specific antidote exists.[81,86] GHB was classified as a schedule I drug that currently has no accepted medical use for treatment in the United States. Recent large-scale, double-blind, placebo-controlled clinical trials in the United States, however, led to reestablish sodium oxybate (the sodium salt of GHB) as a first-line treatment of narcolepsy-cataplexy.[79–81,87] In the United States, sodium oxybate is the approved formula of GHB and is classified as a schedule III compound. The compound is especially useful in patients with severe insomnia and cataplexy who do not tolerate antidepressant medication well because of its side effects on sexual potency. Although improvement in sleepiness occurs quickly, anticataplectic effects appeared 1 week to 2 weeks after the initiation of the treatment. Sodium oxybate has demonstrated statistically significant improvements in both symptoms, EDS and cataplexy, either as a monotherapy or in combination with modafinil, in clinical trials.[88] According to the meta-analysis, sodium oxybate was superior to placebo in increasing MWT (5.18 minutes; 95% CI, 2.59–7.78) and reducing weekly sleep attacks (−9.65 times; 95% CI, −17.72–1.59).[89] From these wake-promoting effects (on the day after the intake of compound at night), some researchers try to classify sodium oxybate as a CNS stimulant, but the mode of action of wake-promoting effects of sodium oxybate is unknown. Patients first need to take liquid sodium oxybate before they go to bed, and then they need to take the second dose 2.5 hours to 4 hours after the first dose. This is because

of the short half-life (0.5–1 hour in the body) and short duration of action (2–4 hours) of sodium oxybate.[90] The recommended starting dose is 4.5 g a night divided into 2 equal doses of 2.25 g, which may be adjusted up to a maximum of 9 g per night in increments of 1.5 g per night with 1-week to 2-week intervals. The benefit was significant after 4 weeks, highest after 8 weeks, and maintained during long-term therapy.[91] The side effects of sodium oxybate are nausea, insomnia, headache, dizziness, vomiting, weight loss, psychiatric complications, and sleep apnea[92] (see **Table 2**).

Because of the abuse potency of the compound, the Risk Evaluation and Mitigation Strategies program operated by the US FDA mandates prescriber/patient education for safe use and registration to prescribe sodium oxybate.[93] There are also economic drawbacks to using sodium oxybate for the treatment of narcolepsy. The cost of sodium oxybate is expensive, at up to $143,604 per 1 year.[94] The patent will expire in 2024, and the cost of sodium oxybate is likely to be more economical after 2024.

The mechanism of how sodium oxybate works has not been fully understood and it may have multiple mechanisms of action in the brain. A series of experimental evidence suggests that sodium oxybate may work as an agonist on γ-aminobutryic acid (GABA)$_B$ receptors.[95] Sodium oxybate is one of the precursors of GABA, and a portion of it may be converted to GABA and stimulate GABA receptors.[96] Several researchers also claimed that sodium oxybate has its own receptor (GHB receptor),[97] but functional roles of this receptor are still largely unknown (**Fig. 2**).

Despite these new findings, the physiologic significance of the brain GHB signaling pathway,

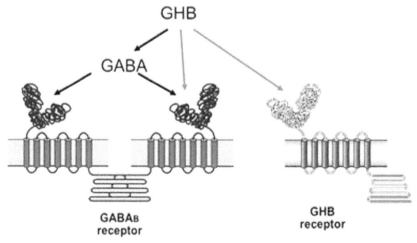

Fig. 2. The GHB receptor.

especially for the therapeutic effects against EDS and cataplexy, is still unknown. One of the possible modes of action is mediating the regulation of activities of adrenergic locus coeruleus (LC) neurons. The activity of the LC is essential for the maintenance of muscle tone, and the LC ceases to fire during cataplectic attacks.[98] GHB may prevent a cataplectic attack by dampening the tone of LC neurons via the stimulation of inhibitory extrasynaptic GABA receptors in the LC, thus increasing the threshold for autoinhibition.[99] Worsening of periodic leg movements in narcoleptic patients by sodium oxybate may suggest dopaminergic involvements in the drug action.

Pitolisant (H₃ inverse agonist)

Histamine has long been implicated in the control of vigilance, and H_1 antagonists are strongly sedative. The downstream effects of hypocretins on the histaminergic system (hcrtr2 excitatory effects) are likely important in mediating the wake-promoting properties of hypocretin.[100] Although centrally injected histamine or histaminergic H_1 agonists promote wakefulness, systemic administrations of these compounds induce various unacceptable side effects via peripheral H_1 receptor stimulation. In contrast, the histaminergic H_3 receptors are regarded as inhibitory autoreceptors and are enriched in the CNS. H_3 antagonists or inverse agonist enhance wakefulness in normal rats and cats[101] and in narcoleptic mice models.[102] Histaminergic H_3 antagonists might be a useful as wake-promoting compounds for the treatment of EDS or as cognitive enhancers,[103] and several histaminergic H_3 receptor antagonists/inverse agonists are currently being investigated. Pitolisant (previously called BF2.649 and tiprolisant; Bioprojet, Wakix, Paris, France) was the first clinically used inverse agonist of the histamine H_3 autoreceptor and increases histamine release in the hypothalamus and cortex. In a pilot single-blind study on 22 patients with narcolepsy/cataplexy, pitolisant (40 mg in the morning) reduced EDS.[104] Recent double-blind phase III trials on 95 narcoleptic subjects in 32 sleep disorder centers in 5 European countries revealed that pitolisant (10 mg, 20 mg, or 40 mg) once a day was efficacious on the 2 major symptoms of narcolepsy, EDS and cataplexy, compared with placebo and was better tolerated compared with twice-a-day modafinil (100 mg, 200 mg, or 400 mg).[105] If these findings are substantiated in further ongoing studies, H_3-receptor inverse agonists, including pitolisant, could offer a new treatment option for patients with narcolepsy.

Pitolisant is currently only available in Europe. The side effects are gastrointestinal pain, increased appetite, weight gain, headache, insomnia, and anxiety.[106] The initial dose of pitolisant is 9 mg, taken as a single dose in the morning. The maximum dose is up to 36 mg.

Combination strategy

Combination therapy of some stimulants is also recommended when the administration of a single type of stimulant is not effective against EDS of narcolepsy patients.

The recommended combinations of stimulants are sodium oxybate + modafinil/armodafinil, pitolisant, or methylphenidate + sodium oxybate, and modafinil or methylphenidate + pitolisant.

Other stimulants

Amphetamine and dextroamphetamine (amphetamines, dose 5–60 mg/d), mazindol (a weak DA releaser with DA and NE reuptake inhibitor, dose 2–8 mg/d), pemoline (amphetamine-like stimulant, dose 37.5–112.5 mg/d), and bupropion (DA uptake inhibitor with wake-promotion, dose 150–300 mg/d) are occasionally used if the first-line and second-line medications turn out to be insufficient.

Pharmacotherapy of Rapid Eye Movement Sleep–Related Symptoms in Narcolepsy

The pharmacotherapy of REM sleep–related symptoms in narcolepsy is briefly discussed. Besides sodium oxybate, tricyclic antidepressants; serotonin–NE reuptake inhibitors, such as milnacipran; and selective serotonin reuptake inhibitors, such as paroxetine and fluvoxamine, are recommended for patients suffering from cataplexy, hypnagogic hallucinations, and sleep paralysis.[107] Side effects of these antidepressants include dry mouth, obesity, sexual dysfunction, type 2 diabetes, and suicidal tendencies.[108] Antidepressants suppress cataplexy, hypnagogic hallucinations, and sleep paralysis, and this effect seems due to suppression of REM sleep or prolongation of REM sleep latency.[21,109]

Idiopathic Hypersomnia

With the clear definition of narcolepsy (cataplexy and dissociated manifestations of REM sleep), it became apparent that some patients with hypersomnia suffer from a different disorder. In the late 1950s and early 1960s, Bedrich Roth[110] first described a syndrome characterized by EDS, prolonged sleep, and sleep drunkenness, and by the absence of sleep attacks, cataplexy, sleep paralysis, and hallucinations. The terms, *independent sleep drunkenness* and *hypersomnia with sleep drunkenness* were initially suggested, but now this syndrome is categorized as idiopathic hypersomnia with and without long sleep time.[42]

In the absence of systematic studies, the prevalence of idiopathic hypersomnia is unknown. Nosologic uncertainty causes difficulty in determining the epidemiology of the disorder. Recent reports from large sleep centers reported the ratio of idiopathic hypersomnia to narcolepsy to be 1:10.[111] The age of onset of symptoms varies, but it is frequently between 10 years and 30 years. The condition usually develops progressively over several weeks or months. Once established, symptoms are generally stable and long lasting, but spontaneous improvement in EDS may be observed in up to one-quarter of patients.[111]

The pathogenesis of idiopathic hypersomnia is unknown. Hypersomnia usually starts insidiously. Occasionally, EDS is first experienced after transient insomnia, abrupt changes in sleep-wake habits, overexertion, general anesthesia, viral illness, or mild head trauma.[111] Despite reports of an increase in HLA-DQ1, DQ11, DR5, Cw2, and DQ3 and decrease in Cw3, no consistent findings have emerged.[111]

The most recent attempts to understand the pathophysiology of idiopathic hypersomnia relate to the investigation of potential role of the hypocretins. Most studies suggest, however, normal CSF levels of hypocretin-1 in idiopathic hypersomnia.[41,112]

Patients of idiopathic hypersomnia have less sleep paralysis (20% of patients with idiopathic hypersomnia) and sleep hallucinations (25%) than narcolepsy. Among idiopathic hypersomnia patients, sleep drunkenness and long nocturnal sleep times without fragmentation are common, and the effects and duration of naps are unrefreshing and long compared with narcolepsy patients.[15,113,114]

There is no FDA-approved medicine to treat EDS caused by idiopathic hypersomnia. In the clinical setting, modafinil is used off-label to treat EDS in idiopathic hypersomnia, as in narcolepsy.[115,116] If EDS is irresistible and resistant to modafinil, methylphenidate and amphetamine-like compounds are also used. A recent article has shown that sodium oxybate improves the sleepiness of idiopathic patients as much as it improves sleepiness in narcolepsy type 1; however, sodium oxybate has strong side effects and dependency, as discussed preivously.[116,117]

Hypersomnia due to a Medical Disorder

The prevalence of symptomatic narcolepsy (ie, narcolepsy due to a medical disorder) is likely small, and only approximately 120 of such cases have been reported in the literature in the past 30 years.[118] The prevalence of symptomatic (ie, hypersomnia due to a medical disorder) hypersomnia, however, may be much higher. For example, several million subjects in the United States suffer from chronic brain injury; 75% of these patients have sleep problems and approximately half of them claim sleepiness.[119] Patients with hypersomnia due to a medical disorder have EDS caused by coexisting medical or neurologic disorders. Daytime sleepiness of this disorder may be similar to that of narcolepsy or idiopathic hypersomnia.[15,114] Common disorders are discussed later, and in any secondary hypersomnia, it is important to treat the underlying disease besides providing symptomatic therapies.

Posttraumatic Hypersomnia

According to a meta-analysis research, the prevalence of EDS among posttraumatic brain injury patients is 27%.[120] CSF hypocretin-1 levels are low in most of patients with moderate to severe traumatic brain injury in their acute injury phase.[121] Regarding treatment, the effectiveness of modafinil is still under controversy. A randomized controlled trial (RCT) has shown that modafinil improves the Epworth Sleepiness Scale (ESS) score significantly compared with placebo at 6 treatment weeks.[122] Another RCT shows, however, that modafinil did not consistently improve the ESS score compared with the placebo at 10 treatment weeks.[123] Another RCT has demonstrated that armodafinil do not improve the ESS score compared with placebo at 12 treatment weeks.[124]

Hypersomnia Secondary to Parkinson Disease

Like narcolepsy and idiopathic hypersomnia, daytime sleepiness is measured by ESS and MSLT. Among Parkinson disease patients, 20% to 50% are said to have EDS.[125–127]

The effect of modafinil on this disorder is still controversial. There are some studies that have shown that modafinil improves the EDS in Parkinson disease patients,[128,129] whereas there are other articles that have shown that modafinil does not improve the EDS in Parkinson disease patients.[129,130] An article has also shown that sodium oxybate can improve the EDS in Parkinson disease patients.[131]

Common Stimulants in Daily Life

Caffeine is probably the most popular and widely consumed CNS stimulant in the world. Caffeine is digested from foods, drinks, and sometimes chocolate, coffee, energy drinks, soft drinks, and so forth. Caffeine is a xanthine derivative and acts as an adenosine A_1 and adenosine A_{2A}

receptor agonist.[132] Adenosine content is increased in the basal forebrain after sleep deprivation. Adenosine has thus been proposed as a sleep-inducing substance accumulating in the brain during prolonged wakefulness.[133] Side effects of caffeine are often overlooked; however, sometimes they are crucial. A variety of side effects of caffeine are well known, which are headache, stomach upset, nervousness, and so forth. For the common side effects of caffeine in terms of sleep, caffeine typically prolongs sleep latency, reduces total sleep time and sleep efficiency, and worsens perceived sleep quality.[132] An average cup of coffee contains 50 mg to 150 mg of caffeine. Caffeine is also available over the counter (NoDoz, 200 mg caffeine [GlaxoSmithKline plc, Middlesex, United Kingdom]; Vivarin, 200 mg caffeine [Meda Consumer Healthcare Inc, NJ]). This suggests that stimulant effects of caffeine tablets are not strong enough to manage pathologic sleepiness, but narcoleptic patients often take caffeine before they are diagnosed. According to a recent review, moderate caffeine intake (400 mg/d) is not associated with adverse effects.[134] The average cup of ground roasted coffee contains 85 mg of caffeing, and instant coffee contains 60 mg of caffeing.[135] Drinking fewer than 5 cups of ground roasted coffee per day is better for health.

FUTURE TREATMENT OPTIONS
Hypocertin-Based Treatments

Because a large majority of human narcolepsy patients are hypocretin ligand deficient, hypocretin replacement therapy may be a new therapeutic option. This may be effective for both sleepiness (ie, fragmented sleep/wake pattern) and cataplexy. Animal experiments using ligand-deficient narcoleptic dogs suggest that stable and centrally active hypocretin analogs (possibly nonpeptide synthetic hypocretin ligands) need to be developed to be peripherally effective.[136,137] This is also substantiated by a mice study that found normalization of sleep/wake patterns and behavioral arrest episodes (equivalent to cataplexy and REM sleep onset) in hypocretin-deficient mice knockout models supplemented by central administration of hypocretin-1.[138] In addition, orexin gene therapy (injection of an aden-oassociated viral vector coding for prepro-orexin plus a red fluorescence protein into the mediobasal hypothalamus) markedly improved the MWT in orexin/ataxin-3 narcoleptic mice.[139] These results demonstrate that cell transplantations and gene therapy may be developed in the future. One of the concerns for this option is that the hypocretin

peptides do not cross the blood-brain barrier (BBB) well. Intranasal delivery is a noninvasive method of bypassing the BBB to deliver therapeutic agents to the brain and spinal cord. Although developments of small molecule nonpeptide hypocretin receptor agonists are in progress and shown effective in mouse models,[140] these are still not available for clinical use. The toxicity/side effects of systemic administration of hypocretin receptor agonists are also unknown.

Recent reports in both rhesus monkeys and humans show some effects using intranasal hypocretin-1 administration.[141,142] A recent double-blind, randomized, placebo-controlled crossover design study on 7 patients with narcolepsy/cataplexy and matched healthy controls showed that intranasal hypocretin-1 restores olfactory function in narcolepsy/cataplexy patients.[141] But unfortunately, no data exist concerning potential effects on daytime sleepiness and cataplexy at this time.

Immune-Based Treatments

Type 1 narcolepsy is currently thought to be an autoimmune disorder targeting hypothalamus hypocretin neurons. An autoimmune basis for the hypocretin cell loss in narcolepsy has been suspected due to its strong DQB1*0602 association and association with T-cell receptor polymorphisms.[143] Based on the autoimmune hypothesis of narcolepsy, immune-based therapy, such as steroids (in 1 patient), intravenous immunoglobulins, and plasmapheresis have been proposed, with some promising results in a few cases.[144,145] Recently, a case of narcolepsy with cataplexy with undetectable CSF hypocretin-1 level that completely reversed shortly after disease onset was reported.[144] Although needing replication in well-designed trials, these results suggest that immune-based therapy could become a new treatment option for patients with narcolepsy/cataplexy at disease onset.

Other Possible Treatments of Interests (Non–Hypocretin-Based Treatments)

In addition to hypocretin replacement, preclinical and clinical trials for new classes of compounds are also in progress.

More than a decade ago, Osamu Hayaishi[146] and his group claimed that prostaglandin (PG) D2 is an endogenous sleep substance, and a series of animal studies by his group reported that PGD2 or PGD2 receptor (DP1) agonists promote sleep in animals (see Huang and colleagues[147]). The same research group also reported that PG DP1 potently promotes wakefulness. This suggests the possibility use of PG DP1 antagonists as wake-promoting compounds. This may also be clinically important because it is reported that increased serum lipocalin-type PGD synthase (beta-trace) levels correlate with EDS associated with narcolepsy.[148] Wake-promoting effects of a DP1 antagonist, ONO-4127, were evaluated in a mouse model of narcolepsy (ie, orexin/ataxin-3 transgenic mice) and compared with effects of modafinil.[149] ONO-4127 perfused in the basal forebrain area potently promoted wakefulness in both wild-type and narcoleptic mice, and the wake-promoting effects of ONO-4127 at 2.93×10^{-4} M approximately corresponded to those of modafinil at 100 mg/kg, orally; ONO-4127 reduced DREM (direct transitions from wake to REM sleep), an electro-encephalogram/electromyogram assessment of behavioral cataplexy, in narcoleptic mice, suggesting ONO-4127 is likely to have anticataplectic effects; DP1 antagonists may be a new class of compounds for the treatment of narcolepsy-cataplexy.

Another possible area that currently gathers less pharmaceutical interest is the use of thyrotropin-releasing hormone (TRH) direct or indirect agonists. TRH itself is a small peptide, which penetrates the BBB at very high doses. Small molecules with agonistic properties and increased BBB penetration (ie, CG3703, CG3509, or TA0910) have been developed, partially thanks to the small nature of the starting peptide.[150] TRH (at a high dose of several milligrams/kilogram) and TRH agonists increase alertness and have been shown to be wake promoting and anticataplectic in the narcoleptic canine model,[151,152] and these effects might be related to the excitatory effects of TRH on motoneurons.[153] Initial studies had demonstrated that TRH enhances DA and NE neurotransmission,[154,155] and these properties may partially contribute to the wake-promoting and anticataplectic effects of TRH. Recent studies have suggested that TRH may promote wakefulness by directly interacting with the thalamocortical network; TRH itself and TRH receptor type 2 are abundant in the reticular thalamic nucleus.[156] Local application of TRH in the thalamus abolishes spindle wave activity,[157] and in the slice preparations, TRH depolarized thalamocortical and reticular/perigenuculate neurons by inhibition of leak K+ conductance.[157]

Other pathways with possible applications in the development of novel stimulant medications include the adenosinergic system (more selective receptor antagonists than caffeine), the dopaminergic/adrenergic system (for example, DA/NE-reuptake inhibitors), the GABAergic system (for example, inverse benzodiazepine agonists), and the glutamatergic system (ampakines).[158]

SUMMARY

This article overviews pharmacotherapy of EDS associated with narcolepsy type 1, narcolepsy type 2, idiopathic hypersomnia, and hypersomnia due to a medical disorder.

Narcolepsy-cataplexy is most commonly caused by a loss of hypocretin-producing cells in the hypothalamus (ie, type 1 narcolepsy). Low CSF hypocretin-1 levels can be used to diagnose the condition. The disorder is tightly associated with HLA-DQB1*0602, suggesting that the cause in most patients may be autoimmune destruction of these cells. The treatment of EDS includes the use of amphetamine-like CNS stimulants, modafinil and its R-enantiomer armodafinil. Methylphenidate is the most commonly prescribed amphetamine-like stimulant in the United States, and this compound is efficacious and well tolerated by most narcoleptic patients. Because of its safety and low side-effect profile, modafinil became the first-line treatment of choice for EDS associated with narcolepsy. These wake-promoting compounds, however, do not improve cataplexy and dissociated manifestations of REM sleep, so antidepressants (monoamine uptake inhibitors) are additionally used to treat these aspects. Sodium oxybate (a sodium salt of GHB, available in the United States), when given at night, improves EDS and cataplexy, Therefore, the number of US patients treated with sodium oxybate is increasing, and it has become the first-line treatment of narcolepsy. Combination therapy with some stimulants is also recommended when the administration of single stimulant type is not effective against EDS of narcolepsy patients.

There is no FDA-approved medicine to treat EDS associated with idiopathic hypersomnia. In the clinical setting, modafinil is used off-label to treat EDS in idiopathic hypersomnia. If EDS is irresistible and resistant to modafinil, methylphenidate and amphaemine-like compounds are also used.

Treatments of EDS associated with symptomatic hypersomnia (ie, hypersomnias due to a medical disorder) are more complex because these conditions are heterogeneous, and hypocretin involvements are seen in some disease conditions but not in all. Specific brain structures that have been damaged and mechanisms involved in the EDS are likely varied. Unresponsiveness to stimulant treatments may occur depending on the underlying pathophysiologic mechanism. In this regard, development of new types of wake-promoting compounds would likely benefit these patients.

Emerging treatments undergoing investigation include histaminergic compounds (pitolisant, an H_3 inverse agonist, is available in Europe), TRH agonists, DP1 antagonists, hypocretin replacement/supplement therapies, and immunomodulation as prevention.

There are many potential approaches for narcolepsy; compounds and new therapies, such as hypocretin transplant or gene technology, are being developed.[159] The development of small molecular synthetic hypocretin receptor agonists, however, is likely the next step for this therapeutic option in humans, because hypocretin peptides themselves do not penetrate the brain effectively. If ligand replacement therapy is demonstrated as effective in hypocretin-deficient narcolepsy, hypocretin cell transplant or gene therapy technology may also be applicable in the near future. These therapies, however, are many years away, and the efficacy of exogenously administered hypocretin analogs (nonpeptide agonists) in humans should be established first.

To prevent hypoceretin neuronal loss (ie, narcolepsy type 1), immune-based treatments is promising, but accumulation of much cases is needed to prove the efficacy of this approach.

REFERENCES

1. Arand D, Bonnet M, Hurwitz T, et al. The clinical use of the MSLT and MWT. Sleep 2005;28(1):123–44.
2. Pagnin D, de Queiroz V, Carvalho YT, et al. The relation between burnout and sleep disorders in medical students. Acad Psychiatry 2014;38(4):438–44.
3. Swanson LM, Arnedt JT, Rosekind MR, et al. Sleep disorders and work performance: findings from the 2008 National Sleep Foundation Sleep in America poll. J Sleep Res 2011;20(3):487–94.
4. Young TB. Epidemiology of daytime sleepiness: definitions, symptomatology, and prevalence. J Clin Psychiatry 2004;65(Suppl 16):12–6.
5. Wu S, Wang R, Ma X, et al. Excessive daytime sleepiness assessed by the Epworth Sleepiness Scale and its association with health related quality of life: a population-based study in China. BMC Public Health 2012;12:849.
6. Plante DT, Finn LA, Hagen EW, et al. Longitudinal associations of hypersomnolence and depression in the Wisconsin sleep cohort study. J Affect Disord 2017;207:197–202.
7. Roth T. Effects of excessive daytime sleepiness and fatigue on overall health and cognitive function. J Clin Psychiatry 2015;76(9):e1145.
8. Garbarino S, Durando P, Guglielmi O, et al. Sleep apnea, sleep debt and daytime sleepiness are independently associated with road accidents. A cross-sectional study on truck drivers. PLoS One 2016;11(11):e0166262.
9. Murray BJ. A practical approach to excessive daytime sleepiness: a focused review. Can Respir J 2016;2016:4215938.
10. Doyle JB, Daniels LE. Symptomatic treatment for narcolepsy. J Am Med Assoc 1931;96(17):1370–2.
11. Akimoto H, Honda Y, Takahashi Y. Pharmacotherapy in narcolepsy. Dis Nerv Syst 1960;21:704–6.
12. Guilleminault C, Carskadon M, Dement WC. On the treatment of rapid eye movement narcolepsy. Arch Neurol 1974;30(1):90–3.
13. Parkes JD, Baraitser M, Marsden CD, et al. Natural history, symptoms and treatment of the narcoleptic syndrome. Acta Neurol Scand 1975;52(5):337–53.
14. Passouant P, Billiard M. [Narcolepsy]. Rev Prat 1976;26(27):1917–23.
15. ICSD-3. International classification of sleep disorders. 3rd edition. Rochester (MN): American Sleep Disorders Association; 2014. Medicine AAoS.
16. Arnulf I. Kleine-levin syndrome. Sleep Med Clin 2015;10(2):151–61.
17. Medicine AAoS. International classification of sleep disorders. 3rd edition. Daren (IL): American Academy of Sleep Medicine; 2014.
18. Hublin C, Kaprio J, Partinene M, et al. The prevalence of narcolepsy: an epidemiological study of the Finnish twin cohort. Ann Neurol 1994;35:709–16.
19. Tashiro T, Kanbayashi T, Hishikawa Y. An epidemiological study of narcolepsy in Japanese. Paper presented at: The 4th International Symposium on Narcolepsy. Tokyo, Japan, June 16–17, 1994. p. 13.
20. Dauvilliers Y, Montplaisir J, Molinari N, et al. Age at onset of narcolepsy in two large populations of patients in France and Quebec. Neurology 2001;57(11):2029–33.
21. Nishino S, Mignot E. Pharmacological aspects of human and canine narcolepsy. Prog Neurobiol 1997;52(1):27–78.
22. Pizza F, Contardi S, Mondini S, et al. Daytime sleepiness and driving performance in patients with obstructive sleep apnea: comparison of the MSLT, the MWT, and a simulated driving task. Sleep 2009;32(3):382–91.
23. Littner MR, Kushida C, Wise M, et al. Practice parameters for clinical use of the multiple sleep latency test and the maintenance of wakefulness test. Sleep 2005;28(1):113–21.
24. Sullivan SS, Kushida CA. Multiple sleep latency test and maintenance of wakefulness test. Chest 2008;134(4):854–61.
25. Scammell TE. Narcolepsy. N Engl J Med 2015;373(27):2654–62.
26. Dauvilliers Y, Billiard M, Montplaisir J. Clinical aspects and pathophysiology of narcolepsy. Clin Neurophysiol 2003;114(11):2000–17.

27. Guilleminault C, Kryger MH, Roth T, et al. Narcolepsy syndrome. Principles and Practice of Sleep Medicine. 2nd edition. Philadelphia: WB Saunders; 1994. p. 549–61.

28. Juji T, Satake M, Honda Y, et al. HLA antigens in Japanese patients with narcolepsy. All the patients were DR2 positive. Tissue Antigens 1984;24(5): 316–9.

29. Gelb M, Guilleminault C, Kraemer H, et al. Stability of cataplexy over several months–information for the design of therapeutic trials. Sleep 1994;17(3):265–73.

30. Hishikawa Y, Wakamatsu H, Furuya E, et al. Sleep satiation in narcoleptic patients. Electroencephalogr Clin Neurophysiol 1976;41:1–18.

31. Broughton R, Dunham W, Newman J, et al. Ambulatory 24 hour sleep-wake monitoring in narcolepsy-cataplexy compared to matched control. Electroencephalogr Clin Neurophysiol 1988; 70:473–81.

32. Montplaisir J, Billard M, Takahashi S, et al. Twenty-four-hour recording in REM-narcoleptics with special reference to nocturnal sleep disruption. Biol Psychiatry 1978;13(1):78–89.

33. Godbout R, Montplaisir J. Comparison of sleep parameters in narcoleptics with and without periodic movements of sleep. In: Koella WP, Ruther E, Schulz H, editors. Sleep '84. New York: Gustav Fischer Verlag; 1985. p. 380–2.

34. Mosko SS, Shampain DS, Sassin JF. Nocturnal REM latency and sleep disturbance in narcolepsy. Sleep 1984;7:115–25.

35. Mayer G, Pollmächer T, Meier-Ewert K, et al. Zur Einschätzung des Behinderungsgrades bei Narkolepsie. Gesundheitswesen 1993;55:337–42.

36. Schenck CH, Mahowald MW. Motor dyscontrol in narcolepsy: Rapid-Eye-Movement (REM) sleep without atonia and REM sleep behavior disorder. Ann Neurol 1992;32(1):3–10.

37. Chokroverty S. Sleep apnea in narcolepsy. Sleep 1986;9(1):250–3.

38. Guilleminault C, Dement WC, Passouant P, editors. Narcolepsy. New York: Spectrum Publications; 1976. Advances in Sleep Research; No. 3.

39. Juji T, Matsuki K, Tokunaga K, et al. Narcolepsy and HLA in the Japanese. Ann N Y Acad Sci 1988;540:106–14.

40. Nishino S, Ripley B, Overeem S, et al. Hypocretin (orexin) deficiency in human narcolepsy. Lancet 2000;355(9197):39–40.

41. Mignot E, Lammers GJ, Ripley B, et al. The role of cerebrospinal fluid hypocretin measurement in the diagnosis of narcolepsy and other hypersomnias. Arch Neurol 2002;59(10):1553–62.

42. ICSD-2. ICSD-2-International classification of sleep disorders. In: Sateia MJ, editor. Diagnostic and coding manual. 2nd edition. Westchester (IL): American Academy of Sleep Medicine; 2005. p. 38–43.

43. Mignot E, Hayduk R, Black J, et al. HLA DQB1*0602 is associated with cataplexy in 509 narcoleptic patients. Sleep 1997;20(11): 1012–20.

44. Dauvilliers Y, Maret S, Bassetti C, et al. A monozygotic twin pair discordant for narcolepsy and CSF hypocretin-1. Neurology 2004;62(11):2137–8.

45. Ripley B, Fujiki N, Okura M, et al. Hypocretin levels in sporadic and familial cases of canine narcolepsy. Neurobiol Dis 2001;8(3):525–34.

46. Thannickal TC, Nienhuis R, Siegel JM. Localized loss of hypocretin (orexin) cells in narcolepsy without cataplexy. Sleep 2009;32(8):993–8.

47. Garma L, Marchand F. Non-pharmacological approaches to the treatment of narcolepsy. Sleep 1994;17(8 Suppl):S97–102.

48. Roehrs T, Zorick F, Wittig R, et al. Alerting effects of naps in patients with narcolepsy. Sleep 1986;9(1): 194–9.

49. Rogers AE. Problems and coping strategies identified by narcoleptic patients. J Neurosurg Nurs 1984;16(6):326–34.

50. Morgenthaler TI, Kapur VK, Brown T, et al. Practice parameters for the treatment of narcolepsy and other hypersomnias of central origin. Sleep 2007; 30(12):1705–11.

51. Hirai N, Nishino S. Recent advances in the treatment of narcolepsy. Curr Treat Options Neurol 2011;13(5):437–57.

52. Mitler MM, Aldrich MS, Koob GF, et al. Narcolepsy and its treatment with stimulants. ASDA standards of practice. Sleep 1994;17(4):352–71.

53. Mitler MM, Hajdukovic R. Relative efficacy of drugs for the treatment of sleepiness in narcolepsy. Sleep 1991;14(3):218–20.

54. Rogers AE, Aldrich MS, Berrios AM, et al. Compliance with stimulant medications in patients with narcolepsy. Sleep 1997;20(1):28–33.

55. Auger RR, Goodman SH, Silber MH, et al. Risks of high-dose stimulants in the treatment of disorders of excessive somnolence: a case-control study. Sleep 2005;28(6):667–72.

56. Nishino S, Okuro M. Armodafinil for excessive daytime sleepiness. Drugs Today (Barc) 2008;44(6): 395–414.

57. Darwish M, Kirby M, Hellriegel ET, et al. Armodafinil and modafinil have substantially different pharmacokinetic profiles despite having the same terminal half-lives: analysis of data from three randomized, single-dose, pharmacokinetic studies. Clin Drug Investig 2009;29(9):613–23.

58. Randomized trial of modafinil for the treatment of pathological somnolence in narcolepsy. US Modafinil in Narcolepsy Multicenter Study Group. Ann Neurol 1998;43(1):88–97.

59. Randomized trial of modafinil as a treatment for the excessive daytime somnolence of narcolepsy: US

Modafinil in Narcolepsy Multicenter Study Group. Neurology 2000;54(5):1166–75.

60. Harsh JR, Hayduk R, Rosenberg R, et al. The efficacy and safety of armodafinil as treatment for adults with excessive sleepiness associated with narcolepsy. Curr Med Res Opin 2006;22(4):761–74.

61. United States Department of Justice. Drug Enforcement Administration. Drug Scheduling. Available at: https://www.dea.gov/druginfo/ds.shtml. Accessed February 10, 2017.

62. Roth T, Schwartz JR, Hirshkowitz M, et al. Evaluation of the safety of modafinil for treatment of excessive sleepiness. J Clin Sleep Med 2007; 3(6):595–602.

63. U.S. Food & Drug Administration. Drug Safety. Medication Guide. Available at: http://www.fda.gov/downloads/drugs/drugsafety/ucm231722.pdf. Accessed February 11, 2017.

64. Schwartz JR, Feldman NT, Bogan RK, et al. Dosing regimen effects of modafinil for improving daytime wakefulness in patients with narcolepsy. Clin Neuropharmacol 2003;26(5):252–7.

65. Cephalon, Inc. FDA approval of NUVIGIL. Available at: https://www.sec.gov/Archives/edgar/data/873364/000110465907048203/a07-16834_1ex99d1.htm. Accessed February 11, 2017.

66. Mignot E, Nishino S, Guilleminault C, et al. Modafinil binds to the dopamine uptake carrier site with low affinity. Sleep 1994;17(5):436–7.

67. Nishino S, Mao J, Sampathkumaran R, et al. Increased dopaminergic transmission mediates the wake-promoting effects of CNS stimulants. Sleep Res Online 1998;1(1):49–61.

68. Dopheide MM, Morgan RE, Rodvelt KR, et al. Modafinil evokes striatal [(3)H]dopamine release and alters the subjective properties of stimulants. Eur J Pharmacol 2007;568(1–3):112–23.

69. Wisor JP, Nishino S, Sora I, et al. Dopaminergic role in stimulant-induced wakefulness. J Neurosci 2001;21(5):1787–94.

70. Qu WM, Huang ZL, Xu XH, et al. Dopaminergic D1 and D2 receptors are essential for the arousal effect of modafinil. J Neurosci 2008;28(34):8462–9.

71. Volkow ND, Fowler JS, Logan J, et al. Effects of modafinil on dopamine and dopamine transporters in the male human brain: clinical implications. JAMA 2009;301(11):1148–54.

72. Yoss RE, Daly D. Treatment of narcolepsy with ritalin. Neurology 1959;9(3):171–3.

73. Kuczenski R, Segal DS. Neurochemistry of amphetamine, in psychopharmacology, toxicology and abuse. San Diego (CA): Academic Press; 1994. p. 81–113.

74. Leonard BE, McCartan D, White J, et al. Methylphenidate: a review of its neuropharmacological, neuropsychological and adverse clinical effects. Hum Psychopharmacol 2004;19(3):151–80.

75. Schenk JO. The functioning neuronal transporter for dopamine: kinetic mechanisms and effects of amphetamines, cocaine and methylphenidate. Prog Drug Res 2002;59:111–31.

76. Nissen SE. ADHD drugs and cardiovascular risk. N Engl J Med 2006;354(14):1445–8.

77. Cooper WO, Habel LA, Sox CM, et al. ADHD drugs and serious cardiovascular events in children and young adults. N Engl J Med 2011;365(20): 1896–904.

78. Broughton R, Mamelak M. The treatment of narcolepsy-cataplexy with nocturnal gamma-hydroxybutyrate. Can J Neurol Sci 1979;6(1):1–6.

79. Group USXMS. A randomized, double blind, placebo-controlled multicenter trial comparing the effects of three doses of orally administered sodium oxybate with placebo for the treatment of narcolepsy. Sleep 2002;25(1):42–9.

80. Group USXMS. A 12-month, open-label, multicenter extension trial of orally administered sodium oxybate for the treatment of narcolepsy. Sleep 2003;26(1):31–5.

81. Group USXMS. Sodium oxybate demonstrates long-term efficacy for the treatment of cataplexy in patients with narcolepsy. Sleep Med 2004;5(2): 119–23.

82. Mamelak M, Scharf MB, Woods M. Treatment of narcolepsy with gamma-hydroxybutyrate. A review of clinical and sleep laboratory findings. Sleep 1986;9(1 Pt 2):285–9.

83. Plazzi G, Pizza F, Vandi S, et al. Impact of acute administration of sodium oxybate on nocturnal sleep polysomnography and on multiple sleep latency test in narcolepsy with cataplexy. Sleep Med 2014;15(9):1046–54.

84. Mack RB. Love potion number 8 1/2. Gamma-hydroxybutyrate poisoning. N C Med J 1993; 54(5):232–3.

85. Wong CG, Gibson KM, Snead OC 3rd. From the street to the brain: neurobiology of the recreational drug gamma-hydroxybutyric acid. Trends Pharmacol Sci 2004;25(1):29–34.

86. Nicholson KL, Balster RL. GHB: a new and novel drug of abuse. Drug Alcohol Depend 2001;63(1): 1–22.

87. Black J, Houghton WC. Sodium oxybate improves excessive daytime sleepiness in narcolepsy. Sleep 2006;29(7):939–46.

88. Robinson DM, Keating GM. Sodium oxybate: a review of its use in the management of narcolepsy. CNS Drugs 2007;21(4):337–54.

89. Alshaikh MK, Tricco AC, Tashkandi M, et al. Sodium oxybate for narcolepsy with cataplexy: systematic review and meta-analysis. J Clin Sleep Med 2012; 8(4):451–8.

90. Thorpy MJ. Update on therapy for narcolepsy. Curr Treat Options Neurol 2015;17(5):347.

91. Palatini P, Tedeschi L, Frison G, et al. Dose-dependent absorption and elimination of gamma-hydroxybutyric acid in healthy volunteers. Eur J Clin Pharmacol 1993;45(4):353–6.

92. Wang YG, Swick TJ, Carter LP, et al. Safety overview of postmarketing and clinical experience of sodium oxybate (Xyrem): abuse, misuse, dependence, and diversion. J Clin Sleep Med 2009; 5(4):365–71.

93. Administration tUSFaD. Available at: http://www.fda.gov/Drugs/DrugSafety/PostmarketDrugSafetyInformationforPatientsandProviders/ucm332408.htm. Accessed February 9, 2017.

94. Saini P, Rye DB. Hypersomnia: evaluation, treatment, and social and economic aspects. Sleep Med Clin 2017;12(1):47–60.

95. Maitre M, Klein C, Mensah-Nyagan AG. Mechanisms for the specific properties of gamma-hydroxybutyrate in brain. Med Res Rev 2016; 36(3):363–88.

96. Pardi D, Black J. γ-hydroxybutyrate/sodium oxybate. CNS drugs 2006;20(12):993–1018.

97. Andriamampandry C, Taleb O, Viry S, et al. Cloning and characterization of a rat brain receptor that binds the endogenous neuromodulator gamma-hydroxybutyrate (GHB). Faseb J 2003;17(12): 1691–3.

98. Wu MF, Gulyani SA, Yau E, et al. Locus coeruleus neurons: cessation of activity during cataplexy. Neuroscience 1999;91(4):1389–99.

99. Szabadi E. GHB for cataplexy: possible mode of action. J Psychopharmacol 2015;29(6):744–9.

100. Nishino S, Ripley B, Mignot E, et al. CSF hypocretin-1 levels in schizophrenics and controls: relationship to sleep architecture. Psychiatry Res 2002;110(1):1–7.

101. Shiba T. Wake promoting effects of thioperamide, a histamine H3 antagonist in orexin/ataxin-3 narcoleptic mice. Sleep 2004;27(Suppl):A241–2.

102. Parmentier R, Anaclet C, Guhennec C, et al. The brain H3-receptor as a novel therapeutic target for vigilance and sleep-wake disorders. Biochem Pharmacol 2007;73(8):1157–71.

103. Lin JS, Dauvilliers Y, Arnulf I, et al. An inverse agonist of the histamine H(3) receptor improves wakefulness in narcolepsy: studies in orexin-/-mice and patients. Neurobiol Dis 2008;30(1):74–83.

104. Dauvilliers Y, Bassetti C, Lammers GJ, et al. Pitolisant versus placebo or modafinil in patients with narcolepsy: a double-blind, randomised trial. Lancet Neurol 2013;12(11):1068–75.

105. Sharif NA, To ZP, Whiting RL. Analogs of thyrotropin-releasing hormone (TRH): receptor affinities in brains, spinal cords, and pituitaries of different species. Neurochem Res 1991;16(2):95–103.

106. Leu-Semenescu S, Nittur N, Golmard JL, et al. Effects of pitolisant, a histamine H3 inverse agonist, in drug-resistant idiopathic and symptomatic hypersomnia: a chart review. Sleep Med 2014;15(6): 681–7.

107. Swick TJ. Treatment paradigms for cataplexy in narcolepsy: past, present, and future. Nat Sci Sleep 2015;7:159–69.

108. Santarsieri D, Schwartz TL. Antidepressant efficacy and side-effect burden: a quick guide for clinicians. Drugs Context 2015;4:212290.

109. Thase ME. Depression, sleep, and antidepressants. J Clin Psychiatry 1998;59(Suppl 4):55–65.

110. Roth B. Narkolepsie und hypersomnie. Berlin: VEB Verlag Volk und Gesundheit; 1962.

111. Bassetti C, Aldrich MS. Idiopathic hypersomnia. A series of 42 patients. Brain 1997;120(Pt 8): 1423–35.

112. Bassetti C, Gugger M, Bischof M, et al. The narcoleptic borderland: a multimodal diagnostic approach including cerebrospinal fluid levels of hypocretin-1 (orexin A). Sleep Med 2003;4(1):7–12.

113. Vernet C, Leu-Semenescu S, Buzare MA, et al. Subjective symptoms in idiopathic hypersomnia: beyond excessive sleepiness. J Sleep Res 2010; 19(4):525–34.

114. International classification of sleep disorders: diagnostic and coding manual. 3rd edition. Westchester (IL): American Academy of Sleep Medicine; 2014.

115. Mayer G, Benes H, Young P, et al. Modafinil in the treatment of idiopathic hypersomnia without long sleep time–a randomized, double-blind, placebo-controlled study. J Sleep Res 2015;24(1):74–81.

116. Billiard M, Sonka K. Idiopathic hypersomnia. Sleep Med Rev 2016;29:23–33.

117. Leu-Semenescu S, Louis P, Arnulf I. Benefits and risk of sodium oxybate in idiopathic hypersomnia versus narcolepsy type 1: a chart review. Sleep Med 2016;17:38–44.

118. Nishino S, Kanbayashi T. Symptomatic narcolepsy, cataplexy and hypersomnia, and their implications in the hypothalamic hypocretin/orexin system. Sleep Med Rev 2005;9(4):269–310.

119. Verma A, Anand V, Verma NP. Sleep disorders in chronic traumatic brain injury. J Clin Sleep Med 2007;3(4):357–62.

120. Mathias JL, Alvaro PK. Prevalence of sleep disturbances, disorders, and problems following traumatic brain injury: a meta-analysis. Sleep Med 2012;13(7):898–905.

121. Baumann CR, Stocker R, Imhof HG, et al. Hypocretin-1 (orexin A) deficiency in acute traumatic brain injury. Neurology 2005;65(1):147–9.

122. Kaiser PR, Valko PO, Werth E, et al. Modafinil ameliorates excessive daytime sleepiness after traumatic brain injury. Neurology 2010;75(20):1780–5.

123. Jha A, Weintraub A, Allshouse A, et al. A randomized trial of modafinil for the treatment of fatigue and

excessive daytime sleepiness in individuals with chronic traumatic brain injury. J Head Trauma Rehabil 2008;23(1):52–63.

124. Menn SJ, Yang R, Lankford A. Armodafinil for the treatment of excessive sleepiness associated with mild or moderate closed traumatic brain injury: a 12-week, randomized, double-blind study followed by a 12-month open-label extension. J Clin Sleep Med 2014;10(11):1181–91.

125. Braga-Neto P, da Silva-Junior FP, Sueli Monte F, et al. Snoring and excessive daytime sleepiness in Parkinson's disease. J Neurol Sci 2004;217(1):41–5.

126. Gjerstad MD, Alves G, Wentzel-Larsen T, et al. Excessive daytime sleepiness in Parkinson disease: is it the drugs or the disease? Neurology 2006;67(5):853–8.

127. Verbaan D, van Rooden SM, Visser M, et al. Nighttime sleep problems and daytime sleepiness in Parkinson's disease. Mov Disord 2008; 23(1):35–41.

128. Adler CH, Caviness JN, Hentz JG, et al. Randomized trial of modafinil for treating subjective daytime sleepiness in patients with Parkinson's disease. Mov Disord 2003;18(3):287–93.

129. Hogl B, Saletu M, Brandauer E, et al. Modafinil for the treatment of daytime sleepiness in Parkinson's disease: a double-blind, randomized, crossover, placebo-controlled polygraphic trial. Sleep 2002; 25(8):905–9.

130. Ondo WG, Fayle R, Atassi F, et al. Modafinil for daytime somnolence in Parkinson's disease: double blind, placebo controlled parallel trial. J Neurol Neurosurg Psychiatr 2005;76(12): 1636–9.

131. Ondo WG, Perkins T, Swick T, et al. Sodium oxybate for excessive daytime sleepiness in Parkinson disease: an open-label polysomnographic study. Arch Neurol 2008;65(10):1337–40.

132. Fisone G, Borgkvist A, Usiello A. Caffeine as a psychomotor stimulant: mechanism of action. Cell Mol Life Sci 2004;61(7–8):857–72.

133. Porkka-Heiskanen T, Strecker RE, Thakkar M, et al. Adenosine: a mediator of the sleep-inducing effects of prolonged wakefulness. Science 1997; 276(5316):1265–8.

134. Nawrot P, Jordan S, Eastwood J, et al. Effects of caffeine on human health. Food Addit Contam 2003;20(1):1–30.

135. Barone JJ, Roberts HR. Caffeine consumption. Food Chem Toxicol 1996;34(1):119–29.

136. Mieda M, Willie JT, Hara J, et al. Orexin peptides prevent cataplexy and improve wakefulness in an orexin neuron-ablated model of narcolepsy in mice. Proc Natl Acad Sci U S A 2004;101(13): 4649–54.

137. Schatzberg SJ, Cutter-Schatzberg K, Nydam D, et al. The effect of hypocretin replacement therapy in a 3-year-old Weimaraner with narcolepsy. J Vet Intern Med 2004;18(4):586–8.

138. Kantor S, Mochizuki T, Janisiewicz AM, et al. Orexin neurons are necessary for the circadian control of REM sleep. Sleep 2009;32(9):1127–34.

139. Deadwyler SA, Porrino L, Siegel JM, et al. Systemic and nasal delivery of orexin-A (Hypocretin-1) reduces the effects of sleep deprivation on cognitive performance in nonhuman primates. J Neurosci 2007;27(52):14239–47.

140. Nagahara T, Saitoh T, Kutsumura N, et al. Design and synthesis of non-peptide, selective orexin receptor 2 agonists. J Med Chem 2015;58(20): 7931–7.

141. Baier PC, Hallschmid M, Seeck-Hirschner M, et al. Effects of intranasal hypocretin-1 (orexin A) on sleep in narcolepsy with cataplexy. Sleep Med 2011;12(10):941–6.

142. Mishima K, Fujiki N, Yoshida Y, et al. Hypocretin receptor expression in canine and murine narcolepsy models and in hypocretin-ligand deficient human narcolepsy. Sleep 2008;31(8):1119–26.

143. Kawashima M, Lin L, Tanaka S, et al. Anti-Tribbles homolog 2 (TRIB2) autoantibodies in narcolepsy are associated with recent onset of cataplexy. Sleep 2010;33(7):869–74.

144. Dauvilliers Y, Abril B, Mas E, et al. Normalization of hypocretin-1 in narcolepsy after intravenous immunoglobulin treatment. Neurology 2009;73(16): 1333–4.

145. Dauvilliers Y, Carlander B, Rivier F, et al. Successful management of cataplexy with intravenous immunoglobulins at narcolepsy onset. Ann Neurol 2004;56(6):905–8.

146. Ueno R, Honda K, Inoue S, et al. Prostaglandin D2, a cerebral sleep-inducing substance in rats. Proc Natl Acad Sci U S A 1983;80(6):1735–7.

147. Huang ZL, Urade Y, Hayaishi O. Prostaglandins and adenosine in the regulation of sleep and wakefulness. Curr Opin Pharmacol 2007;7(1): 33–8.

148. Jordan W, Tumani H, Cohrs S, et al. Narcolepsy increased L-PGDS (beta-trace) levels correlate with excessive daytime sleepiness but not with cataplexy. J Neurol 2005;252:1372–8.

149. Sagawa Y, Sato M, Sakai N, et al. Wake-promoting effects of ONO-4127Na, a prostaglandin DP1 receptor antagonist, in hypocretin/orexin deficient narcoleptic mice. Neuropharmacology 2016; 110(Part A):268–76.

150. Riehl J, Honda K, Kwan M, et al. Chronic oral administration of CG-3703, a thyrotropin releasing hormone analog, increases wake and decreases cataplexy in canine narcolepsy. Neuropsychopharmacology 2000;23(1):34–45.

151. Nicoll RA. Excitatory action of TRH on spinal motoneurones. Nature 1977;265(5591):242–3.

152. Nishino S, Arrigoni J, Shelton J, et al. Effects of thyrotropin-releasing hormone and its analogs on daytime sleepiness and cataplexy in canine narcolepsy. J Neurosci 1997;17(16):6401–8.

153. Sharp T, Bennett GW, Marsden CA. Thyrotrophin-releasing hormone analogues increase dopamine release from slices of rat brain. J Neurochem 1982;39(6):1763–6.

154. Heuer H, Schafer MK, O'Donnell D, et al. Expression of thyrotropin-releasing hormone receptor 2 (TRH-R2) in the central nervous system of rats. J Comp Neurol 2000;428(2):319–36.

155. Keller HH, Bartholini G, Pletscher A. Enhancement of cerebral noradrenaline turnover by thyrotropin-releasing hormone. Nature 1974;248(448):528–9.

156. Broberger C. Neurotransmitters switching the thalamus between sleep and arousal: functional effects and cellular mechanism. New Frontiers in Neuroscience Research. Showa University International Symposium for Life Science. 1st Annual Meeting Showa University Kamijo Hall. Tokyo, August 31, 2004.

157. Mignot E, Nishino S. Emerging therapies in narcolepsy-cataplexy. Sleep 2005;28(6):754–63.

158. Okura M, Riehl J, Mignot E, et al. Sulpiride, a D2/D3 blocker, reduces cataplexy but not REM sleep in canine narcolepsy. Neuropsychopharmacology 2000;23(5):528–38.

159. Nishino S, Mignot E. Narcolepsy and cataplexy. Handb Clin Neurol 2011;99:783–814.

Nonpharmacologic Management of Excessive Daytime Sleepiness

Matthew R. Ebben, PhD

KEYWORDS

- Excessive daytime sleepiness • Behavioral management • Sleep restriction • Sleep need
- Sleep extension • Sleep debt • Sleep banking • Sleep deprivation

KEY POINTS

- A sleep duration of 7 to 8 hours has been associated with the lowest risk of mortality. At a population level, this information is important; however, for individuals reporting excessive daytime sleepiness, determining personal sleep need is likely to provide the most clinical benefit.
- Excessive daytime sleepiness has been linked to reduced performance, increased work-related accidents, and motor vehicle crashes. Therefore, treating sleepiness is critically important.
- Increasing time in bed before a period of sleep deprivation may help to moderate performance decrements during short periods of reduced sleep.
- Progressively increasing time in bed can help reduce excessive daytime sleepiness in those with chronic partial sleep deprivation. However, care should be taken not to increase time in bed too much at one time because this may result in reduced sleep efficiency.

INTRODUCTION

The focus of this article is to investigate behavioral strategies for improving daytime sleepiness. Other high-quality reviews on this topic have been published in the last several years, including one published in this publication in 2012.[1] In general, previous reviews have focused on sleepiness or hypersomnia secondary to conditions such as sleep apnea, circadian rhythm disorders, narcolepsy, and depression. However, somnolence is so commonly present in these conditions that, often, residual sleepiness is more a function of inadequate treatment of the primary disorder than a separate symptom that needs to be treated independently. Therefore, the goal of this article is to look mainly at sleepiness not stemming from another medical or psychological condition. The only caveat I make to this theme is to briefly discuss behavioral options to address sleepiness associated with narcolepsy because this group of patients develops a unique pattern of somnolence over the course of the day, which makes behavioral management more challenging.

To achieve the goal of understanding behavioral management of sleepiness, it is necessary to first define how nighttime sleep is thought to impact daytime somnolence and performance. Therefore, the literature investigating and discussing optimal sleep in terms of sleep duration, sleep insufficiency, and sleep need is reviewed. This review is followed by prophylactic measures that can be implemented when reduced nighttime sleep is anticipated for short periods of time (banking sleep). As mentioned earlier, behavioral treatment of narcolepsy, including sleep extension and prophylactic naps, is discussed and followed by a description of a technique I have been developing

Disclosure Statement: The author has nothing to disclose.
Department of Neurology, Center for Sleep Medicine, Weill Cornell Medical College of Cornell University, 425 East 61st Street, 5th Floor, New York, NY 10065, USA
E-mail address: mae2001@med.cornell.edu

Sleep Med Clin 12 (2017) 479–487
http://dx.doi.org/10.1016/j.jsmc.2017.03.020
1556-407X/17/© 2017 Elsevier Inc. All rights reserved.

in clinical practice to determine sleep need in individuals in order to optimize subjective daytime alertness.

EXCESSIVE DAYTIME SLEEPINESS

Excessive daytime sleepiness (EDS) is a condition characterized by a pressure to sleep during the day, which causes either social or occupational problems for the individual. This condition is different from (idiopathic) hypersomnia, which involves daytime somnolence despite 11 hours or more of sleep.[2] Excessive sleepiness can be defined both objectively with tests, such as the multiple sleep latency test (MSLT)[3] and/or the maintenance for wakefulness test (MWT),[4] or with questionnaires either focused exclusively on sleepiness, such as the Epworth Sleepiness Scale,[5] the Stanford Sleepiness Scale,[6] or the Karolinska Sleepiness Scale,[7] or with questions regarding somnolence imbedded in other surveys. According to the National Sleep Foundation's 2008 Sleep in America poll, 18% of American's are excessively sleepy.[8]

Daytime sleepiness has been investigated in several studies throughout the world, with prevalence ranging from 9% to 26%.[9] This wide range in prevalence of sleepiness is likely due as much to differences in study design and method used to query sleepiness as it is to true differences in the underlying alertness of populations. However, cultural differences in patterns of sleep, genetic variation, work schedules, and social activities in different countries may also play a role in level of sleepiness. Nonetheless, sleepiness is a major public health concern worldwide and has been found to significantly affect performance when induced experimentally.[10–13] Moreover, sleepiness has been linked to increased motor vehicle and work place accidents.[14–17] A study investigating the optimal duration of sleep to prevent deficits in psychomotor vigilance found that an average of 8.2 hours is needed per night for peak performance.[18] However, the US Department of Health and Human Services estimates that only 65% of Americans get a healthy amount of sleep.[19]

OPTIMAL SLEEP (SLEEP NEED VERSUS SLEEP DURATION VERSUS SLEEP INSUFFICIENCY)

In this section, 3 different but related concepts are examined in relation to optimal sleep. These concepts are sleep duration, sleep insufficiency, and sleep need. Understanding the differences in the terminology used to describe ideal sleep is critical to comprehending the previous research in this

area, which can otherwise seem contradictory. Moreover, appreciating these distinctions is necessary to develop a thoughtful treatment approach to behaviorally induced chronic partial sleep deprivation, which seems to be a substantial source of daytime sleepiness.

Sleep duration refers to the total amount of sleep obtained without factoring in whether or not individuals feel rested. More research has been done in this area than in sleep insufficiency or sleep need because questions related to sleep duration are more common than inquiries about whether the current total sleep amount is acceptable in existing large-scale data sets. Sleep duration is also easier to define both objectively and subjectively than other terminology related to optimal sleep.

Several studies have looked at the relationship between sleep length and death. Two relatively recent systematic reviews have shown a U-shaped curve for the association between sleep duration and all-cause mortality.[20,21] The lowest risk of death was found in individuals sleeping 7 to 8 hours per night. Those sleeping more or less than this amount showed an increased risk of mortality. More specifically, coronary heart disease, hypertension, and problems with glucose metabolism have been found to be linked to both short and long sleepers.[22–26] In one study, very short sleep of less than 5 hours per night was associated with increased risk for hypertension, hyperlipidemia, diabetes, and obesity.[27] Interestingly, this study did not find an elevated risk for any of these outcomes for the group self-reporting sleep duration of greater than 9 hours. A study by Altman and colleagues[28] found a significant relationship between sleep duration of less than 5 hours and body mass index, obesity, hypertension, myocardial infarction, and stroke. However, a sleep duration greater than 9 hours was only significantly associated with myocardial infarction and stroke.

A study performed by Van Dongen and colleagues[18] in which subjects were experimentally sleep restricted to 4, 6, or 8 hours in bed found that over the course of 14 days those in the 4- and 6-hour groups had significant decrements in cognitive performance. In fact, the investigators of this study state that 2 weeks of chronic partial sleep deprivation is equivalent to 2 days of total sleep deprivation. This finding is consistent with other studies, which have shown the cumulative effects of sleep restriction on psychomotor performance, mood, and objective measures of daytime sleepiness.[29–31]

In contrast to sleep duration, sleep insufficiency describes when the current amount of sleep is inadequate regardless of total sleep time. For example, someone may sleep 9 hours per night but feel that 10 hours is necessary to feel fully refreshed. Therefore, this person would be considered to have insufficient sleep. On the other hand, another individual may sleep 5 hours per night and feel that their sleep is adequate. As a result, this individual would not be considered to have sleep insufficiency. Sleep need is the most difficult concept out of the 3 to describe. Although not well defined in the literature, within this article it is used to describe the amount of sleep a person needs to feel refreshed and alert during the day. In other words, sleep need describes the amount of sleep a person needs to prevent sleep insufficiency. Admittedly, even this straightforward definition leads to ambiguity between whether alertness should be defined subjectively through questionnaires or objectively with tests, such as the MSLT or MWT. Nonetheless, the treatment approach described later in this article is based on determining subjective sleep need in patients complaining of EDS.

The relationship between an individual's optimal sleep requirement and health and cognitive function is more elusive and not as well publicized as the research focused exclusively on duration. From an epidemiologic perspective, the difference between sleep need and duration is simply a function of the population's degree of chronic sleep deprivation. However, from the perspective of an individual, knowing the average sleep duration or need of the population in which they live, although interesting, does not necessarily help them to understand their personal sleep need. Ursin and colleagues[32] calculated a normal distribution of subjective sleep need in middle-aged adults and found a mean for both men and women between 7.0 and 7.5 hours, respectively, with a range of 4 to 10 hours. The standard deviation of sleep need in this study was approximately 1 hour. However, subjective sleepiness has been found to poorly predict objective alertness.[33] Therefore, it is unclear if subjective sleep need is a good indication of biological sleep need.

A few studies have sought to investigate the risks associated with unmet sleep need. In a study by Altman and colleagues,[28] sleep duration alone, sleep insufficiency alone, and the combined effect of sleep duration and insufficiency were examined. The goal of this study was to see if the deleterious effects of sleep duration is moderated by the subjective impression of inadequate sleep. When examined together, sleep insufficiency accounted for an increased risk of hyperlipidemia; duration alone accounted for elevated risk of stroke, myocardial infraction, and obesity.

In a study by Hwangbo and colleagues, daytime sleepiness was investigated based on habitual sleep duration alone and separately controlling for unmet sleep need. The overall prevalence of EDS in their study population was 12%, despite 32% of those studied reporting less than 7 hours of sleep per night. Interestingly, habitual sleep duration was not predictive of EDS when unmet sleep need was taken into account. This study supports the theory that individual sleep need is more important for daytime alertness than overall sleep duration. Unfortunately, overall health status was not explored in this study.

SLEEP DEBT AND BANKING SLEEP

If biological sleep need is not satisfied, sleep pressure will accrue; this process has been termed sleep debt.[34] Several studies have found that when sleep deprivation occurs (and during wakefulness in general), drive to offload slow-wave activity (SWA) and rapid eye movement (REM) sleep amasses such that, once sleep does ensue, increased SWA and REM sleep is seen.[34–36] (Usually sleep pressure is thought to relate to SWA, and REM sleep is thought to be regulated by a combination of circadian and sleep-related forces; but REM sleep also shows rebound when deprived.) In fact, the homeostatic process described in Borbely's[37] 2-process model of sleep regulation defines sleep drive as a buildup of homeostatic pressure (process S) during wakefulness, which is measured by the amount of SWA that occurs during the subsequent sleep period. The length of wakefulness is proportional to the amount of SWA discharged.[35] The effects of sleep pressure were initially studied by looking at rebound from periods of either partial or full sleep deprivation.[34–36] More recently, sleep extension protocols have looked at the effects of chronic partial sleep debt.[38–40]

One of the first studies examining extended sleep was performed in the early 1970s by Taub and colleagues.[41] In this study, the sleep of a group of 12 healthy male volunteers was extended from approximately 7 to 9 hours per night. Interestingly, performance on vigilance and pinball tasks decreased after a 1-day recovery period. More recently, Roehrs and colleagues[39] extended the sleep of a group of both sleepy and alert normal subjects, whose group determination was based on MSLT score. The sleepy subjects showed an immediate increase in MSLT sleep latency after sleep extension. However, the alert subjects initially had a decrease in sleep latency; only after 6 days of extended sleep did mean sleep latency on the MSLT increase greater than the baseline level. Although, performance on a divided attention task improved in both groups throughout the extension period.

In 1999, Rupp and colleagues[42] performed a study looking at the effects of extended sleep during a subsequent period of sleep deprivation. On this study, subjects were assigned to either extended time in bed (10 hours) or habitual time in bed (7 hours) for 1 week. This was followed by a week of sleep restricted to 3 hours of time in bed. The extended-sleep group performed significantly better than the habitual-time-in-bed group on psychomotor vigilance tasks and had higher sleep latencies on the MWT. As a result, the term *banking sleep* was coined to describe extending sleep to more than the habitual time in bed in order to improve performance during future episodes of sleep deprivation. Arnal and colleagues[38] performed a follow-up study investigating the benefits of extending sleep before a period of total sleep deprivation. Like Rupp and colleagues,[42] Arnal and colleagues[38] found that sleep extension resulted in enhanced psychomotor vigilance task performance and improved MSLT scores during periods of sleep deprivation. However, some have speculated that sleep extension improves performance and decreases sleepiness during sleep deprivation by decreasing baseline sleep debt instead of truly banking sleep for later use.[43]

Nonetheless, both Rupp and colleagues[42] and Arnal and colleagues[38] show that relieving sleep pressure by extending time in bed to more than habitual time in bed before a period of reduced sleep will result in improved performance during the deprivation period. Therefore, individuals can moderate the discomfort associated with impending reduced sleep by an anticipatory period of extended sleep. Additional studies are required to see if these findings extend to the reduced performance seen with shift workers, who not only have reduced sleep but also battle the effects of being awake during disadvantageous phases of the circadian cycle. Arguably, this group of workers would benefit more from banking sleep than any other group because they can often predict times of reduced sleep based on their work schedule.

BEHAVIORAL TREATMENT OF SLEEPINESS ASSOCIATED WITH NARCOLEPSY

Narcolepsy is a disorder of REM sleep characterized by EDS, hypnogogic and/or hypnopompic hallucinations, sleep paralysis, and cataplexy (in some but not all cases).[2] It is typically diagnosed through a combination of clinical history and objective testing, which includes a polysomnogram followed by a MSLT. A sleep latency of 8 minutes or less with 2 or more REM sleep episodes on the MSLT (or one sleep-onset REM episode on the nighttime study followed by at least one REM episode on the MSLT) is considered diagnostic of narcolepsy.[2] A clinical history of cataplexy is pathognomonic of narcolepsy. However, 15% to 36% of narcoleptic patients do not have cataplexy.[2]

Behavioral treatment of sleepiness associated with narcolepsy has been investigated by a few groups. The most common methods tested for improving daytime sleepiness includes sleep extension and daytime naps (although additional cognitive-behavioral approaches have been investigated to treat other problems associated with narcolepsy). One study extended sleep in narcoleptic patients from 8 to 12 hours and found a significant increase in sleep latency after the extended sleep condition.[11] However, a recent review of studies on sleep satiation in narcoleptic patients found little benefit overall in extending sleep.[44] Narcoleptic patients tend to have fragmented nighttime sleep, but most feel alert on awakening in the morning. However, as the day progresses, they begin to experience sleepiness at a faster rate than those without narcolepsy,[45] which may explain why sleep extension is not an effective treatment approach.

Studies have generally found daytime napping to improve alertness in narcoleptic patients.[44] A study by Helmus and colleagues[45] prescribed naps of either 15 or 120 minutes and found the longer naps to be more beneficial to daytime alertness. However, regardless of nap length, sleepiness returned when tested 3 hours later, suggesting that multiple brief naps throughout the day are likely to be more helpful than isolated long naps. However, Rogers and colleagues[46] studied the effects of two 15-minute naps on daytime alertness and did not find an overall benefit from the naps alone. Yet, when the scheduled naps were paired with regular bedtimes, daytime alertness was improved. Therefore, a combination of a consistent sleep schedule with multiple daytime naps seems to be the best behavioral strategy to improve alertness in narcoleptic patients.

A NEW BEHAVIORAL APPROACH TO TREAT EXCESSIVE DAYTIME SLEEPINESS (AND DETERMINING SUBJECTIVE SLEEP NEED)

The behavioral approach the author describes stems from his work in sleep restriction therapy (SRT). SRT is one of the elements of cognitive-behavioral therapy for insomnia (CBT-I). This therapy is a collection of nonpharmacologic treatments used to improve nighttime sleep quality in patients complaining of difficulty sleeping. SRT was originally developed by Art Spielman and colleagues[47] in the mid 1980s and involves restricting time in bed in order to increase the likelihood that patients will sleep during the night.

SRT begins by first determining the treatment schedule for patients. This task is done by giving patients sleep logs to fill out for a couple weeks (**Fig. 1**). Once completed, the clinician reviews the logs to determine a new sleep schedule, which is typically done by averaging total sleep time over the period of time tracked by the patients.[48] The patients are then advised to reduce time in bed to approximate their current total sleep time. Therefore, if patients are only sleeping 6.5 hours per night, but they are spending 9 hours in bed, they are advised to reduce the time in bed to 6.5 hours. Ideally, once patients have been on the schedule for 2 to 3 weeks, they have an increase in sleep efficiency and a decrease in sleep latency.

The initial phase of SRT treatment is remarkably successful in improving nighttime sleep quality.[49] However, in many cases, sleepiness remains. When this occurs, patients are advised to increase their time in bed by 15 minutes. They can add this additional time to either their wake time or sleep time. For example, if patients currently have a sleep schedule of 11:00 PM to 5:30 AM, they can extend their time in bed by either going to sleep at 10:45 PM or sleeping in until 5:45 AM (but not both). They are asked to sleep on the new schedule for at least 5 days before making an additional adjustment in the schedule. This allows time for patients to gradually catch up on sleep.

Although a 5-day time period was developed through clinical trial and error, this time period comports with Kitamura and colleagues'[50] recent finding that it takes 4 days of sleep extension to recover from a 1-hour sleep debt. If too much time in bed is given at once, patients may initially be able to generate additional sleep to fill this much larger time in bed but may not be able to sustain the new schedule over the long-term, thus, causing them to develop insomnia once again. The idea that too much time in bed can reduce nighttime sleep quality is evidenced by the sleep extension studies. These studies have consistently shown decreased sleep efficiency and increased latency to sleep during periods of extended sleep.[38–40]

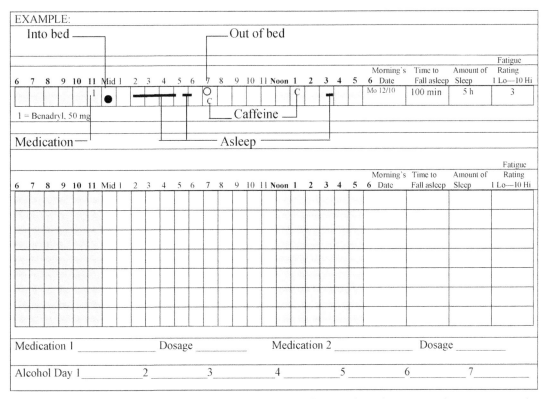

Fig. 1. Sleep log. (*Adapted from* Ebben MR, Spielman AJ. Non-pharmacological treatments for insomnia. J Behav Med 2009;32(3):248; with permission.)

Interestingly, the author has found this same technique of extending sleep used in SRT very useful in patients complaining of EDS, who do not report subjective difficulty sleeping at night. Moreover, other elements of CBT-I can also be useful when assessing the likely cause of daytime sleepiness. This subject is described in more detail later.

Behavioral treatment of sleepy patients should begin with a through screening for likely medical and/or psychological causes of the sleepiness (**Fig. 2** for the treatment decision tree). These causes include (but are not limited to) sleep apnea, narcolepsy, thyroid dysfunction, nutritional/vitamin deficiency, gastroesophageal reflux disease, depression, and/or anxiety. If a clinical history suggests that patients have one of these conditions, that issue is the focus of investigation until it is either ruled out or successfully treated.

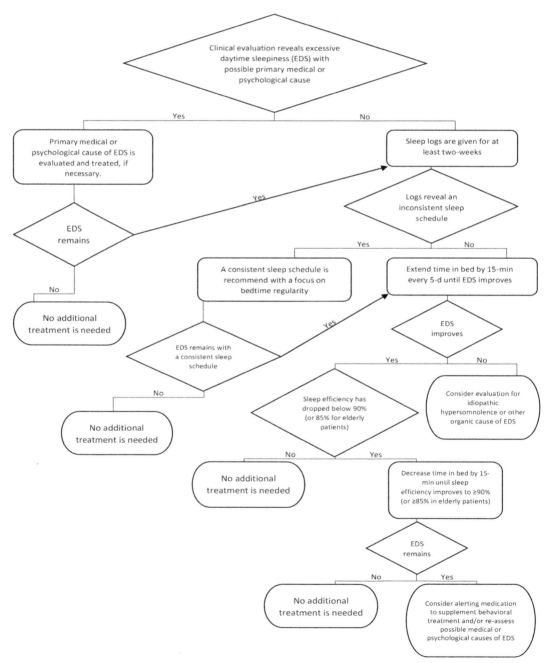

Fig. 2. Algorithm for behavioral management of EDS.

Once cleared for treatment, as with SRT, sleepy patients are asked to fill out sleep logs for at least 2 weeks. When these logs are reviewed, particular attention is paid to sleep efficiency, timing of sleep, sleepiness/fatigue ratings, and weekend versus weekday schedule. Usually behavioral treatment of sleepy patients involves a few phases after the initial sleep logs are reviewed. The first phase of management involves looking at the consistency of the sleep schedule over time. It is known that a variable sleep/wake schedule can cause a misalignment of homeostatic and circadian features of sleep resulting in increased daytime sleepiness. This theory is informed by the 2-process model of sleep regulation.[37] Therefore, if significant variations in sleep timing is seen on the patients' sleep dairies, this should be addressed. Regularization of the sleep schedule alone without sleep extension has been shown to improve daytime sleepiness.[51] Unlike with SRT, much of the focus on the sleep schedule of sleepy patients is on a consistent bedtime. Wake time in most of these cases is determined by work schedule on weekdays, and weekends are often spent catching up on sleep. Once patients have been on a consistent sleep schedule for at least a couple weeks, if sleepiness remains, the next phase of treatment is begun. If patients are no longer feeling sleepy during the day on the more consistent sleep schedule, no additional treatment is necessary.

Sleeping longer on weekends versus weekdays, despite a consistent bedtime, is a good indication of chronic sleep deprivation during the week. Therefore, if a patient's sleep log indicates longer bouts of sleep on weekends, the best way to address this issue is to increase total sleep time until the patient feels rested. Using SRT as a model, time in bed is increased by 15 minutes every 5 days until daytime alertness improves. If sleep efficacy is decreased without an increase in alertness, patients are advised to reduce time in bed by 15 minutes. In general, the focus is to increase sleep during the nighttime sleep period because those working during the day may find it difficult to find a place or opportunity to nap. Nonetheless, in those able, additional sleep time can also be added in the form of daytime naps. Adding daytime naps is particularly useful for individuals who have a longer-than-normal sleep need. In some cases, behavioral management alone will not sufficiently treat daytime sleepiness and other treatment approaches to improve alertness may need to be attempted.

The ultimate goal of the sleep extension protocol described earlier is to extend total sleep time on a consistent basis until patients feel alert during the day. Care is also taken to ensure that sleep efficiency is not significantly decreased in this process, as we do not want patients to develop insomnia. Through this process of increasing sleep time without decreasing quality of sleep, we hope to establish the individual sleep need of patients. Once discovered, patients now know how much sleep is needed to feel alert and refreshed during the day. Interestingly, often after determining their sleep need, patients will choose a schedule without sufficient sleep, resulting in mild sleepiness, although at least they know the reason for their somnolence and how to relieve it, if desired.

SUMMARY

The effects of sleep duration on mortality and other important health indicators is well established.[20–26] However, less is known about how the sleep need of the individual moderates the importance of overall sleep duration. Nonetheless, in clinical practice patients are sometimes encountered that cannot generate 7 to 8 hours of sleep or report EDS with the recommended amount of habitual sleep. Assuming, like most other biological systems, that sleep need is normally distributed,[32] it is not surprising that many persons' sleep need will fall outside of the optimal range of sleep duration. Given what is known about the risks associated with long and short sleep duration, there is a natural drive to help patients achieve sleep within this ideal range. However, for those with either long or short biological sleep needs, this task is nearly impossible without the use of hypnotic or alerting medication, which have their own set of risks that likely counteract any benefit obtained by optimizing sleep duration.

Instead of focusing on sleep duration, a more reasonable approach is to attempt to discover the persons' individual sleep need. A recent investigation by Kitamura and colleagues[50] outlines a laboratory-based approach for determining sleep need through a fixed sleep extension protocol. Alternatively, in this article, a clinically based approach to determine sleep need is outlined with an emphasis on increasing daytime alertness without significantly decreasing sleep efficiency and/or increasing sleep latency. However, it is important to note that the method described in this article, although found to be effective clinically in the author's practice is New York City, has never been empirically evaluated. Although given the limited options available for behavioral interventions in patients with EDS, this approach seems to be a safer alternative to a purely pharmacologic approach.

REFERENCES

1. Conroy DA, Novick DM, Swanson LM. Behavioral management of hypersomnia. Sleep Med Clin 2012;7(2):325–31.
2. American Academy of Sleep Medicine. International classification of sleep disorders. 3rd edition. Darien (IL): American Academy of Sleep Medicine; 2014.
3. Carskadon MA, Dement WC, Mitler MM, et al. Guidelines for the multiple sleep latency test (MSLT): a standard measure of sleepiness. Sleep 1986;9(4):519–24.
4. Mitler MM, Gujavarty KS, Browman CP. Maintenance of wakefulness test: a polysomnographic technique for evaluation treatment efficacy in patients with excessive somnolence. Electroencephalogr Clin Neurophysiol 1982;53(6):658–61.
5. Johns MW. A new method for measuring daytime sleepiness: the Epworth sleepiness scale. Sleep 1991;14(6):540–5.
6. Hoddes E, Dement W, Zarcone V. The development and use of the Stanford sleepiness scale (SSS). Psychophysiology 1972;9:150.
7. Akerstedt T, Gillberg M. Subjective and objective sleepiness in the active individual. Int J Neurosci 1990;52(1–2):29–37.
8. Swanson LM, Arnedt JT, Rosekind MR, et al. Sleep disorders and work performance: findings from the 2008 National Sleep Foundation sleep in America poll. J Sleep Res 2011;20(3):487–94.
9. Ohayon MM. From wakefulness to excessive sleepiness: what we know and still need to know. Sleep Med Rev 2008;12(2):129–41.
10. Banks S, Dinges DF. Behavioral and physiological consequences of sleep restriction. J Clin Sleep Med 2007;3(5):519–28.
11. Cohen DA, Wang W, Wyatt JK, et al. Uncovering residual effects of chronic sleep loss on human performance. Sci Transl Med 2010;2(14):14ra13.
12. Goel N, Rao H, Durmer JS, et al. Neurocognitive consequences of sleep deprivation. Semin Neurol 2009;29(4):320–39.
13. Leproult R, Colecchia EF, Berardi AM, et al. Individual differences in subjective and objective alertness during sleep deprivation are stable and unrelated. Am J Physiol Regul Integr Comp Physiol 2003; 284(2):R280–90.
14. Horne JA, Reyner LA. Driver sleepiness. J Sleep Res 1995;4(S2):23–9.
15. Horne JA, Reyner LA. Sleep related vehicle accidents. BMJ 1995;310(6979):565–7.
16. Ozer C, Etcibasi S, Ozturk L. Daytime sleepiness and sleep habits as risk factors of traffic accidents in a group of Turkish public transport drivers. Int J Clin Exp Med 2014;7(1):268–73.
17. Melamed S, Oksenberg A. Excessive daytime sleepiness and risk of occupational injuries in non-shift daytime workers. Sleep 2002;25(3):315–22.
18. Van Dongen HP, Maislin G, Mullington JM, et al. The cumulative cost of additional wakefulness: dose-response effects on neurobehavioral functions and sleep physiology from chronic sleep restriction and total sleep deprivation. Sleep 2003; 26(2):117–26.
19. Liu Y, Wheaton AG, Chapman DP, et al. Prevalence of healthy sleep duration among adults–United States, 2014. MMWR Morb Mortal Wkly Rep 2016; 65(6):137–41.
20. Cappuccio FP, D'Elia L, Strazzullo P, et al. Sleep duration and all-cause mortality: a systematic review and meta-analysis of prospective studies. Sleep 2010;33(5):585–92.
21. Gallicchio L, Kalesan B. Sleep duration and mortality: a systematic review and meta-analysis. J Sleep Res 2009;18(2):148–58.
22. Ayas NT, White DP, Manson JE, et al. A prospective study of sleep duration and coronary heart disease in women. Arch Intern Med 2003;163(2):205–9.
23. Shankar A, Koh WP, Yuan JM, et al. Sleep duration and coronary heart disease mortality among Chinese adults in Singapore: a population-based cohort study. Am J Epidemiol 2008;168(12):1367–73.
24. Nakajima H, Kaneita Y, Yokoyama E, et al. Association between sleep duration and hemoglobin A1c level. Sleep Med 2008;9(7):745–52.
25. Zizi F, Pandey A, Murrray-Bachmann R, et al. Race/ethnicity, sleep duration, and diabetes mellitus: analysis of the National Health interview survey. Am J Med 2012;125(2):162–7.
26. Kachi Y, Ohwaki K, Yano E. Association of sleep duration with untreated diabetes in Japanese men. Sleep Med 2012;13(3):307–9.
27. Grandner MA, Chakravorty S, Perlis ML, et al. Habitual sleep duration associated with self-reported and objectively determined cardiometabolic risk factors. Sleep Med 2014;15(1):42–50.
28. Altman NG, Izci-Balserak B, Schopfer E, et al. Sleep duration versus sleep insufficiency as predictors of cardiometabolic health outcomes. Sleep Med 2012;13(10):1261–70.
29. Carskadon MA, Dement WC. Cumulative effects of sleep restriction on daytime sleepiness. Psychophysiology 1981;18(2):107–13.
30. Dinges DF, Pack F, Williams K, et al. Cumulative sleepiness, mood disturbance, and psychomotor vigilance performance decrements during a week of sleep restricted to 4-5 hours per night. Sleep 1997;20(4):267–77.
31. Belenky G, Wesensten NJ, Thorne DR, et al. Patterns of performance degradation and restoration during sleep restriction and subsequent recovery: a sleep dose-response study. J Sleep Res 2003; 12(1):1–12.
32. Ursin R, Bjorvatn B, Holsten F. Sleep duration, subjective sleep need, and sleep habits of 40- to

45-year-olds in the Hordaland health study. Sleep 2005;28(10):1260–9.

33. Richardson GS, Drake CL, Roehrs TA, et al. Habitual sleep time predicts accuracy of self-reported alertness. Sleep 2002;25:A145.

34. Webb WB, Agnew HW. The effects on subsequent sleep of an acute restriction of sleep length. Psychophysiology 1975;12(4):367–70.

35. Dijk DJ, Beersma DG, Daan S. EEG power density during nap sleep: reflection of an hourglass measuring the duration of prior wakefulness. J Biol Rhythms 1987;2(3):207–19.

36. Nakazawa Y, Kotorii M, Ohsima M, et al. Study on the partial differential REM deprivation (PDRD). Folia Psychiatr Neurol Jpn 1977;31(1):1–7.

37. Borbely AA. A two process model of sleep regulation. Hum Neurobiol 1982;1(3):195–204.

38. Arnal PJ, Sauvet F, Leger D, et al. Benefits of sleep extension on sustained attention and sleep pressure before and during total sleep deprivation and recovery. Sleep 2015;38(12):1935–43.

39. Roehrs T, Timms V, Zwyghuizen-Doorenbos A, et al. Sleep extension in sleepy and alert normals. Sleep 1989;12(5):449–57.

40. Wehr TA, Moul DE, Barbato G, et al. Conservation of photoperiod-responsive mechanisms in humans. Am J Physiol 1993;265(4 Pt 2):R846–57.

41. Taub JM, Globus GG, Phoebus E, et al. Extended sleep and performance. Nature 1971;233(5315):142–3.

42. Rupp TL, Wesensten NJ, Bliese PD, et al. Banking sleep: realization of benefits during subsequent sleep restriction and recovery. Sleep 2009;32(3):311–21.

43. Axelsson J, Vyazovskiy VV. Banking sleep and biological sleep need. Sleep 2015;38(12):1843–5.

44. Marin Agudelo HA, Jimenez Correa U, Carlos Sierra J, et al. Cognitive behavioral treatment for narcolepsy: can it complement pharmacotherapy? Sleep Sci 2014;7(1):30–42.

45. Helmus T, Rosenthal L, Bishop C, et al. The alerting effects of short and long naps in narcoleptic, sleep deprived, and alert individuals. Sleep 1997;20(4):251–7.

46. Rogers AE, Aldrich MS, Lin X. A comparison of three different sleep schedules for reducing daytime sleepiness in narcolepsy. Sleep 2001;24(4):385–91.

47. Spielman AJ, Caruso LS, Glovinsky PB. A behavioral perspective on insomnia treatment. Psychiatr Clin North Am 1987;10(4):541–53.

48. Ebben MR, Spielman AJ. Non-pharmacological treatments for insomnia. J Behav Med 2009;32(3):244–54.

49. Morin CM, Culbert JP, Schwartz SM. Nonpharmacological interventions for insomnia - a meta-analysis of treatment efficacy. Am J Psychiatry 1994;151(8):1172–80.

50. Kitamura S, Katayose Y, Nakazaki K, et al. Estimating individual optimal sleep duration and potential sleep debt. Sci Rep 2016;6:35812.

51. Manber R, Bootzin RR, Acebo C, et al. The effects of regularizing sleep-wake schedules on daytime sleepiness. Sleep 1996;19(5):432–41.

Hypersomnolence and Traffic Safety

 CrossMark

Ravi Gupta, MD, PhD[a], Seithikurippu R. Pandi-Perumal, MSc[b],
Aljohara S. Almeneessier, MD, ABFM[c], Ahmed S. BaHammam, MD, FRCP[d],*

KEYWORDS

- Drivers • Drowsiness • Sleepiness • Narcolepsy • Obstructive sleep apnea

KEY POINTS

- Drowsiness is a major cause of motor vehicle accidents.
- Common sleep problems implicated in hypersomnolence are sleep deprivation, obstructive sleep apnea, and central hypersomnias.
- The optimal management of sleep disorders and sleep deprivation can improve vigilance, thereby reducing the odds of having an accident.
- Diagnostic tests are available to measure sleepiness and these tests may be used to assess fitness-to-drive.
- Physicians, particularly family physicians and general practitioners, should be educated regarding the risk of sleepy driving and the importance of routine assessment of fitness-to-drive among patients.
- Legislation should be drafted to assess hypersomnolence before granting driver's licenses.

INTRODUCTION

Motor vehicle accidents (MVAs) are a leading cause of mortality and morbidity worldwide and are expected to be the fourth leading cause of death in 2030.[1,2] Approximately 1.3 million people die per year worldwide because of MVAs, and another 20 to 50 million sustain nonfatal injuries that lead to significant disability.[1] The available data suggest that fatigue and sleepiness are major risk factors for MVAs.[3] Although it is difficult to estimate the number of MVAs that involve drowsy drivers, some modeling studies have estimated that the rate for fatal accidents is 15% to 33%.[4] Drowsiness results in several types of neurologic dysfunction, such as reduced reaction time, decreased attention, and impaired decision-making skills.[4] A French study of 4774 drivers reported that 11.8% of the sample had Epworth Sleepiness Scale (ESS) scores of 11 or higher, 28.6% reported experiencing sleepiness at the wheel severe enough to require stopping, and 46.8% and 39.4% reported feeling sleepy during night-time and daytime driving, respectively. Moreover, 10.7% reported a near-miss accident during the previous year (46% of which were reportedly sleep-related) and 5.8% reported having an accident (5.2% of which of were sleep-related).[5] The Centers for Disease

Funding: This work was partially supported by a grant from the National Plan for Science and Technology Program by the King Saud University Project in Saudi Arabia. The sponsor had no role in the design or conduct of this research.
^a Department of Psychiatry & Sleep Clinic, Himalayan Institute of Medical Sciences, Swami Ram Nagar, Doiwala, Dehradun, India; ^b Somnogen Canada Inc, College Street, Toronto, Ontario M6H 1C5, Canada; ^c Department of Family and Community Medicine, College of Medicine, King Saud University, Riyadh 11324, Saudi Arabia; ^d University Sleep Disorders Center, Department of Medicine, College of Medicine, King Saud University, Box 225503, Riyadh 11324, Saudi Arabia
* Corresponding author.
E-mail addresses: ashammam2@gmail.com; ashammam@ksu.edu.sa

sleep.theclinics.com

Control and Prevention reported that drowsy drivers were responsible for nearly 72,000 accidents, 44,000 injuries, and 800 deaths in 2013.[6] However, this report further mentions that this major risk factor is grossly underreported. Moreover, the report indicates that certain groups of drivers are prone to experience drowsiness during driving. People at risk are those who do not get adequate sleep (for any reason); drivers who operate commercial vehicles, including trucks and buses; drivers who use substances that promote drowsiness (eg, sleeping pills, alcohol, and opiates); and those who are suffering from sleep disorders.[6] This report specifies that people who sleep less than 6 hours per day and those who snore are at higher risk of falling asleep at the wheel.[6] A short period of sleeping during the night and a long duration of driving have been found to increase the chances of rear-end collisions, as well as accidents involving a single vehicle.[7] In addition, nighttime driving increases the chances of accidents.[8]

This article discusses the available evidence that relates MVAs with drowsiness, sleep deprivation, or sleep disorders. Moreover, it explores the legislative position of sleep-related factors in terms of issuing driving licenses in different countries. It further examines the evidence regarding the effect of sleep disorder treatment on MVAs.

SLEEP DEPRIVATION

Sleep deprivation can be acute or chronic. Acute sleep deprivation refers to a condition in which one is unable to sleep for a whole night or a major portion of it. Chronic sleep deprivation is defined when a person is not getting sufficient daily sleep for a few days to several weeks. This type of sleep deprivation also has a cumulative effect; thus, the person is chronically deprived of sleep after a few days. Both types of sleep deprivation have ill effects on health. In the United States, it has been estimated that 56,000 accidents per year are related to sleep deprivation.[9] A similar link between sleep deprivation and an increased risk of MVAs has been reported in other countries.[10,11] It has been found that after 17 hours of continuous wakefulness, cognitive functions (eg, reaction time and hand-eye-coordination) are greatly impaired and an increasing number of errors are made.[12] Attention, as well as the ability to process the information, is also drastically impaired.[12] After 17 hours of continuous wakefulness, cognitive and psychomotor performance decreases to a level comparable to the performance impairment detected among those with a blood alcohol concentration of 0.05%, which is not safe for industrial and driving work.[12] Another study examined the

impact of the length of wakefulness on performance impairment during simulated afternoon and midnight driving in a group of healthy people with normal sleep duration (7 hours) before they took the test.[13] The results suggested that nighttime driving was associated with increased sleepiness and enhanced risk of accidents, owing to the longer period of wakefulness despite normal sleep duration on prior nights.[7,13,14] Whether 6 to 7 hours of sleep is enough for a daytime driving is also questionable.[7,15] Adolescents obtaining 6.5 hours of nighttime sleep for 5 days were found to perform worse on simulated driving than those who had 10 hours of nighttime sleep when the test was taken during the daytime.[15] While on duty, long-haul truck drivers frequently cut down their sleep up to 4 hours per day and thus become sleep deprived, increasing the chances of an MVA.[16] Another study reported that approximately half of truck drivers worked unrealistic schedules, with more than 50 hours of driving per week, and 27% of drivers reported poor sleep quality.[17] A higher prevalence of sleep debt has been reported in professional drivers compared with control participants.[18] These examples show the effects of chronic partial sleep deprivation on the risk of MVAs. An increased duration of wakefulness, when combined with alcohol use, has been found to impair driving performance, even during the elimination phase of ethanol consumption.[19]

The impact of sleep deprivation on the risk of MVAs seems to be influenced by age. In a counterbalanced design study that assessed the effect of sleep restriction for the preceding 5 hours on prolonged (2 hours) afternoon simulated driving in 20 younger (mean age 23 years) and 19 older (mean age 67 years) healthy drivers revealed that after sleep restriction, young drivers exhibited significantly more sleepiness-related lane deviations and greater low-frequency electroencephalography (EEG) power (4–11 Hz), indicating sleepiness.[20]

OBSTRUCTIVE SLEEP APNEA AND SAFE DRIVING

Snoring is a sign of obstructive sleep apnea (OSA), a common sleep disorder that affects between 6% and 17% of the population.[21] OSA is associated with poor performance on the psychomotor vigilance test.[22] Several studies have shown that, compared with controls, OSA patients have a higher risk of falling asleep while driving and are 3 times more likely to cause MVAs.[3,23,24] However, there is no compelling evidence to restrict driving in patients with OSA, unless they have a history of MVA.[25] The American Thoracic Society defines a high-risk driver as one who has moderate to severe daytime sleepiness and a recent unintended motor vehicle crash or near-miss attributable to sleepiness, fatigue, or inattention.[25] **Table 1** shows a summary of studies that assessed OSA, sleepiness, and risk of MVA in different countries. Using studies published between 1980 and 2003, as well as data from the National Safety Council, it has been estimated that OSA was responsible for approximately 810,000 collisions, resulting in the loss of 1400 lives and 16 billion dollars in damages per year in the United States.[26] However, the association between OSA and decreased performance is not universal, and some studies did not identify an association between OSA and MVAs.[22,27,28] Nevertheless, it has been argued that reporting MVAs due to OSA may negatively affect an individual's employment and ability to keep their driver's license.[29] Hence, drivers with OSA may underreport MVAs to their treating physicians.

It is likely that the effect of OSA on driving performance is related to OSA severity.[22,27] Accident rates are related to the severity of OSA, and the risk increases with increasing severity because of increasing daytime sleepiness.[30,31] A study revealed that apnea-hypopnea index (AHI) values (AHI $\geq$40) and ESS scores (ESS $\geq$11: [OR = 1.87, 95% CI: 0.099–3.53, P = .05] and ESS $\geq$16: [OR = 3.56, 95% CI: 1.85–6.84, P<.001]) of 616 Japanese drivers were correlated with an increased risk of dozing off at the wheel, as well as a higher risk of being involved in an MVA.[32] A systematic review of published studies reported that noncommercial drivers with OSA had a significantly increased risk of involvement in MVAs (2-fold to 3-fold greater accident rate).[33] Increased sleepiness is a risk factor for a MVA among OSA patients. The European sleep apnea database of 8476 drivers with OSA revealed that an ESS score greater than 16, driving more than 15,000 km per year, sleeping less than 5 hours per day, and use of hypnotics were the main risk factors for MVA, with increasing numbers of risk factors across the spectrum of OSA severity.[34] Other data suggest that daytime sleepiness increases the risk for MVAs among OSA patients, as well those with simple snoring.[16,35–38] Early diagnostic evaluation and treatment of OSA and education of the patient and family about the risk of sleepy driving are likely to decrease the prevalence of sleepiness-related crashes in patients with OSA.[25]

CENTRAL DISORDERS OF HYPERSOMNOLENCE AND MOTOR VEHICLE ACCIDENTS

Patients with central causes of hypersomnolence have an increased risk of MVAs.[39–42] However, a limited number of studies have addressed this topic. A recent French study showed that central disorders causing hypersomnolence (narcolepsy and primary hypersomnia) increased the odds of having MVAs.[43] The chances of having MVAs were a function of daytime sleepiness.[43] The risk of MVAs was high in both treated and untreated subjects at study inclusion (untreated, odds ratio [OR] 2.21, 95% CI 1.30–3.76; treated OR 2.04, 95% CI 1.26–3.30). However, the risk of MVAs for subjects treated for at least 5 years was not different from the risk for healthy subjects (OR 1.23, 95% CI 0.56–2.69), suggesting that the risk of MVAs is potentially reversed by long-term treatment.[43]

MEDICATIONS AND RISK OF MOTOR VEHICLE ACCIDENTS

Several studies have shown that subjects with insomnia and those who were on various sleep medications had an increased risk of accidents owing to fatigue, reduced alertness, and sleepiness at the wheel.[44–46] Several studies examined the residual effects of hypnotic drugs on driving performance. Participants received a hypnotic tablet at bedtime and driving performance was tested the next day. The results of these studies showed that benzodiazepine hypnotics and zopiclone significantly worsened driving performance, whereas zolpidem and zaleplon had less impact on driving performance.[47–49] Ramelteon, a melatonin receptor antagonist, has been shown to significantly impair next-morning driving performance.[50]

The findings of these studies concur with epidemiologic data showing an increased risk of accidents among those who use benzodiazepine hypnotics and zopiclone.[51]

COUNTERMEASURES THAT MAY REDUCE SLEEPINESS WHILE DRIVING

Considering that sleepiness is an important cause of MVAs, it is important to assess the countermeasures that may prevent sleepiness and reduce the risk of MVAs. Several countermeasures can be taken to reduce the sleepiness among sleep-deprived drivers or during vehicle driving at odd hours. Building rumble strips in the middle of the road, especially on narrow roads, has been found to awaken sleepy drivers.[52] Modafinil (300 mg) taken at approximately 3:00 AM has been found to reduce lane-deviation in sleep-deprived subjects, without any effect of vehicle speed beyond prescribed limits when tested 2 hours after ingestion.[53] However, modafinil can induce euphoria, compromising one's ability to realistically assess the risk of driving

Table 1
A summary of studies that addressed obstructive sleep apnea and motor vehicle accidents among drivers

Authors	Country	Type of Study	Study Population	Results
Hanning & Welsh,[94] 1996	United Kingdom	Questionnaire-based survey	2247 drivers with no claim history. Questioned for history of accidents, snoring, and daytime sleepiness	Snorers were more likely to report daytime sleepiness and having had to pull off from the road while driving
Pack et al,[22] 2006	USA	Questionnaire followed by actigraphy and in-laboratory polysomnography (PSG). Experimental study	1329 drivers: 247 at high risk for OSA and 159 at low risk for OSA	Short sleep duration and severe OSA were associated with sleepiness and poor performance on the road. Of the study population, 29% had OSA, with severe OSA in 5%
Ozoh et al,[27] 2013	Lagos	Descriptive cross-sectional study using questionnaires	500 male commercial drivers	Of the study population, 49% had a high risk for OSA and 14.4% had daytime sleepiness. No relationship was observed between OSA, daytime sleepiness and past history of MVAs
Dogan et al,[95] 2006	Turkey	Descriptive cross-sectional study using questionnaire	340 drivers	Of the study population, 41.2% had habitual snoring. Habitual snorers had odds ratio (OR) 1.6 (1.03–2.53) for accidents
Lloberes et al,[35] 2000	Spain	Case-control study with PSG	172 subjects with OSA and 40 controls	Self-reported sleepiness among OSA subjects increased the chance of accidents (OR 5, 95% CI 2.3–10.9)
Perez-Chada et al,[16] 2005	Argentina	Questionnaire-based study	738 long-haul truck drivers	Snoring more than 3 times a week (OR 1.73, 95% CI 1.23–2.44), sleepiness while driving (OR 1.92, 95% CI 1.08–1.96), and ESS score >10 (OR 2.53, 95% CI 1.61–3.97) predicted accidents or near-miss accidents
Akkoyunlu et al,[36] 2013	Turkey	Questionnaire-based study	520 city drivers	The accident rate was predicted by daytime sleepiness among those at high risk for OSA
Masa et al,[37] 2000	Spain	Case-control study using PSG	145 habitually sleepy drivers and controls	Those with a history of MVA had a higher respiratory disturbance index (OR 8.5, 95% CI 1.2–59)
Shiomi et al,[38] 2002	Japan	Case-control study using PSG	448 subjects with OSA and 106 simple snorers	The accident rates were higher in subjects with severe OSA. Sleepiness among OSA and snorers predicted risk of MVA
Braeckman et al,[17] 2011	Belgium	Cross-sectional cohort study using questionnaires	476 truck drivers	Of the study population (21.5%) were at high risk for OSA and 18% had scores >10 on ESS
BaHammam et al,[11] 2014	Saudi Arabia	Cross-sectional study using questionnaires	1219 city drivers	The prevalence of a high risk for OSA was higher among drivers who had MVAs in the past 6 mo

in such conditions.[53] Caffeine (200 mg) and napping have been found to reduce errors during nighttime driving without influencing subsequent sleep.[54,55] The effects of 3 stimulants, modafinil (400 mg), caffeine (600 mg), and dextroamphetamine (20 mg), on alertness and vigilance were compared after 64 hours of continuous wakefulness. Caffeine showed an immediate effect, whereas dextroamphetamine showed long-lasting effects, and modafinil was found to be comparable with placebo.[56] The maximum rate of adverse effects was reported in the caffeine group, whereas dextroamphetamine adversely affected post-test sleep.[56] In-car blue light during nighttime driving has been found to be useful in some studies.[57] Scheduled naps during nighttime driving have also been found to improve alertness and to reduce errors.[58]

EFFECT OF SLEEP DISORDER TREATMENT ON THE RISK OF MOTOR VEHICLE ACCIDENTS

One major question is whether treatment of sleep disorders prevent MVAs. It has been repeatedly reported in the literature that optimal and proper treatment of sleep disorders can improve alertness and reduce the chances of accidents.[59,60] Treating narcolepsy and primary hypersomnia has been found to reduce the risk of MVAs.[43,61] A systematic review and meta-analysis on OSA, continuous positive airway pressure (CPAP), and accidents found that CPAP use reduced the accident risk in drivers with moderate to severe OSA (relative risk [RR] 0.278, 95% CI 0.22–0.35, P<.001); self-reported sleepiness, a symptom of OSA, was also decreased.[23]

A survey examined the opinion of sleep physicians regarding fitness-to-drive in patients with sleep disorders.[62] Most sleep physicians indicated that patients with untreated OSA, narcolepsy, and insomnia are not fit to drive unless they receive treatment.[62] In the opinion of these professionals, excessive daytime sleepiness was the major limiting factor for driving.[62] The evidence for the management of sleep disorders and driving performance is given in **Table 2**.

MONITORING OF HYPERSOMNOLENCE

Various tools for evaluating hypersomnolence have been developed. (See Renee Monderer and colleagues' article, "Evaluation of the Sleepy Patient: Differential Diagnosis," in this issue.) Some of the more commonly used tools include

1. Sleep questionnaires: Several questionnaires have been designed to assess hypersomnolence, such as the ESS, the Stanford Sleepiness scale, the Pittsburgh Sleep Quality Index, and the Karolinska Sleepiness Scale.[63–65] Unfortunately, subjective assessments of sleepiness do not correlate with objective measures. Moreover, none of those tools have been validated against MVA risk.
2. Optalert (OPTALERT, Optalert Pty Ltd, Melbourne, Australia) (system of infrared reflectance oculography): Optalert is a new method to monitor eye and eyelid movements by infrared reflectance oculography. Transducers are attached to a glass frame and measure drowsiness continuously using a new scale (Johns Drowsiness Scale) during driving tasks.[66,67]
3. Multiple sleep latency test[68–70]: This test assesses the propensity to sleep in a comfortable position, a factor that is commonly used in the diagnosis of narcolepsy. Patients with mean sleep latencies less than 5 minutes are considered to have pathologic sleepiness and should be warned about their increased risk for industrial or MVAs.[71]
4. Maintenance of wakefulness test (MWT)[70,72]: This test assesses an individual's ability to stay awake. A study revealed that an MWT mean sleep latency of 0 to 19 minutes is associated with simulated driving impairment.[73] However, more studies are necessary to confirm that pathologic MWT scores are associated with actual driving impairment.
5. The Oxford sleep resistance test[74]: This test combines elements of the MWT and psychomotor testing.
6. Pupillography: This test evaluates the diameter and variability of the pupil and the relationship of these measures with subjective sleepiness complaints.[75,76]
7. Actigraphy: This device assesses sleep duration and circadian rhythm disorders and may be used to infer hypersomnia.[70,77]
8. Polysomnography (the gold standard for diagnosing OSA), is the most commonly used test to evaluate sleep and its disorders.[78–80]

These survey instruments and physiologic tests are very important for accurately diagnosing sleep disorders and their symptoms so that driver errors and accidents, which may affect public health, can be avoided. Nevertheless, none of these tools can accurately predict the degree of impairment and the risk of MVAs.[39,40] Moreover, available methods of simulated driving cannot accurately predict the risk of accidents but can predict who may have a low chance of being in an MVA.[81,82]

ROLE OF THE TREATING PHYSICIANS

Daytime sleepiness has been found in several studies to be associated with an increased risk of

Table 2
A summary of studies that assessed the effects of treatment on the risk of motor vehicle accidents in subjects with hypersomnolence

Authors	Type of Study	Intervention	Study Population	Results
Philip et al,[61] 2014	Randomized, crossover, double-blind placebo-controlled trial	Modafinil 400 mg/d or placebo for 5 d before a driving test	13 subjects with narcolepsy and 14 with idiopathic hypersomnia	Modafinil improved wakefulness and reduced inappropriate line crossing and the standard deviation of the lateral position of vehicle
Hirshkowitz et al,[96] 2007	Randomized double-blind study	Armodafinil 150 mg/d	Subjects with OSA on nasal CPAP (nCPAP) having residual excessive daytime sleepiness (EDS)	Armodafinil improved wakefulness and reduced fatigue
Hack et al,[97] 2001	Case-control study	nCPAP for OSA and sleep for sleep-deprived subjects	26 subjects with OSA before and after nCPAP; 12 healthy subjects after sleep deprivation and after normal sleep or before and after alcohol intoxication	nCPAP for OSA, normal sleep in sleep-deprived subjects and removal of alcohol reversed impaired driving; The effects of OSA are related to sleep fragmentation or sleep deprivation, whereas alcohol induces impairment through impaired cognitive performance
Cassel et al,[98] 1996	Cohort study	nCPAP for OSA subjects	59 subjects using nCPAP for 1 y	Spells of sleepiness, daytime sleep onset latency, fatigue, and vigilance test reaction time improved with nCPAP, thus reducing the number of MVAs
Horstmann et al,[30] 2000	Cohort study	nCPAP for OSA	85 subjects with obstructive sleep apnea hypopnea syndrome (OSAHS) using nCPAP	nCPAP reduced the number of accidents from 10.6 to 2.7 per million kilometers

MVAs.[16,35,36,83] Drivers are often not able to predict their level of alertness before driving or their performance during driving.[84] MVAs result in a very large economic and social burden. Therefore, regular health checks should be put in place before acquiring or renewing a driver's license, especially in patients with sleep disorders. Physicians should also keep this risk in mind when assessing patients with sleep disorders or those with medical conditions or medications that may increase daytime sleepiness.[85] Whether physicians have a legal responsibility to assess of their patients' medical fitness-to-drive is a matter of debate.[86,87] Although some countries hold physicians legally accountable for failing to report certain medical conditions to the local traffic authorities,[88,89] other countries do not.[85] Moreover, the level of awareness regarding the importance of this issue is high among physicians in some countries, whereas there is lack of perceived responsibility among physicians in other countries. In a survey conducted in Canada, 72% of family physicians believed that they should be held legally responsible for alerting traffic authorities regarding patients who are unfit to drive.[90] In contrast, a study in Saudi Arabia showed that only 15% of the surveyed sample considered that it was their responsibility to report patients as being unfit to drive to the local traffic authorities.[85]

LEGISLATIVE ISSUES

Several European countries, in addition to Canada, Australia, and several US states, have detailed traffic laws that prohibit patients with sleep disorders, such as OSA and narcolepsy, from driving or obtaining a driver's license until the disorder is medically treated.[28,91,92] Several European countries (Belgium, Netherlands, Finland, Spain, Sweden, France, and the United Kingdom) have imposed legal restrictions on issuing a driving license to patients suffering from OSA and narcolepsy.[92] However, in other countries (particularly developing countries), there are no traffic regulations that govern sleepy driving. Regulations must be implemented to reduce the risk of sleepy driving. Regulations should hold sleepy drivers accountable for the risks that they take and the damage that they cause if they do not seek medical advice.[93] Moreover, clear regulations are needed to determine the legal responsibilities of the treating physicians in regards to patients with hypersomnolence.

SUMMARY

Considering that data obtained around the world support hypersomnolence and sleep disorders as important causes of industrial and road accidents, there is a need to include sleep-related parameters in the screening of at least commercial drivers (if not all drivers). This screening should be a part of the initial medical work-up before drivers are granted a commercial license. Moreover, these drivers should be subjected to annual health monitoring. Drivers should be encouraged to seek help from sleep physicians and to follow the advice they receive. Additionally, drivers should be educated about the importance of getting adequate sleep before driving and using effective countermeasures for sleepiness. Moreover, physicians, particularly family physicians and general practitioners, should be educated regarding the risk of sleep driving and the importance of routine assessments of fitness-to-drive.

REFERENCES

1. WHO. Global plan for the decade of action for road safety 2011-2020. Geneva, Switzerland: World Health Organization; 2010.
2. Mulgrew AT, Nasvadi G, Butt A, et al. Risk and severity of motor vehicle crashes in patients with obstructive sleep apnoea/hypopnoea. Thorax 2008; 63(6):536–41 [Research Support, Non-U.S. Gov't].
3. Rodenstein D. Sleep apnea: traffic and occupational accidents–individual risks, socioeconomic and legal implications [review]. Respiration 2009;78(3):241–8.
4. Centers for Disease Control and Prevention (CDC). Drowsy driving - 19 states and the District of Columbia, 2009-2010. MMWR Morb Mortal Wkly Rep 2013;61(51–52):1033–7.
5. Sagaspe P, Taillard J, Bayon V, et al. Sleepiness, near-misses and driving accidents among a representative population of French drivers. J Sleep Res 2010;19(4):578–84.
6. Centers of Disease Control and Prevention. Drowsy driving: asleep at the wheel 2015 [updated November 5, 2015; cited February 5, 2017]; Available at: http://www.cdc.gov/features/dsdrowsydriving.
7. Abe T, Komada Y, Nishida Y, et al. Short sleep duration and long spells of driving are associated with the occurrence of Japanese drivers' rear-end collisions and single-car accidents. J Sleep Res 2010; 19(2):310–6 [Research Support, Non-U.S. Gov't].
8. Rice TM, Peek-Asa C, Kraus JF. Nighttime driving, passenger transport, and injury crash rates of young drivers. Inj Prev 2003;9(3):245–50 [Research Support, U.S. Gov't, P.H.S.].
9. National Highway Traffic Safety Administration (NHTSA). An analysis of the significant decline in motor vehicle traffic fatalities in 2008. Ann Emerg Med 2011;58(4):377–8.
10. Leechawengwongs M, Leechawengwongs E, Sukying C, et al. Role of drowsy driving in traffic

accidents: a questionnaire survey of Thai commercial bus/truck drivers. J Med Assoc Thai 2006; 89(11):1845–50.

11. BaHammam AS, Alkhunizan MA, Lesloum RH, et al. Prevalence of sleep-related accidents among drivers in Saudi Arabia. Ann Thorac Med 2014; 9(4):236–41.

12. Williamson AM, Feyer AM. Moderate sleep deprivation produces impairments in cognitive and motor performance equivalent to legally prescribed levels of alcohol intoxication. Occup Environ Med 2000; 57(10):649–55 [Clinical Trial Randomized Controlled Trial Research Support, Non-U.S. Gov't].

13. Akerstedt T, Hallvig D, Anund A, et al. Having to stop driving at night because of dangerous sleepiness–awareness, physiology and behaviour. J Sleep Res 2013;22(4):380–8 [Research Support, Non-U.S. Gov't].

14. Anund A, Kecklund G, Kircher A, et al. The effects of driving situation on sleepiness indicators after sleep loss: a driving simulator study. Ind Health 2009; 47(4):393–401 [Research Support, Non-U.S. Gov't].

15. Garner AA, Miller MM, Field J, et al. Impact of experimentally manipulated sleep on adolescent simulated driving. Sleep Med 2015;16(6):796–9 [Research Support, N.I.H., Extramural Research Support, Non-U.S. Gov't Research Support, U.S. Gov't, P.H.S.].

16. Perez-Chada D, Videla AJ, O'Flaherty ME, et al. Sleep habits and accident risk among truck drivers: a cross-sectional study in Argentina. Sleep 2005; 28(9):1103–8.

17. Braeckman L, Verpraet R, Van Risseghem M, et al. Prevalence and correlates of poor sleep quality and daytime sleepiness in Belgian truck drivers. Chronobiol Int 2011;28(2):126–34 [Research Support, Non-U.S. Gov't].

18. Carter N, Ulfberg J, Nystrom B, et al. Sleep debt, sleepiness and accidents among males in the general population and male professional drivers. Accid Anal Prev 2003;35(4):613–7 [Comparative Study Research Support, Non-U.S. Gov't].

19. Arnedt JT, Wilde GJ, Munt PW, et al. Simulated driving performance following prolonged wakefulness and alcohol consumption: separate and combined contributions to impairment. J Sleep Res 2000;9(3):233–41.

20. Filtness AJ, Reyner LA, Horne JA. Driver sleepiness-comparisons between young and older men during a monotonous afternoon simulated drive. Biol Psychol 2012;89(3):580–3 [Comparative Study].

21. Senaratna CV, Perret JL, Lodge CJ, et al. Prevalence of obstructive sleep apnea in the general population: a systematic review [review]. Sleep Med Rev 2016. [Epub ahead of print].

22. Pack AI, Maislin G, Staley B, et al. Impaired performance in commercial drivers: role of sleep apnea and short sleep duration. Am J Respir Crit Care Med 2006;174(4):446–54 [Research Support, N.I.H., Extramural Research Support, Non-U.S. Gov't].

23. Tregear S, Reston J, Schoelles K, et al. Obstructive sleep apnea and risk of motor vehicle crash: systematic review and meta-analysis. J Clin Sleep Med 2009;5(6):573–81 [Meta-Analysis Research Support, U.S. Gov't, Non-P.H.S. Review].

24. Amra B, Dorali R, Mortazavi S, et al. Sleep apnea symptoms and accident risk factors in Persian commercial vehicle drivers. Sleep Breath 2012;16(1): 187–91.

25. Strohl KP, Brown DB, Collop N, et al. An official American Thoracic Society clinical practice guideline: sleep apnea, sleepiness, and driving risk in noncommercial drivers. An update of a 1994 Statement [review]. Am J Respir Crit Care Med 2013; 187(11):1259–66.

26. Sassani A, Findley LJ, Kryger M, et al. Reducing motor-vehicle collisions, costs, and fatalities by treating obstructive sleep apnea syndrome. Sleep 2004; 27(3):453–8 [Research Support, Non-U.S. Gov't].

27. Ozoh OB, Okubadejo NU, Akanbi MO, et al. High-risk of obstructive sleep apnea and excessive daytime sleepiness among commercial intra-city drivers in Lagos metropolis. Niger Med J 2013;54(4):224–9.

28. de Mello MT, Narciso FV, Tufik S, et al. Sleep disorders as a cause of motor vehicle collisions. Int J Prev Med 2013;4(3):246–57.

29. Kales SN, Straubel MG. Obstructive sleep apnea in North American commercial drivers [review]. Ind Health 2014;52(1):13–24.

30. Horstmann S, Hess CW, Bassetti C, et al. Sleepiness-related accidents in sleep apnea patients. Sleep 2000;23(3):383–9.

31. Cui R, Tanigawa T, Sakurai S, et al. Relationships between sleep-disordered breathing and blood pressure and excessive daytime sleepiness among truck drivers. Hypertens Res 2006;29(8):605–10 [Research Support, Non-U.S. Gov't].

32. Komada Y, Nishida Y, Namba K, et al. Elevated risk of motor vehicle accident for male drivers with obstructive sleep apnea syndrome in the Tokyo metropolitan area. Tohoku J Exp Med 2009;219(1):11–6.

33. Ellen RL, Marshall SC, Palayew M, et al. Systematic review of motor vehicle crash risk in persons with sleep apnea [review]. J Clin Sleep Med 2006;2(2): 193–200.

34. Karimi M, Hedner J, Lombardi C, et al. Driving habits and risk factors for traffic accidents among sleep apnea patients–a European multi-centre cohort study. J Sleep Res 2014;23(6):689–99 [Multicenter Study Research Support, Non-U.S. Gov't].

35. Lloberes P, Levy G, Descals C, et al. Self-reported sleepiness while driving as a risk factor for traffic accidents in patients with obstructive sleep apnoea syndrome and in non-apnoeic snorers. Respir Med 2000;94(10):971–6.

36. Akkoyunlu ME, Kart L, Uludag M, et al. Relationship between symptoms of obstructive sleep apnea syndrome and traffic accidents in the city drivers. Tuberk Toraks 2013;61(1):33–7 [in Turkish].

37. Masa JF, Rubio M, Findley LJ. Habitually sleepy drivers have a high frequency of automobile crashes associated with respiratory disorders during sleep. Am J Respir Crit Care Med 2000;162(4 Pt 1): 1407–12 [Research Support, Non-U.S. Gov't].

38. Shiomi T, Arita AT, Sasanabe R, et al. Falling asleep while driving and automobile accidents among patients with obstructive sleep apnea-hypopnea syndrome. Psychiatry Clin Neurosci 2002;56(3):333–4.

39. Kotterba S, Mueller N, Leidag M, et al. Comparison of driving simulator performance and neuropsychological testing in narcolepsy. Clin Neurol Neurosurg 2004;106(4):275–9 [Clinical Trial Comparative Study Controlled Clinical Trial].

40. George CF, Boudreau AC, Smiley A. Comparison of simulated driving performance in narcolepsy and sleep apnea patients. Sleep 1996;19(9): 711–7 [Comparative Study Research Support, Non-U.S. Gov't].

41. Bartels EC, Kusakcioglu O. Narcolepsy: a possible cause of automobile accidents. Lahey Clin Found Bull 1965;14(1):21–6.

42. Grubb TC. Narcolepsy and highway accidents. JAMA 1969;209(11):1720.

43. Pizza F, Jaussent I, Lopez R, et al. Car crashes and central disorders of hypersomnolence: a French study. PLoS One 2015;10(6):e0129386 [Research Support, Non-U.S. Gov't].

44. Leger D, Massuel MA, Metlaine A. Professional correlates of insomnia. Sleep 2006;29(2):171–8 [Research Support, Non-U.S. Gov't].

45. Daley M, Morin CM, LeBlanc M, et al. Insomnia and its relationship to health-care utilization, work absenteeism, productivity and accidents. Sleep Med 2009;10(4):427–38 [Research Support, Non-U.S. Gov't].

46. Williamson A, Lombardi DA, Folkard S, et al. The link between fatigue and safety [review]. Accid Anal Prev 2011;43(2):498–515.

47. Verster JC, Veldhuijzen DS, Volkerts ER. Residual effects of sleep medication on driving ability [review]. Sleep Med Rev 2004;8(4):309–25.

48. Verster JC, Veldhuijzen DS, Patat A, et al. Hypnotics and driving safety: meta-analyses of randomized controlled trials applying the on-the-road driving test. Curr Drug Saf 2006;1(1):63–71 [Meta-analysis].

49. Verster JC, Spence DW, Shahid A, et al. Zopiclone as positive control in studies examining the residual effects of hypnotic drugs on driving ability. Curr Drug Saf 2011;6(4):209–18.

50. Mets MA, de Vries JM, de Senerpont Domis LM, et al. Next-day effects of ramelteon (8 mg), zopiclone (7.5 mg), and placebo on highway driving performance, memory functioning, psychomotor performance, and mood in healthy adult subjects. Sleep 2011; 34(10):1327–34 [Randomized Controlled Trial Research Support, Non-U.S. Gov't].

51. Barbone F, McMahon AD, Davey PG, et al. Association of road-traffic accidents with benzodiazepine use. Lancet 1998;352(9137):1331–6 [Comparative Study Research Support, Non-U.S. Gov't].

52. Anund A, Ahlstrom C, Kecklund G, et al. Rumble strips in centre of the lane and the effect on sleepy drivers. Ind Health 2011;49(5):549–58 [Research Support, Non-U.S. Gov't].

53. Gurtman CG, Broadbear JH, Redman JR. Effects of modafinil on simulator driving and self-assessment of driving following sleep deprivation. Hum Psychopharmacol 2008;23(8):681–92 [Randomized Controlled Trial].

54. Philip P, Taillard J, Moore N, et al. The effects of coffee and napping on nighttime highway driving: a randomized trial. Ann Intern Med 2006;144(11): 785–91 [Randomized Controlled Trial].

55. Sagaspe P, Taillard J, Chaumet G, et al. Aging and nocturnal driving: better with coffee or a nap? A randomized study. Sleep 2007;30(12):1808–13 [Comparative Study Randomized Controlled Trial Research Support, Non-U.S. Gov't].

56. Killgore WD, Rupp TL, Grugle NL, et al. Effects of dextroamphetamine, caffeine and modafinil on psychomotor vigilance test performance after 44 h of continuous wakefulness. J Sleep Res 2008; 17(3):309–21 [Comparative Study Randomized Controlled Trial].

57. Taillard J, Capelli A, Sagaspe P, et al. In-car nocturnal blue light exposure improves motorway driving: a randomized controlled trial. PLoS One 2012;7(10):e46750 [Randomized Controlled Trial Research Support, Non-U.S. Gov't].

58. Signal TL, Gander PH, Anderson H, et al. Scheduled napping as a countermeasure to sleepiness in air traffic controllers. J Sleep Res 2009;18(1):11–9 [Research Support, Non-U.S. Gov't].

59. George CF. Reduction in motor vehicle collisions following treatment of sleep apnoea with nasal CPAP. Thorax 2001;56(7):508–12.

60. Gurubhagavatula I, Nkwuo JE, Maislin G, et al. Estimated cost of crashes in commercial drivers supports screening and treatment of obstructive sleep apnea. Accid Anal Prev 2008;40(1):104–15 [Research Support, N.I.H., Extramural Research Support, Non-U.S. Gov't Research Support, U.S. Gov't, Non-P.H.S.].

61. Philip P, Chaufton C, Taillard J, et al. Modafinil improves real driving performance in patients with hypersomnia: a randomized double-blind placebo-controlled crossover clinical trial. Sleep 2014;37(3): 483–7 [Randomized Controlled Trial Research Support, Non-U.S. Gov't].

62. Mets MA, Alford C, Verster JC. Sleep specialists' opinion on sleep disorders and fitness to drive a car: the necessity of continued education. Ind Health 2012;50(6):499–508 [Research Support, Non-U.S. Gov't].

63. Buysse DJ, Reynolds CF 3rd, Monk TH, et al. The Pittsburgh Sleep Quality Index: a new instrument for psychiatric practice and research. Psychiatry Res 1989;28(2):193–213 [Research Support, U.S. Gov't, P.H.S.].

64. Johns MW. A new method for measuring daytime sleepiness: the Epworth sleepiness scale. Sleep 1991;14(6):540–5.

65. Kaida K, Takahashi M, Akerstedt T, et al. Validation of the Karolinska sleepiness scale against performance and EEG variables. Clin Neurophysiol 2006; 117(7):1574–81 [Comparative Study Validation Studies].

66. Johns M, Tucker A, Chapman R, et al. Monitoring eye and eyelid movements by infrared reflectance oculography to measure drowsiness in drivers. Somnologie 2007;11:234–42.

67. Johns M, Chapman R, Crowley K, et al. A new method for assessing the risks of drowsiness while driving. Somnologie 2008;12:66–74.

68. Carskadon MA, Dement WC, Mitler MM, et al. Guidelines for the multiple sleep latency test (MSLT): a standard measure of sleepiness. Sleep 1986;9(4):519–24.

69. Zwyghuizen-Doorenbos A, Roehrs T, Schaefer M, et al. Test-retest reliability of the MSLT. Sleep 1988; 11(6):562–5 [Research Support, U.S. Gov't, P.H.S.].

70. Mathis J, Hess CW. Sleepiness and vigilance tests [review]. Swiss Med Wkly 2009;139(15–16):214–9.

71. Richardson GS, Carskadon MA, Flagg W, et al. Excessive daytime sleepiness in man: multiple sleep latency measurement in narcoleptic and control subjects. Electroencephalogr Clin Neurophysiol 1978; 45(5):621–7.

72. Mitler MM, Gujavarty KS, Browman CP. Maintenance of wakefulness test: a polysomnographic technique for evaluation treatment efficacy in patients with excessive somnolence. Electroencephalogr Clin Neurophysiol 1982;53(6):658–61 [Research Support, U.S. Gov't, P.H.S.].

73. Sagaspe P, Taillard J, Chaumet G, et al. Maintenance of wakefulness test as a predictor of driving performance in patients with untreated obstructive sleep apnea. Sleep 2007;30(3):327–30 [Research Support, Non-U.S. Gov't].

74. Mazza S, Pepin JL, Deschaux C, et al. Analysis of error profiles occurring during the OSLER test: a sensitive mean of detecting fluctuations in vigilance in patients with obstructive sleep apnea syndrome. Am J Respir Crit Care Med 2002;166(4):474–8 [Research Support, Non-U.S. Gov't Validation Studies].

75. Wilhelm B, Giedke H, Ludtke H, et al. Daytime variations in central nervous system activation measured by a pupillographic sleepiness test. J Sleep Res 2001;10(1):1–7 [Clinical Trial Research Support, Non-U.S. Gov't].

76. Balkin TJ, Bliese PD, Belenky G, et al. Comparative utility of instruments for monitoring sleepiness-related performance decrements in the operational environment. J Sleep Res 2004;13(3):219–27 [Comparative Study Research Support, U.S. Gov't, Non-P.H.S. Research Support, U.S. Gov't, P.H.S.].

77. Sack RL, Auckley D, Auger RR, et al. Circadian rhythm sleep disorders: part I, basic principles, shift work and jet lag disorders. An American academy of sleep medicine review [review]. Sleep 2007;30(11):1460–83.

78. Berry RB, Brooks R, Gamaldo CE, et al. The AASM manual for the scoring of sleep and associated events: rules, terminology and technical specifications, version 2.2. Darien (IL): American Academy of Sleep Medicine; 2015.

79. Morgenthaler T, Lee-Chiong T, Alessi C, et al. Practice parameters for the clinical evaluation and treatment of circadian rhythm sleep disorders. An American academy of sleep medicine report. Sleep 2007;30(11):1445–59. Standards of Practice Committee of the AASM.

80. Sack RL, Auckley D, Auger RR, et al. Circadian rhythm sleep disorders: part II, advanced sleep phase disorder, delayed sleep phase disorder, free-running disorder, and irregular sleep-wake rhythm. An American academy of sleep medicine review [review]. Sleep 2007;30(11):1484–501.

81. Carmona Bernal C, Capote Gil F, Botebol Benhamou G, et al. Assessment of excessive daytime sleepiness in professional drivers with suspected obstructive sleep apnea syndrome. Arch Bronconeumol 2000;36(8):436–40 [Clinical Trial Comparative Study]. [in Spanish].

82. Turkington PM, Sircar M, Allgar V, et al. Relationship between obstructive sleep apnoea, driving simulator performance, and risk of road traffic accidents. Thorax 2001;56(10):800–5 [Research Support, Non-U.S. Gov't].

83. Powell NB, Schechtman KB, Riley RW, et al. Sleepy driving: accidents and injury. Otolaryngol Head Neck Surg 2002;126(3):217–27 [Research Support, Non-U.S. Gov't].

84. Verster JC, Roth T. Drivers can poorly predict their own driving impairment: a comparison between measurements of subjective and objective driving quality. Psychopharmacology 2012;219(3):775–81 [Clinical Trial Comparative Study Research Support, Non-U.S. Gov't].

85. Alkharboush GA, Al Rashed FA, Saleem AH, et al. Assessment of patients' medical fitness-to-drive by primary care physicians: a cross-sectional study. Traffic Inj Prev 2017. [Epub ahead of print].

86. Adams AJ. Rebuttal: should family physicians assess fitness to drive?: yes. Can Fam Physician 2010;56(12):e411.

87. Laycock KM. Rebuttal: should family physicians assess fitness to drive?: no. Can Fam Physician 2010;56(12):e412.

88. Reuben DB, St George P. Driving and dementia California's approach to a medical and policy dilemma. West J Med 1996;164(2):111–21.

89. Berger JT, Rosner F, Kark P, et al. Reporting by physicians of impaired drivers and potentially impaired drivers. J Gen Intern Med 2000;15(9):667–72.

90. Jang RW, Man-Son-Hing M, Molnar FJ, et al. Family physicians' attitudes and practices regarding assessments of medical fitness to drive in older persons. J Gen Intern Med 2007;22(4):531–43.

91. Krieger J. Sleep apnoea and driving: how can this be dealt with? Eur Respir Rev 2007;16(106):189–95.

92. Masullo A, Feola A, Marino V, et al. Sleep disorders and driving licence: the current Italian legislation and medico-legal issues. Clin Ter 2014;165(5): e368–72.

93. Powell NB, Chau JK. Sleepy driving. Sleep Med Clin 2011;6:117–24.

94. Hanning CD, Welsh M. Sleepiness, snoring and driving habits. J Sleep Res 1996;5(1):51–4 [Comparative Study].

95. Dogan OT, Dal U, Ozsahin SL, et al. The prevalence of sleep related disorders among the drivers and it's relation with traffic accidents. Tuberk Toraks 2006; 54(4):315–21 [in Turkish].

96. Hirshkowitz M, Black JE, Wesnes K, et al. Adjunct armodafinil improves wakefulness and memory in obstructive sleep apnea/hypopnea syndrome. Respir Med 2007;101(3):616–27 [Multicenter Study Randomized Controlled Trial Research Support, Non-U.S. Gov't].

97. Hack MA, Choi SJ, Vijayapalan P, et al. Comparison of the effects of sleep deprivation, alcohol and obstructive sleep apnoea (OSA) on simulated steering performance. Respir Med 2001;95(7): 594–601 [Clinical Trial Comparative Study Randomized Controlled Trial Research Support, Non-U.S. Gov't].

98. Cassel W, Ploch T, Becker C, et al. Risk of traffic accidents in patients with sleep-disordered breathing: reduction with nasal CPAP. Eur Respir J 1996; 9(12):2606–11 [Research Support, Non-U.S. Gov't].

Moving?

Printed and bound by CPI Group (UK) Ltd, Croydon, CR0 4YY

03/10/2024

01040304-0001

.